"This is a valuable collection of essays offering a critical analysis of the complex and often conflicted intersection of geopolitics, public health, and crisis management in the context of a global pandemic. The collection of essays provides deep, multi-disciplinary insight on the delicate and often contentious relationship of strict government control designed to protect and provide care on the one hand and the socio-political dynamics and restrictive consequences of biopower on the other."

Joseph Alter, *Professor and Director of the Asian Studies Center, Department of Anthropology, University of Pittsburgh, USA*

"This remarkable collection clearly proves that we must put Taiwan at the center of the study of global epidemic control. The twelve theoretically informed chapters probe the intersection of democracy, surveillance, resistance, and health in startlingly fresh and sophisticated ways. *Taiwan's COVID-19 Experience* will be a must-read for academics, medical professionals, and policy-makers alike."

Ruth Rogaski, *Associate Professor of History and Asian Studies, Department of History, Vanderbilt University, USA*

"In the rapidly growing scholarship on global COVID-19 experiences, this book distinguishes itself with its wealth of empirical analysis and broad historical and theoretical perspectives."

Guobin Yang, *Grace Lee Boggs Professor of Sociology and Communication and Director of Center on Digital Culture and Society, University of Pennsylvania, USA*

Taiwan's COVID-19 Experience

This book explores and develops the ongoing conversation about how Taiwan navigated through the COVID-19 pandemic.

Emphasizing the themes of governance and governmentality, it moves the foci of the discussion from COVID policies to the social and political orders undergirding the statecraft of pandemic management. Furthermore, it analyzes how the pandemic fostered a historical moment at which new forms of governance and governmentality were beginning to take root. It also situates Taiwan's precarious nationhood in its global context, thereby challenging a prevalent methodological nationalism – the assumption that the nation is a natural unit of analysis whose borders are more or less unquestioned – and contributing to decolonizing Western theories with perspectives from the Global South.

Presenting rich original materials on the legal and public debates, individual reflections, and grassroots campaigns during COVID, this book will be essential reading for students and scholars of Taiwan's governance and social health policy, as well as medical anthropology and sociology.

Ming-Cheng M. Lo is Professor of Sociology at the University of California, Davis, USA. Lo's research addresses the cultures of democracy in East Asia, as well as the sense-making processes regarding illnesses, disasters, and cultural traumas.

Yu-Yueh Tsai is Associate Research Fellow at the Institute of Sociology, Academia Sinica, Taiwan, working in the fields of medical sociology, science, technology, and society (STS), and race and ethnicity studies.

Michael Shiyung Liu is Distinguish Professor of the History of Science and Medicine at Shanghai Jiao Tong University and Professor of History affiliated to the Asian Studies Center, University of Pittsburgh, USA. His research interests include Japanese colonial medicine, East Asian environmental history, and modern history of public health in East Asia.

Routledge Research on Taiwan Series
Series Editor: Dafydd Fell, SOAS, UK

The *Routledge Research on Taiwan Series* seeks to publish quality research on all aspects of Taiwan studies. Taking an interdisciplinary approach, the books will cover topics such as politics, economic development, culture, society, anthropology and history.

This new book series will include the best possible scholarship from the social sciences and the humanities and welcomes submissions from established authors in the field as well as from younger authors. In addition to research monographs and edited volumes, general works or textbooks with a broader appeal will be considered.

The Series is advised by an international Editorial Board and edited by *Dafydd Fell* of the Centre of Taiwan Studies at the School of Oriental and African Studies.

40 Taiwan During the First Administration of Tsai Ing-wen
Navigating in Stormy Waters
Edited by Gunter Schubert and Chun-yi Lee

41 The Social Construction of the Ocean and Modern Taiwan
Kuang-hao Hou

42 Social Forces in the Re-Making of Cross-Strait Relations
Hegemony and Social Movements in Taiwan
Kuang-hao Hou

43 Switching Diplomatic Recognition Between Taiwan and China
Economic and Social Impact
Chien-Huei Wu

44 Taiwan's COVID-19 Experience
Governance, Governmentality, and the Global Pandemic
Edited by Ming-Cheng M. Lo, Yu-Yueh Tsai and Michael Shiyung Liu

For more information about this series, please visit: https://www.routledge.com/Routledge-Research-on-Taiwan-Series/book-series/RRTAIWAN

Taiwan's COVID-19 Experience

Governance, Governmentality, and the Global Pandemic

Edited by
Ming-Cheng M. Lo, Yu-Yueh Tsai
and Michael Shiyung Liu

Routledge
Taylor & Francis Group
LONDON AND NEW YORK

First published 2024
by Routledge
4 Park Square, Milton Park, Abingdon, Oxon OX14 4RN

and by Routledge
605 Third Avenue, New York, NY 10158

Routledge is an imprint of the Taylor & Francis Group, an informa business

British Library Cataloguing-in-Publication Data
A catalogue record for this book is available from the British Library

Library of Congress Cataloging-in-Publication Data
Names: Lo, Ming-Cheng M., editor. | Tsai, Yu-Yueh, editor. | Liu, Michael Shiyung, editor.
Title: Taiwan's COVID-19 experience : governance, governmentality, and the global pandemic / edited by Ming-Cheng M. Lo, Yu-Yueh Tsai and Michael Shiyung Liu.
Description: Abingdon, Oxon ; New York, NY : Routledge, 2024. | Series: Routledge research on Taiwan series | Includes bibliographical references and index.
Identifiers: LCCN 2024005534 (print) | LCCN 2024005535 (ebook) | ISBN 9781032572208 (hardback) | ISBN 9781032572215 (paperback) | ISBN 9781003438380 (ebook)
Subjects: LCSH: COVID-19 (Disease)—Taiwan. | COVID-19 (Disease)—Government policy—Taiwan. | Medical policy—Taiwan.
Classification: LCC RA644.C67 T3445 2024 (print) | LCC RA644.C67 (ebook) | DDC 362.1962/41440951249—dc23/eng/20240405
LC record available at https://lccn.loc.gov/2024005534
LC ebook record available at https://lccn.loc.gov/2024005535

ISBN: 978-1-032-57220-8 (hbk)
ISBN: 978-1-032-57221-5 (pbk)
ISBN: 978-1-003-43838-0 (ebk)

DOI: 10.4324/9781003438380

Typeset in Times New Roman
by codeMantra

Contents

Figures

Tables

Contributors

Ta-Chien Chan is Research Fellow at Research Center for Humanities and Social Sciences, Academia Sinica, Taiwan.

Li-Chi Chen is Research Fellow at Massachusetts General Hospital, Boston, MA, USA.

Po-Hsun Chen is PhD candidate at the Centre for the History of Science, Technology and Medicine, the University of Manchester, UK. He is physician in biomedicine and traditional Chinese medicine, Taiwan.

Shun-Ling Chen is Associate Research Professor and Co-Director of Information Law Center at Institutum Iurisprudentiae, Academia Sinica, Taiwan.

Tzung-wen Chen is Professor in the Department of Sociology, National Chengchi University, Taiwan.

Ying-Yu Chen is Assistant Professor in the Department of Communication and Technology, National Yang Ming Chiao Tung University, Taiwan.

Yawen Cheng is Professor at the Institute of Health Policy and Management, College of Public Health, National Taiwan University, Taipei, Taiwan.

Mei-Fang Fan is Distinguished Professor at the Institute of Science, Technology and Society, National Yang Ming Chiao Tung University, Taiwan.

Yu-Ling Huang is Associate Professor in the Department of Humanities and Social Medicine, School of Medicine, National Cheng-Kung University, Taiwan.

Hsuan-Wei Lee is Assistant Research Fellow at the Institute of Sociology, Academia Sinica, Taiwan.

Chih-Han Leng is Graduate Student in the Department of Psychology, National Taiwan University, Taiwan.

Michael Shiyung Liu is Professor of History at Asian Studies Center, University of Pittsburgh, USA.

Ming-Cheng M. Lo is Professor of Sociology at the University of California, Davis, USA.

Mei-Lin Pan is Professor and Chairperson in the Department of Humanities and Social Sciences, National Yang Ming Chiao Tung University, Taiwan.

Sung-Yueh Perng is Associate Professor at the Institute of Science, Technology and Society, National Yang Ming Chiao Tung University, Taiwan.

Yu-Hui Tai is Associate Professor in the Department of Communication and Technology, National Yang Ming Chiao Tung University, Taiwan.

Chi-Shiun Tsai is Graduate Student at Heinz College, Carnegie Mellon University, USA.

Hsin-Yi Sandy Tsai is Associate Professor in the Institute of Telecommunications Management, National Cheng Kung University, Taiwan.

Yu-Yueh Tsai is Associate Research Fellow at the Institute of Sociology, Academia Sinica, Taiwan.

Fan-Tzu Tseng is Associate Research Fellow at the Institute of Sociology, Academia Sinica, Taiwan.

Chuan-Feng Wu is Associate Research Professor and Director of Information Law Center at Institutum Iurisprudentiae, Academia Sinica, Taiwan.

Ming-Jui Yeh is Assistant Professor at the Institute of Health Policy and Management, College of Public Health, National Taiwan University, Taiwan.

Acknowledgments

The production of this book has been a truly collaborative process. We are grateful to our authors for engaging with our multiple rounds of comments and suggestions, always with patience and good humor. Along the way, our own vision for this book was both sharpened and broadened by these conversations.

Reflecting upon Taiwan's COVID-19 experiences, in many ways, represents a solemn moment in our academic careers. The enormity of the human sufferings caused by this global pandemic has defined the context in which we situate our inquiries, with the humble hope that this edited volume will make a small contribution to better conceptualizing the possibilities of good pandemic governance. The global nature of this disaster has made us keenly aware that no human is an island and that, now more than ever, the island nation of Taiwan must be better understood by the world. We are grateful that Dr. Dafydd Fell, the series editor for Routledge Research on Taiwan, shares and endorses this vision. We appreciate the anonymous reviewers for providing such helpful comments, and we thank Andrew Leach for judiciously guiding us through the production process at Routledge.

Yu-Yueh thanks Director Chih-Jou Chen and the Institute of Sociology, Academia Sinica (Taiwan) for providing support and funding for the conference "COVID-19, Global, and Taiwan's Governance," held during January 26–27, 2022, which ushered in the inception of this project. The research assistance offered by Yi-Hsuan Kuo, Audrey Chen, and Michelle Chen is also acknowledged. She is grateful for the financial support provided by the Individual Thematic Research Program of Academia Sinica Research Grants (AS-TP-111-H02).

Michael acknowledges the support of Dr. James A. Cook and the staff at the Asian Studies Center, University of Pittsburgh, as well as friends and family in Shanghai and Pittsburgh. Without their help and understanding, his frequent travels for collecting data and writing could not have been completed as planned.

Ming-Cheng presented an earlier version of the Introduction to this volume at the 2023 American Sociological Association annual meetings. She is indebted to her fellow panelists, including Bin Xu, Shai Drome, and Gianpaolo Baiocchi, as well as the audience, for their astute comments. She thanks Hsin-Yi Hsieh for her research assistance. She is grateful that her family put up with her habit of bringing tasks related to "the COVID book" on multiple family vacations.

Finally, as editors, we would like to thank one another. None of us would have wanted to take on this project alone. Yet together, we brought to bear upon this book our diverse perspectives rooted in different institutions, academic backgrounds, and lived experiences. We are grateful for the teamwork that has brought us across the finishing line.

Introduction

Pandemic Governance and Governmentality in Taiwan

Ming-Cheng M. Lo

Despite its international isolation, Taiwan has become increasingly important geopolitically, a phenomenon observed by both scholars and politicians. Many point to Taiwan as a successful latecomer to democratization; others highlight the island's outsized role in the confrontations between the competing visions of the world order championed by the opposing global powers. In this context, how Taiwan navigated the COVID-19 pandemic has prompted a lively discussion, with researchers in the social and health sciences not only documenting Taiwan's strong COVID containment record and analyzing its relatively successful pandemic intervention strategies, but also elaborating on the implications of Taiwan's COVID experience for rethinking, and indeed refuting, the "authoritarian advantage" in crisis management (Lo and Hsieh 2020; Wang et al. 2020).

The chapters in this collection seek to broaden and deepen these conversations about Taiwan's COVID experience. Specifically, we move the foci of the discussion from COVID policies to the social and political orders undergirding the statecraft of pandemic management, while also analyzing how "fighting COVID" itself became a process that challenged these existing orders. The analyses in this book remain empirically grounded in concrete policies and practices; however, the volume as whole also addresses more general questions about how to best comprehend – and hold in tension – the protective *and* restrictive powers of the state and, furthermore, how to productively situate Taiwan, especially its experiences as a marginalized nation, in the conversations about the global challenges facing liberal democracy, many of which were accentuated during the public health and social crises brought on by the pandemic. From this angle, and following Lupton's (2022) insightful perspectives about theorizing COVID, this edited volume seeks to locate Taiwan's COVID story within its socio-political context, as well as to unpack its theoretical implications by addressing the tensions between local specifics and globalizing forces.

Two concepts, governance and governmentality, are helpful in our inquiry. The notion of governance serves to frame COVID policies as informed by the legal bureaucratic authority institutionalized in the state and consolidated through civil society, with debates centering on what counts as rational state action. Discussions about COVID policies along these lines, implicitly or explicitly, draw on the concept of a Weberian "managerial state" (or versions of it) that highlights

DOI: 10.4324/9781003438380-1

effectiveness and accountability (Evans and Rauch 1999). In addition, informed by the scholarship on the welfare state and social citizenship, researchers also emphasize the protection of marginalized and vulnerable groups as an important aspect of pandemic governance (Choi, Kühner, and Shi 2022; Sachs et al. 2022). In contrast, the concept of governmentality sensitizes us to how, during the pandemic, new categories of health risks and medical needs were constructed by the state and internalized by its citizenry. Often engaging with Foucauldian theories, these discussions highlight a repressive "soft power" of the state, which is exercised through the very process of delivering what its population supposedly desires (Hannah and Schemann 2020). In very broad terms, discussions of pandemic governance generally focus on whether, and how, the state effectively and justly provides protection for its citizens' lives and livelihood, whereas writings on pandemic governmentality analyze how such state protection can be accompanied by subtle forms of repression.

In what follows, I first offer a general discussion of pandemic governance, including how the expansion of neoliberal and post-liberal trends partially accounted for the surprisingly poor responses to COVID by many wealthy Western countries. Within this context, I will argue that Taiwan's pandemic governance primarily reflects the institutions and cultural norms of its robust liberal democracy, notwithstanding the local challenges of an immature welfare state, misinformation, and populism. In the second section, after some theoretical sketches of the concepts of biopower and governmentality, I share some reflections about emergent acts of resistance and their potential meanings. Since power is never eliminated, only transformed, I emphasize that it is crucial to observe *what sorts of new power relations* are being ushered in through the resistance against Taiwan's pandemic governmentality. The third section turns to the efforts to attain global health and health justice, prompted by the urgency of the pandemic, that was primarily championed by the WHO. Taiwan's exclusion from the WHO makes it a perfect "deviant case" that exposes the power inequalities and injustices glossed over by noble slogans such as "we are in this together." I close with some thoughts about how studies of Taiwan, as a marginalized nation, may help to advance intellectual debates about these themes, not the least with the subversive and decolonizing potential often found in perspectives from the periphery. An overview of the chapters in this volume is also provided as a roadmap for readers to navigate the main body of the book.

Taiwan's Pandemic Governance from a Global Perspective

Governance, which has been defined in various terms, can be generally viewed as the process through which decisions are made and implemented within a collective (Bevir 2012). The United Nations specifies that good governance should be participatory, consensus-oriented, accountable, transparent, responsive, effective and efficient, equitable and inclusive, and follows the rule of law.[1] In similar terms, the WHO emphasizes strategic policy frameworks, effective regulations and oversight, coalition building, and accountability (WHO 2010). The World Bank's "Worldwide Governance Indicators" include six key indicators, including: political stability and absence of violence/terrorism, government effectiveness, regulatory quality, rule of law, and control of corruption.[2] Zooming in on the pandemic, discussions about COVID governance tend to focus on a few key areas, including: prevention, containment, health services, and equity (Sachs et al. 2022).[3]

The outcomes of (un-)successful pandemic governance reflect the state's capacity to protect the lives and welfare of its citizens, which are generally evaluated by indicators for mortalities, economic losses, social burdens (such as lockdowns or school closures), and whether the physical, economic, and social harms caused by COVID disproportionately impacted particular social groups (Sachs et al. 2022; Tsou et al. 2022; "Tracking covid-19 excess deaths across countries"[4]). By these measures, the governments in many wealthy Western democracies performed their protective roles surprisingly poorly. A 2022 *Lancet* report states that

> the international distribution of COVID-19 death rates is almost the opposite of what might have been expected before the pandemic. On the basis of the 2019 publication of the Global Health Security Index, which ranked the United States first and the UK second in the world in terms of preparedness for pandemics and epidemics, it was widely assumed that the United States and Europe had the strongest pandemic response capacities.
>
> (Sachs et al. 2022)

Defying expectations, COVID-related deaths per 100,000 population were surprisingly high in the US (341.11) and the UK (325.13), compared to the records in countries with more successful containment policies, such as Taiwan (74.2), South Korea (66.50), and Australia (76.88).[5] Of the six WHO regions, the European region has the highest estimated total COVID-related deaths per million population (4144), followed then by the Americas region (4051); in contrast, the same measures of COVID mortality are significantly lower in the Western Pacific (300) and African (1774) regions (Sachs et al. 2022).

Beyond death tolls, the pandemic caused significant economic hardships globally. During 2019–2022, the average GDP growth for the world was 1.5% less than projected, again with large national and regional variations (Sachs et al. 2022). One notable pattern, however, is that within each country, the social and economic burdens caused by COVID and COVID-containment measures often ended up exacerbating existing, and at times creating new, gender, racial, class, and digital inequalities (Choi, Kühner, and Shi 2022; Kruman and Marback 2022; Kylasam and Kuriakose 2023).

There are complex and sometimes competing explanations for the lack of success in pandemic governance in the most resourceful parts of the world. Without adjudicating these arguments, I highlight the expansion of neoliberalism as an underlying macro trend that precipitated the weakening of the state's protective role in many Western countries (see also Lupton 2022). This trend, in turn, can be seen as rooted in the internal tensions of liberalism.

> Liberal institutions emerged … to save unbridled liberalism from itself: from the vagaries of unregulated markets, the rule of tyrannical majorities, and the whims of egoistic individuals. But the rise of neoliberalism … brought

> tensions between individual freedom and institutional constraints increasingly to the fore. The cultural constitution of individuals as dramatically empowered rights-bearing actors, coupled with the erosion of confidence in major institutions that accompanied the neoliberal turn, threatened the liberal order from within.
>
> (Cole, Schofer, and Velasco 2023: 381)

More specifically, the "era of embedded liberalism," spanning roughly from 1945 to 1980, featured policies that balanced free trade and individual autonomy with government interventions that were "designed to stabilize markets, reduce unemployment, and ensure basic welfare.... [as well as] delivering education, managing public health, and performing a host of other functions" (Cole, Schofer, and Velasco 2023: 382; see also Polanyi [1944] 2001). But in the 1980s, embedded liberalism gradually yielded to neoliberalism, with market deregulation, welfare retrenchment, and a general withering of what Bourdieu calls the "left hand of the state." Cultural norms changed accordingly. "A rhetoric of unbridled 'freedom' eclipsed sober liberal notions of citizenship rights coupled with duties and responsibilities" (Cole, Schofer, and Velasco 2023: 382). The economic and cultural impacts of neoliberalism have now brought about the post-liberal era. Having been unembedded from many of the state's protective institutions and instead urged to become self-reliant, citizens distrust governmental and scientific authorities, expecting little protection from, and feeling largely unbeholden to, these institutions. These "highly agentic" individuals prioritize their preferences over the public good – an important explanation for the rise in vaccine hesitancy even *before* the pandemic (Reich 2016; Cole, Schofer, and Velasco 2023). This observation brings us full circle to the poor pandemic governance of many Western countries. According to the 2022 *Lancet* report, effective pandemic responses require an ethical framework of prosociality, which the authors define as both the state's and the public's orientations toward the needs of the society rather than to narrow individual interests, yet for decades in the US, the UK, and many other Western democracies, prosociality has been in continual decline (Sachs et al. 2022).

From this vantage point, the Taiwanese state appeared quite effective in protecting the lives and livelihoods of its citizens during the pandemic. As already mentioned, Taiwan's COVID-related death toll was much less severe compared globally. The 2022 *Lancet* report praises Taiwan, along with New Zealand, Singapore, South Korea, etc., for successfully maintaining low death rates. Taiwan also experienced minimal economic losses during COVID. Taiwan stood out as an exception with its actual GDP growth during the pandemic (4.3%) exceeding what had been previously projected before COVID (2.0%), whereas most of the other major economies failed to meet their projected growth rates during this period (Sachs et al. 2022). A study that evaluates the overall COVID performance of 50 countries using multiple indicators (e.g., mortality, GDP loss, lockdown efficiency) shows that Taiwan outperformed all other countries in the pre-vaccination phase; after the vaccine became widely available, Taiwan received a lower performance score but still ranked well (ranking 13th out of 50 in the study) (Tsou et al. 2022).

Despite these records, the Taiwanese government's ability to equalize the burden of the pandemic, especially by protecting vulnerable social groups, appears more limited. Taiwan, along with Hong Kong and South Korea, devoted less resources to mitigating the negative economic and social impacts of the pandemic compared to other wealthy societies.[6] The OECD countries, on average, spent more than 6% of their GDP on social policies to counter the negative social effects of COVID-19; the US, Canada, the UK, and Japan dispensed an even higher percentage of resources for similar policies (10–14% of GDP). In contrast, the Taiwanese, Hong Kong, and South Korean governments spent around 3% of their GDP on related efforts (Choi, Kühner, and Shi 2022). One potential explanation for this difference is that these three Asian governments spent less on countering the negative impacts of COVID because their death tolls and economic losses were less severe. Alternatively, these figures can also be viewed as signs of an immature welfare state. Indeed, Choi, Kühner, and Shi (2022) explain that, almost as soon as these former East Asian "little dragons" began to transition from developmental states to welfare states, the global trend of deindustrialization introduced additional social risks to these societies. The result is a "superposition between old and new social risks" (Choi, Kühner, and Shi 2022: 262) that is experienced by many societies but is particularly conspicuous in these emerging welfare states, which in part explains their challenges with protecting vulnerable social groups during the pandemic.

In the case of Taiwan, we find some evidence that lends support to Choi, Kühner, and Shi's (2022) concern. For example, while the online economy boomed during the pandemic, dispatch drivers remained vulnerable, with 70% of these workers lacking access to statutory labor insurance (Taiwan Labor Front 2021[7]; see also Soon, Chou, and Shi 2021). Distance learning exposed the digital divide both between the urban and rural areas and across class differences, with insufficient state intervention to remedy the inequality (Choi, Kühner, and Shi 2022). Migrant workers from Southeast Asia were, at times, scapegoated for spreading the virus and, in some instances, locked down in overcrowded dorm rooms, raising concerns about human rights violations (Chang 2021).[8] Shortages of affordable and quality long-term care for the elderly and the chronically ill were exacerbated by the pandemic ("Editorial," 2020).[9] While Taiwan is certainly not the only society that experienced these inequalities and social vulnerabilities during the pandemic, these observations do reveal inadequacies in Taiwan's welfare state.

However, these inequalities do not necessarily indicate that Taiwan has developed post-liberal institutions or cultural norms. Rather, as several chapters in this volume will demonstrate, Taiwan more closely resembles the examples of "embedded liberalism" in Cole, Schofer, and Velasco's (2023) typology described above, with its pandemic governance featuring "centralized and professional leadership, democratic and accountable political culture, vibrant civil society, and broad social participation" (Yeh and Cheng, this volume). Considering Taiwan's postwar history, it makes sense to view the country as an emerging welfare state that is still in the process of weaving and strengthening its social safety net (Liu 2021; Soon, Chou, and Shi 2021), rather than a once mature welfare state now undergoing retrenchment.[10] More broadly speaking, since its democratic transition in the 1990s, social movements and other mobilizations of civil society have produced a strong cultural mandate to make demands on the state to address citizens' concerns and social needs. The Taiwanese government, in turn, is held accountable and put under pressure to be responsive to civil society's demands. As Yeh and Cheng (this volume) observe, "while many countries have seen rising trends in anti-establishments and social polarization in many aspects, the case in Taiwan shows that an accountable government could boost social trust in institutions, making citizens stand together despite their differences to engage with the common dangers."

This process of state-society engagement is evident – and important – for the social formation of public health governance and epidemic responses in Taiwan. After Taiwan experienced the 2003 SARS epidemic, protests and public discussions led to the "societalization" of its pandemic unpreparedness, pushing the government to strengthen its legal framework for swift epidemic responses (e.g., the Communicable Disease Control Act), expand related medical infrastructure (e.g., negative pressure rooms and viral labs) and the stockpiles of medical materials (e.g., personal protective equipment), and establish a coordinated network of hospitals (i.e., the Disease Control Medical Network) designated to contain major outbreaks (Lo and Hsieh 2020; see also Yeh and Cheng, this volume, for further details). Taiwan's National Health Insurance (NHI), recently established in 1996, was not only highly instrumental in the island's COVID containment efforts, but continually enjoys strong public trust and arguably strengthens a sense of communal solidarity in this politically divided nation (Lo 2020; Wang et al. 2020). Regarding cultural norms, Taiwan's polarized civil society came together temporarily at the beginning of the pandemic to foster a discourse of civil interdependence, which promoted the civic duty of mutual protection by wearing masks, following social-distancing guidelines, and adhering to other safety measures (Lo and Hsieh 2020). In short, the Taiwanese public's demands for institutional reforms as well as the state's responsiveness indicate significant mutual engagement between the two, rather than a cynical citizenry or a laissez-faire government, which helps to explain Taiwan's "prosociality" which is absent in most post-liberal societies. Put differently, accountability and responsiveness, as key elements of good governance, presuppose and indeed require broad participation from citizens in monitoring state actions and voicing diverse perspectives (Bevir 2010; WHO[11]). The public and the state in Taiwan have, for the most part, stayed engaged in these (at times contentious) interactions.

To clarify, I am *not* describing Taiwan as a *collectivist* society. In general, such stereotypes are too unrefined to be useful for analyzing institutional or cultural processes. Empirically, for all its "prosociality," Taiwan endures much political fragmentation, is actively targeted by disinformation campaigns, and has been increasingly threatened by populism. During Taiwan's COVID outbreak in 2021, these trends were mobilized by a rightwing opposition party, the KMT (*kuomingtang*), to mount political protests that, without evidence, accused the DPP-led (Democratic Progressive Party) government of having deliberately blocked purchases of COVID vaccines (Lo and Hsieh 2022). These social processes cannot be easily accounted for by the individualism-collectivism dichotomy. Instead, considering both the state's overall performance and the public's political imagination, Taiwan's pandemic governance largely reflected its robust liberal democratic institutions and cultures, while also facing the challenges of an immature welfare state, misinformation, and populism.

Pandemic Biopower, Governmentality, and Resistance

As discussed above, the state's protective measures, held accountable by and including broad participation from its citizenry, are considered key to good pandemic governance. However, some scholars caution that such state care contains dangerously repressive potential (Agamben 2021). Often examined through the Foucauldian frameworks of biopower and governmentality, the citizens' "virtues" of willing adherence to the state's "protective" regulations such as mask-wearing, social-distancing, or vaccination are interpreted as signs of the naturalization of the knowledge/power nexus that sustains existing political orders.

According to Foucault, societies crossed the threshold of biological modernity "when the biological processes characterizing the life of human beings … became a crucial issue for political decision-making, a new 'problem' to be addressed by governments" (Lorenzini 2021: S41). In this new era, biopolitics operates through the state's "pastoral power," or a biopower, over its population,[12] which is rooted in an intimate knowledge of and a commitment to the well-being of each and all (Foucault 2007). Citizens are now not only governed as *political*, but also as *biological* subjects, with the government classifying, measuring, and attempting to satisfy the population's needs in sanitation, nutrition, vaccination, mental health, and so forth. In many ways, these instances of "biopower" seem to be exactly the kinds of praiseworthy practices of good governance discussed in the previous section. Indeed, some scholars "have argued that we should recognize and value more positively the protective logic of biopower," especially considering the ongoing dismantlement of the welfare state today (Hannah and Schemann 2020: 13; see also Ojakangas 2005). What is alarming, though, is that discourses about a population's biological and health "needs" inevitably give rise to social norms that are naturalized and internalized by the majority. Thus, biopower is dangerous if accepted *blindly*, because, among other things, it stifles our ability to act otherwise. Foucault's analyses of governmentality further detail how Western liberal governments have, in the last 200 years, engaged in increasingly palatable and defused practices of biopower, thereby designing "the 'landscapes of possibility' in which … we can be induced to exercise choices 'freely' but in ways that are beneficial both to ourselves and to the maintenance of specific social orders" (Hannah and Schemann 2020: 12). In this context, our capacity to operate freely – the capacity to imagine alternative norms about health and sexuality, alternative needs for our well-being, or more broadly alternative ways of being governed – can only be maintained and animated by critically reflecting upon the standards and goals naturalized in the logic of governmentality.

The pandemic accentuated these concerns about "freedom." Evaluating how governments defined and attempted to address COVID-related risks and public health concerns, scholars have raised questions about the potential of governmentalized state overreach. Are the "temporary" COVID regulations inclined to become normalized and institutionalized from hereon (Prozorov 2023)? Were citizens blindly participating in their own surveillance by the state, even when their privacy and digital rights were at risk (Kruman and Marback 2022; Kylasam and Kuriakose 2023)? How did some social groups become marginalized or stigmatized in the "politics of differential vulnerability" (Lorenzini 2021: S43; see also Kylasam and Kuriakose 2023)? Instead of uncritically following COVID regulations to restore our "normal" ways of life, how might we consider their transformation "in a more equitable and sustainable direction" (Prozorov 2023: 79)?

In considering these questions, it is worthwhile to recall that Foucault maintains that power is ubiquitous and therefore, instead of eliminating power, resistance gives rise to new power dynamics. The emancipatory or repressive potential of a given political order, then, seems best assessed through contextualized empirical analyses (which, incidentally, characterizes Foucault's own works), whereas *a priori* assertations often risk becoming exaggerated, conspiratorial, or simply off the mark (Liu 2023; Prozorov 2023). Here, an emergent body of empirical research is helpful for understanding Taiwan's pandemic biopower. Liu (2023: 46), importantly, depicts Taiwan's COVID responses as a case of "democratic biopolitics" in that they balanced between "a strong form of state governmentality and a flexible process of transparent democracy." Wu (this volume), though not directly discussing biopower, details how the Taiwanese government attempted to maintain what Liu calls "transparent democracy." Instead of issuing emergency decrees, the Taiwanese government asked its legislature "to pass the COVID-19 Special Act, which serves as a legal framework under which democratic processes can function … while ensuring accountability.… [T]he CECC has adopted an open and responsive communication system that aims to actively provide information to the public [and] to improve transparency." Perng and coauthors (this volume) further document how Taiwan's civil society groups debated and challenged the utilization of digital pandemic measures. However imperfect these democratic mechanisms might have been, they rendered it possible for the public to negotiate with state power, including its biopower. The nature of pandemic biopolitics in Taiwan, thus, is markedly different from its counterpart in authoritarian regimes, with China's zero COVID policy serving as a notable contrast.

At the micro-level, there is some evidence of individuals engaging in their own "critical ontology" (Foucault 1984: 47), as they reevaluated their subjectivities in light of their lived experiences. For example, some of the Taiwanese who were placed under quarantine became aware of, and at times acted upon, their impulses to defy the quarantine regulations (Lee et al. this volume). Tseng's qualitative study (this volume) reveals further nuances. Even as most of her interviewees viewed their compliance with the quarantine regulations as a rite of passage to reaffirm their moral standing in the community, some voices still challenged this commonly internalized moral order. It is perhaps too early to tell whether these reflections might eventually encourage alternative discourses of civil solidarity free of state directives (Prozorov 2023) or, by contrast, end up brewing an egotism that "others" everything and everyone deemed inconvenient to the self (as demonstrated in the instances of mask-burning or Asian hatred in the US). We must await future research for more detailed analyses of these still unfolding processes and their aftermaths.

But two developing trends are worth noting. On the one hand, even before the pandemic, Taiwan was a major target of China's disinformation campaigns (Hartnett and Su 2021). Unsurprisingly, "conspiracies around the virology of COVID-19 were rampant in Taiwanese media, social networks, and even academic fields before the spread of the pandemic was known to the Western world" (Liu 2023: 37). Moving forward, if local acts of resistance become widely influenced by such post-truth claims, then political manipulation by the Chinese government's cyber war, rather than emancipation from the Taiwanese government's biopower, is likely to ensue. On the other hand, civil groups targeting misinformation and demanding government transparency have become active, with one of their previous leaders, Audrey Tang, serving as Taiwan's inaugural Minister of Digital Affairs. Among other things, the hacker-turned-minister sought to combat the infodemic with memes, exploring the power of humor to disrupt the thrill often contained in the exaggerated claims of fake news (Cheng, Su, and Su 2023; Liu 2023). More broadly, Tang and others in the g0v movement, which arose in Taiwan in 2012, advocate for exposing and democratizing the processes through which drafts of policies are finalized. If citizens widely develop similar habits to "remix the message" (Cheng, Su, and Su 2023: 227) when encountering misinformation *and*, if more seek to participate in the *process* of policy- and knowledge-making, then they may become more resilient to various forms of manipulation. Hanging in the balance might very well be what freedom comes to mean for the Taiwanese people.

Global Solidarity for Health?

Despite their different theoretical inspirations, much of the research on pandemic governance and governmentality shares an inclination toward methodological nationalism. With assumptions about the nation-state as a natural unit of analysis for social and political processes, these discussions tend to pay insufficient attention to how state power, protective or repressive, is embedded in global power structures. Given the scale of the COVID-19 pandemic, however, key aspects of COVID governance are shown to depend on international cooperation (Sachs et al. 2022), and yet much of this global coordination failed precisely because of nation-centered biases. This irony, as I will argue in this section, has necessitated critical examinations of methodological nationalism and, more broadly, other nation-centered biases, for which Taiwan's contested statehood serves as an illuminating case.

Calls for global solidarity, popular during COVID, seemed to have failed from the very beginning as the world attempted to grapple with the new virus. The WHO, acting under the 2005 IHR (International Health Regulations), repeatedly erred on the side of inaction, failing to heed early warnings about the severity of the situation (Sachs et al. 2022). The WHO argued that it had to rely on "member countries like China to accurately report their findings," but with time, "a growing chorus of government officials, health experts, editorial boards and academics" accused WHO of "being too deferential to Beijing" (Watt 2020).[13] As countries around the world began to roll out COVID containment strategies, regulations for border closures and immigration control often reflected nationalistic or racist attitudes (Kruman and Marback 2022; Surová 2022), which in turn reinforced pre-existing exclusionary tendencies (Bieber 2022). Even policies that claimed to "follow the science" were informed by models of epistemological knowledge that contained biases of methodological nationalism. As Bryonny (2020: 68, emphasis mine) puts it, restricting mobility to halt viral spread "made sound epidemiological sense. Yet restrictions inevitably drew upon pre-existing borders between people and places – *borders that were socially, politically, and historically inscribed before becoming epidemiologically legible.*" Later, after the COVID vaccine became available, its distribution was dictated more by nationalism and wealth than by the logic of international collaboration. Wealthy Western countries were accused of vaccine nationalism, as they hoarded as many dosages as it would take to vaccinate their whole population two or three times, while leaving behind nations in the Global South in the race to immunize against the virus (Riaz et al. 2021).

These nation-centered biases have deep historical roots in how global health governance came to be envisioned and institutionalized. From its establishment in 1948, the WHO viewed health equity and justice as supported by the framework of nation-states. As such, the WHO conceded that nation-states possess "the exclusive capacity to deal with public health emergencies based on sovereign equality against external interference, indicating their primary responsibility for population health and development" (Lee 2023: 46–47). In recent years, there have been increasing calls and efforts to give more weight to subnational and transnational voices in global health governance, especially in response to the spread of HIV and other infectious diseases. Yet, the final version of the IHR 2005 again reaffirmed that nation-states possess the duty and sovereign right to manage their public health (Gostin and Katz 2016).

With its long-term international isolation, Taiwan's experience can uniquely illuminate one of the inherent contradictions in this nation-centered model of global health solidarity. The WHO claims to pursue health equity for all but treats marginalized nations and peoples on terms dictated by *other*, more powerful nations; this is the lived reality in Taiwan and a key factor shaping its experiences of public health crises. As Tsai (this volume) puts it, Taiwan's exclusion shines a spotlight on how the "power of a few sovereign States within WHO can overshadow the universal right to health." During the 2003 SARS epidemic, Taiwan's requests for access to samples and data were denied by the WHO due to China's interference. The IHR 2005 included an appendix containing a statement made by China asserting its sovereignty over Taiwan. Accordingly, "Taiwan was included in the IHR alert system based on China's statement, regardless of the lack of connection between the Chinese and Taiwanese health authorities and information systems" (Lee 2023: 50). During the COVID pandemic, Taiwan's exclusion from the WHO, ironically, protected it from the latter's failed alarm system, as Taiwan devised its early containment policies based on its own data sources (Lo 2020; Wang et al. 2020).

In the Global North, the fate of the 23 million Taiwanese can be and indeed is easily overlooked, but the local experiences on the island bring into sharp relief the dangers of these nation-centered biases. Taiwan's experience calls our attention to how the peoples without states, live under contested statehood, or are oppressed by their own states, are by and large denied protection from global health governance. More broadly, because of this political noise, knowledge about global health and decisions about epidemic responses are also distorted by what Lee (2023: 54) calls epistemic nationalism, which "arbitrarily classifies the units, clusters, data sources, and health outcomes regarding pandemic situations informed by the delimitations of national territories." For example, in much of the data gathered for epidemiology, information about Taiwan is either misrepresented as being part of China or simply omitted. The knowledge systems and decision-making processes based on epistemic nationalism, as such, can be erroneous and misleading. Even though a small nation like Taiwan is not equipped to overcome these biases, its experiences serve to accentuate how such biases are gumming up the system of global health governance.

There are, however, no easy solutions. Lee (2023: 62) accurately observes that "Taiwan's *de facto* independence, which relies on support from powerful states, particularly the US (under the 'Cold War' framework) and Japan (Taiwan's previous colonizer), is not unproblematic. Yet, this seems to be an inevitable strategy for a small nation to resist contemporary China's imperialism and militarized authoritarianism." In a parallel fashion, when Taiwan experienced a COVID vaccine shortage in 2021, it relied on its "global democratic allies," most notably the US and Japan, for vaccine donations, which bought time for Taiwan's government to navigate through China's interference with its vaccine purchases, its uncertain position in the WHO's COVAX initiative, and the general challenges presented by the global vaccine shortage at the time (Lo and Hsieh 2022). Much can be criticized about the geopolitical agendas behind the US' and other nations' vaccine donations to Taiwan, and even more can be said about the poorer and more marginalized people in the Global South that needed these vaccine donations more desperately than Taiwan. The existing model of global health governance, as it was, did not offer any realistic alternatives, nor did the critics who found faults with Taiwan's survival strategy.

In sum, as I hope to have shown in this brief Introduction, Taiwan's pandemic governance and governmentality reflected a robust liberal democracy, which, while having thus far avoided some of the pitfalls of neoliberalism, also faces externally imposed challenges as much as internally emergent hurdles. Taiwan's COVID experience indicates that its liberal democratic cultures and institutions facilitated meaningful mutual engagement between the state and its citizens, which was key to strengthening the state's protective hand against the new virus, while simultaneously keeping in check the repressive potential of its biopower. Yet, due to the nationalistic vision of a neighboring superpower, this small democracy is barred from almost all global governance organizations, including the WHO, which, ironically, exhausted itself with rallying calls for global solidarity during the pandemic. Moving forward, future research would benefit from explicitly considering this global context when discussing the internal challenges facing Taiwan's health governance, crisis management, and its democratic future in general, including, at the macro level, how its emergent welfare state will further develop and, at the micro level, how individuals' "critical ontology" might be unduly influenced by the rampant disinformation campaigns. Joining attempts to provincialize Western scholarships and problematize methodological nationalism, I hope these perspectives grounded in Taiwan's experiences will help advance the ongoing conversations about the lessons from the COVID-19 pandemic.

Organization of the Book

The 12 chapters in this volume are organized into four sections, creating direct and indirect conversations within and, at times, across each section. It is our hope that these dialogues will spark new insights, questions, and a "collective effervescence" for future conversations.

In the section on **Historical and Contemporary Contexts**, Liu's chapter provides an in-depth analysis of the colonial origin and postwar transformation of quarantine policies and practices in Taiwan, detailing the historical making of the Taiwanese population into a "modern" citizenry susceptible to, and self-disciplined with, various public health interventions. Complimenting Liu's historical analysis, Yeh and Cheng's chapter places Taiwan's COVID responses within its contemporary context as a liberal democracy. This chapter offers an overview of Taiwan's COVID policies and framework of public health governance, documenting the key structural factors for its early success in containing the virus.

Situated in the historical and contemporary contexts described in the previous section, **Liberal Democracy and Pandemic Management** presents four chapters that are devoted to analyzing the strengths and weaknesses of Taiwan's pandemic intervention. Chen and Chan's chapter describes how the Taiwanese government utilized digital surveillance technologies to achieve effective border control, contact tracing, quarantine regulations, etc., accentuating both a robust digital infrastructure and a public-private partnership, rather than concentrated state power, as the key in facilitating these efforts. Chen and Huang's research, in contrast, cautions that such emergency measures may outlive their usefulness, allowing the state to prioritize public health over civil liberties during and beyond the pandemic. Using Taiwan's SMS-based contact-tracing system as its primary example, this chapter raises the concern of Taiwan becoming a "public health state" if it normalizes and institutionalizes pandemic control measures in the long term. Taking a legal studies perspective, Wu's chapter offers a robust discussion about the privacy concerns concerning digital surveillance measures, specifically, regarding lawfulness, purpose limitation, data minimization, and transparency. Wu then proceeds to explain why these surveillance measures seemed widely accepted by the public, emphasizing that Taiwan's democratic governance, "which promotes civic participation, fosters consensus building, and facilitates a functioning personal data protection framework," is fundamental for mitigating-related privacy concerns. Focusing on a citizen forum, an expert panel, and other examples, Perng and coauthors document the ways in which civil society groups demanded government accountability on issues related to digital pandemic responses. Public deliberation is highlighted as an important mechanism for communicating and addressing concerns about transparency, privacy, and inclusivity, keeping in check the temptation to prioritize efficiency at all costs during a period of crisis. In this vein, the two chapters by Wu and Perng and coauthors serve to contrast Taiwan's strategies of digital surveillance against measures commonly used in authoritarian states.

The section on **Self-Governance and Individual Citizens** includes three chapters that analyze how and why individual citizens internalized, challenged, or deviated from the measures described in the previous section. Lee and his collaborators offer a statistical analysis of noncompliant impulses and behaviors among those who were placed under quarantine. These authors report that during quarantine, women felt more anxiety, older people experienced greater impulses to leave, and higher-income individuals were more likely to violate the rules. Tseng's chapter delves deeply into how Taiwanese returnees from overseas navigated their risk status and the associated stigma that resulted from government regulations and public imaginations about the virus. She shows that most returnees strengthened their self-governance, which was driven by their concerns for others' well-being, desire for de-stigmatization, and expectation of reintegration into society. While Tseng's theoretical contributions are eloquently articulated through the concept of "risk-stigma assemblage," her chapter can also be read as exemplifying the arts of pandemic governmentality. Dialoguing directly with the literature on governmentality, Tzung-wen Chen's chapter discusses how the state mobilized multiple levels of "truth regimes," utilized various practices of governance, and involved different parts of the social body to not only legitimize but also popularize the "need" for COVID containment efforts. The author contrasts the different rationalities and strategies of biopolitics during two phases of pandemic response in Taiwan – the first relying primarily on NPI (non-pharmaceutical intervention) measures whereas the second focuses on vaccination campaigns, while also demonstrating how citizens internalized the logics of governmentality as they queued up to purchase masks, compared the different COVID vaccines, and debated which groups should be prioritized for vaccination.

The final section, **Nationhood, Nationalism, and Global Health,** explicitly situates Taiwan's COVID experience in a global context. Po-Hsun Chen offers an original analysis of how NRICM101, an herbal remedy for COVID, was marginalized by both the biomedical and the mainstream traditional and complementary medicine (TCM) communities in Taiwan. Only after NRICM101 successfully established a niche market overseas was it able to promote itself with a nationalist narrative of "Taiwan's glory" and become widely accepted on the island. Tracing the interactions of classification, nationalism, and sociotechnical imaginaries,

Chen explains how NRICM101 pivoted away from traditional Chinese medicine and, instead, presented itself as Taiwanese Chinese medicine. Tai's chapter, in turn, focuses on how China's misinformation campaigns posed serious challenges to Taiwan's COVID containment efforts. Analyzing reports about Taiwan from China's government and media outlets during the pandemic, Tai's study shows that these reports not only incited hostility toward Taiwan among their Chinese readers, but also constituted part of China's "cognitive warfare" to influence the Taiwanese public. Finally, concluding this volume, Tsai's chapter confronts Taiwan's exclusion from the WHO – the key organizational actor in global health governance. Tsai documents how the Taiwan case exemplifies the WHO's organizational and institutional limitations in pursuing its stated goal of health for all peoples. After all, Taiwan's exclusion from the WHO's official forums for sharing information and expertise is not only unfair to its population but could also jeopardize the global efforts to contain viruses that are not deterred by these politically constructed barriers.

Notes

1 Banerji, Amitav. 2015. "Global and National Leadership in Good Governance." *UN Chronicle.* https://www.un.org/en/chronicle/article/global-and-national-leadership-good-governance#:~:text=The%20most%20cited%20definition%20has,follows%20the%20rule%20of%20law (Retrieved on July 31, 2023).

2 See https://info.worldbank.org/governance/wgi/ (Retrieved on July 31, 2023).

3 Sachs and coauthors' (2022) report includes a fifth "pillar" of COVID response, which refers to a global dimension of pandemic governance – a point I will return to later in this Introduction.

4 See https://www.economist.com/graphic-detail/coronavirus-excess-deaths-tracker (Retrieved on July 13, 2023).

5 See https://coronavirus.jhu.edu/data/mortality (Retrieved on July 20, 2023).

6 Public health scholars often discuss health inequality in terms of its impacts on morbidity and mortality (Mishra et al. 2021). Our focus here is slightly different, pivoting, instead, toward the *social and economic* inequalities resulting from COVID.

7 Taiwan Labor Front. 2021. Online survey on employment during pandemic. http://labor.ngo.tw/news/news-now/1023-news20201106 (Retrieved on July 20, 2023).

8 Chang, Ya-chun. 2021. "Taiwan's migrant workers scapegoated for spread of COVID." *Taiwan News*, July 3. https://www.taiwannews.com.tw/en/news/4238638 (Retrieved on July 20, 2023).

9 "Editorial: Home care challenges set to worsen." 2020. *The Taipei Times*, December 13. https://www.taipeitimes.com/News/editorials/archives/2020/12/13/2003748610 (Retrieved on July 20, 2023).

10 Liu (2021) highlights Taiwan's democratization as the watershed moment for Taiwan's welfare system. Similarly, Soon, Chou, and Shi (2021: 375) observe that Taiwan's welfare system, though still less extensive than the welfare systems in Japan or Europe, has been expanding over the last two decades: "Japan's social welfare spending rivals that of the OECD average (over 20% of GDP), as opposed to about 10% for China, Korea and Taiwan, but all four countries have seen increased social spending over the period, indicating a growing trend of the state's welfare commitments."

11 WHO, "Promoting participatory governance, social participation and accountability," https://www.who.int/activities/promoting-participatory-governance-social-participation-and-accountability (Retrieved on July 31, 2023).

12 As a general distinction, we can think of biopower as the "basic underlying rationality of cultivating the life of the population," whereas biopolitics refers to "specific measures and techniques … in many different settings to pursue this larger project" (Hannah and Schemann 2020: 5).

13 Watt, Louise. "Taiwan says it tried to warn the world about coronavirus. Here's what it really knew and when." *Times*, May 19. https://time.com/5826025/taiwan-who-trump-coronavirus-covid19/ (Retrieved on July 25, 2023).

References

Agamben, Giorgio. 2021. *Where are We Now? The Epidemic as Politics*. London: Eris Press.

Bevir, Mark. 2010. *Democratic Governance*. Princeton: Princeton University Press.

Bevir, Mark. 2012. *Governance: A Very Short Introduction*. New York: Oxford University Press.

Bieber, Florian. 2022. "Global Nationalism in Times of the COVID-19 Pandemic." *Nationalities Papers* 50: 13–25.

Bryonny, Goodwin-Hawkins. 2020. "The Intimate Borders of Epidemiological Nationalism." *Anthropology in Action* 27: 67–70.

Cheng, Hsin-I, Chiaoning Su, and Chiaochun Su. 2023. "A Conversation with Taiwan's Minister of Digital Affairs Audrey Tang on Communication, Technology, Identity, and Democracy." Pp. 219–236 in *Resistance in the Era of Nationalisms: Performing Identities in Taiwan and Hong Kong*, edited by Hsin-I Cheng and Hsin-i Sydney Yueh. East Lansing: Michigan State University Press.

Choi, Young Jun, Stefan Kühner, and Shih-Jiunn Shi. 2022. "From 'New Social Risks' to 'COVID Social Risks': The Challenges for Inclusive Society in South Korea, Hong Kong, and Taiwan amid the Pandemic." *Policy and Society* 41(2): 260–274.

Cole, Wade M., Evan Schofer, and Kristopher Velasco. 2023. "Individual Empowerment, Institutional Confidence, and Vaccination Rates in Cross-National Perspective, 1995 to 2018." *American Sociological Review* 88(3): 379–417.

Gostin, Lawrence O., and Rebecca Katz. 2016. "The International Health Regulations: The Governing Framework for Global Health Security." *Milbank Quarterly* 94(2): 264–313.

Evans, Peter, and James E. Rauch. 1999. "Bureaucracy and Growth: A Cross-national Analysis of the Effects of 'Weberian' State Structures on Economic Growth." *American Sociological Review* 64(5): 748–765.

Foucault, Michel. 1984. "What is Enlightenment." Pp. 32–50 in *The Foucault Reader*, edited by Paul Rabinow and translated by Catherine Porter. New York: Pantheon.

Foucault, Michel. 2007. *Security, Territory, Population: Lectures at the Collège de France 1977–1978*. Translated by G. Burchell. London: Palgrave Macmillan.

Hannah Matthew, Jan Simon Hutta, and Christoph Schemann. 2020. "Thinking Corona Measures With Foucault." Unpublished Manuscript. https://www.kulturgeo.uni-bayreuth.de/de/news/2020/Thinking-Corona-measures-with-Foucault/Thinking-Corona-measures-with-Foucault.pdf.

Hartnett, Stephen J., and Chiaoning Su. 2021. "Hacking, Debating, and Renewing Democracy in Taiwan in the Age of 'Post-Truth' Communication." *Taiwan Journal of Democracy* 17(1): 21-43.

Kruman, Marc, and Richard Marback. 2022. "Citizenship in Pandemic Times." *Citizenship Studies* 26(8): 1027–1031.

Kylasam Iyer, Deepa, and Francis Kuriakose. 2023. "Becoming Digital Citizens: Covid-19 and Urban Citizenship Regimes in India." *Citizenship Studies* 27(2): 230–246.

Lee, Po-Han. 2023. "Decolonising Global Solidarity: The WHO's Broken Alarm and Epidemiological Nationalism." *Legalities* 3(1): 44–70.

Liu, Hubert C.Y. 2021. "Financing the welfare state system in Taiwan." Pp. 217–242 in *Financing Welfare State Systems in Asia*, edited by Christian Aspalter. London: Routledge.

Liu, Wen. 2023. "Beyond Critique and Conspiracy COVID: Memes as Reparative Practices in Digital Taiwan." Pp. 31–60 in *Resistance in the Era of Nationalisms: Performing Identities in Taiwan and Hong Kong*, edited by Hsin-I Cheng and Hsin-i Sydney Yueh. East Lansing: Michigan State University Press.

Lo, Ming-Cheng M. 2020. "How Taiwan's Precautionary Approach Contained COVID-19." *Contexts* 19(4): 18–21.

Lo, Ming-Cheng M., and Hsin-yi Hsieh. 2020. "The 'Societalization' of Pandemic Unpreparedness: Lessons from Taiwan's COVID Response." *American Journal of Cultural Sociology* 8: 384–404.

Lo, Ming-Cheng M, and Hsin-yi Hsieh. 2022. "Containing Populism Through Emotive Transformation: Lessons from Taiwan's COVID Vaccine Crisis." Conference Paper Annual Meetings of the American Sociological Association, Los Angeles, CA.

Lorenzini, Daniele. 2021. "Biopolitics in the Time of Coronavirus." *Critical Inquiry* 47(S2): S40–S45.

Lupton, Deborah. 2022. *COVID Societies: Theorising the Coronavirus Crisis*. London: Routledge.

Mishra, V., Golnoush Seyedzenouzi, Ahmad Almohtadi, Tasnim Chowdhury, Arwa Khashkhusha, Ariana Axiaq, Wing Yan Elizabeth Wong, and Amer Harky 2021. "Health Inequalities during COVID-19 and their Effects on Morbidity and Mortality." *Journal of Healthcare Leadership* 13: 19–26.

Ojakangas, Mika. 2005. "Impossible Dialogue on Biopower: Agamben and Foucault." *Foucault Studies* 2: 5–28.

Polanyi, Karl. [1944] 2001. *The Great Transformation: The Political and Economic Origins of Our Time*. Boston, MA: Beacon.

Prozorov, Sergei. 2023. "A Farewell to Homo Sacer? Sovereign Power and Bare Life in Agamben's Coronavirus Commentary." *Law and Critique* 34(1): 63–80.

Reich, Jennifer A. 2016. *Calling the Shots: Why Parents Reject Vaccines*. New York: New York University Press.

Riaz, Mehr Muhammad Adeel, Unaiza Ahmad, Anmol Mohan, Ana Carla dos Santos Costa, Hiba Khan, Maryam Salma Babar, Mohammad Mehedi Hasan, Mohammad Yasir Essar, and Ahsan Zil-E-Ali. 2021. "Global Impact of Vaccine Nationalism during COVID-19 Pandemic." *Tropical Medicine and Health* 49: 101.

Sachs, Jeffrey D., Salim S. Abdool Karim, Lara Aknin, Joseph Allen, Kirsten Brosbøl, Francesca Colombo, Gabriela Cuevas Barron, María Fernanda Espinosa, Vitor Gaspar, Alejandro Gaviria, Andy Haines, Peter J. Hotez, Phoebe Koundouri, Felipe Larraín Bascuñán, Jong-Koo Lee, Muhammad Ali Pate, Gabriela Ramos, K. Srinath Reddy, Ismail Serageldin, John Thwaites, Vaira Vike-Freiberga, Chen Wang, Miriam Khamadi Were, Lan Xue, Chandrika Bahadur, Maria Elena Bottazzi, Chris Bullen, George Laryea-Adjei, Yanis Ben Amor, Ozge Karadag, Guillaume Lafortune, Emma Torres, Lauren Barredo, Juliana G. E. Bartels, Neena Joshi, Margaret Hellard, Uyen Kim Huynh, Shweta Khandelwal, Jeffrey V. Lazarus, and Susan Michie. 2022. "The Lancet Commission on Lessons for the Future from the COVID-19 Pandemic." *The Lancet* 400(10359): 1224–1280.

Soon, Suetgiin, Chelsea C. Chou and Shih-Jiunn Shi. 2021. "Withstanding the Plague: Institutional Resilience of the East Asian Welfare State." *Soc Policy Adm* 55(2): 374–387.

Surová, Svetluša. 2022. "Securitization and Militarized Quarantine of Roma Settlements during the First Wave of COVID-19 Pandemic in Slovakia." *Citizenship Studies* 26(8): 1032–1062.

Tsou, Hsiao-Hui, Shu-Chen Kuo, Yu-Hsuan Lin, Chao A. Hsiung, Hung-Yi Chiou, Wei J. Chen, Shiow-Ing Wu, Huey-Kang Sytwu, Pau-Chung Chen, Meng-Hsuan Wu, Ya-Ting Hsu, Hsiao-Yu Wu, Fang-Jing Lee, Shu-Man Shih, Ding-Ping Liu, and Shan-Chwen Chang. 2022. "A Comprehensive Evaluation of COVID-19 Policies and Outcomes in 50 Countries and Territories." *Scientific Reports* 12(1): 8802.

Wang, C. Jason, Chun Y. Ng, and Robert H. Brook. 2020. "Response to COVID-19 in Taiwan: Big Data Analytics, New Technology, and Proactive Testing." *JAMA*, March 3.

WHO. 2010. *Monitoring the Building Blocks of Health Systems: A Handbook of Indicators and their Measurement Strategies*. Geneva: World Health Organization.

Part 1

Historical and Contemporary Contexts

1 Dynamics of Quarantine Control to Epidemic Precaution in Taiwan

A Historical Review

Michael Shiyung Liu

Discipling Colonial Society with Quarantine Codes

Despite Western medicine having appeared in Taiwan around the mid-19th century, a comprehensive public health infrastructure was not established until Japanese colonialization in the period of 1895–1945. During the colonial era, two related processes—the increase of medical resources and the establishment of a public health system—with three components (preventive medicine, laboratories, and new quarantine infrastructures) laid out the foundation to the medical modernization in Taiwan. In the early stage between the 1910s and 1920s, main goals of public health measures were directed at infectious and communicable diseases. That was quarantine control to reduce the risk of diseases transmission, externally and internally. Because of the horrified experience in Taiwan Campaign in 1895, quarantine strategies to control epidemics were obviously the priority for the public health policymakers of the colonial government.

Transforming "the Land of Miasma" into a Healthy Island

Taiwan was called "the land of miasma" by Japanese soldiers during the Taiwan Campaign in 1895. During the campaign, deaths from disease topped battlefield deaths by a ratio of nearly 30 to 1. The Japanese force of just over 50,000 men suffered horrific losses due to epidemics, with 4,642 soldiers dying of disease as opposed to 164 killed in battle and 515 wounded or injured (Davidson, 1903).[1] Since the beginning of the Japanese occupation, various infectious diseases were recorded in military documents while the victims covered from nameless soldiers to honorable family members. To a general image of Taiwan among Japanese soldiers in Taiwan, the epidemics and endemic diseases were always fumigated to this island's environment and poisoned the living creatures there.

During the first move to occupy Taiwan in 1895, epidemic cholera had already caused a high toll of lives during the Sino-Japanese War a few months before (Janetta, 1987). As Japanese forces moved southward onto the island of Taiwan, James W. Davidson, an American war correspondent provided an account of epidemic cholera and other enteric diseases in Zhanghua, a city in middle Taiwan: "An outbreak of fever spread through the [Japanese] army like wild-fire. From the

DOI: 10.4324/9781003438380-3

highest officer to the lowest coolie, all were incapacitated. ...yet within the first few days these numbered 824, of whom 82 died." However, as cholera claimed the most lives of 384 deaths, a higher number of 2,771 soldiers suffered from malaria, a common endemic disease in Taiwan (Davidson, 1903). Although the cause was unconfirmed, a widespread rumor implied that malaria even caused the life of the leader of Japanese force, Imperial Prince Kitashirakawanomiya Yoshihisa, who died near Tainan on October 28 due to complications from an 11-day suffering (Davidson, 1903; Takekoshi, 1907). Harry Lamley first studied how severe epidemics caused so much casualties among Japanese troops. With Lamley's records and archival data, Paul Katz listed four major killers during early Japanese colonization: cholera, malaria, dysentery, and intestinal typhus (Lamley, 1970; 1973). All were epidemics and endemic diseases in filthy environment and unhealthy behaviors. The colonial authority learned lessons from the triable casualties in early occupation. Transforming what they considered to be filthy behaviors among the Taiwanese to improve the overall public health condition was undoubtedly an important means to improve everyone's survival chance in miasmatic Taiwan.

Governmental statistics revealed the real scenario and turning point of the trend of the changing health condition in colonial Taiwan. From 1895 to 1945, the colonial government tried to control major epidemics and improve public health conditions by promoting quarantine strategies and health education. Followed by the efforts on building quarantine and public health infrastructure, the birth rate and mortality rate in colonial Taiwan were getting better over time. According to the population statistics between 1906 and 1942, the total birth rate in Taiwan (including Taiwanese and Japanese nationals in Taiwan) was around 40–45% with a death rate declined from 33% to 16%. This improvement increased the population growth rate from 5% in 1906 to 25% after the 1930s.[2] The declining mortality rate could be an important indicator to reveal the effectiveness of quarantine controls and public health infrastructure. The trend obviously showed that a turning point occurred around the mid-1920s, pairing with the improving mortality rate. Figure 1.1 shows that the gross mortality rate declined from 33% in 1906 to below 20% in 1942. As mortality rate improved, life expectancy of the Taiwanese population was prolonged. In 1906, life expectancy at birth was 29.7 years old, and this increased to 36.1 years old in 1910. Meanwhile, life expectancy of the Taiwanese population in the 1940s improved beyond 44.8 years old (Tu, 1985).

Taking Preston's classification of seven causes of death as the base for recounting mortality, the regrouping of cause-of-death categories examined here indicated that there was a declined in combined effects of all the major infectious diseases obviously associated with the senescent component of mortality (Preston and others, 1972). As Siler's decomposition method is employed to analyze the impact of certain epidemic causes on the change of life expectancy, the result provides a way to check how and when the long-term effects of quarantine controls and public health precaution could have an impact on the general mortality trend in colonial Taiwan (Siler, 1979) (Figure 1.2).

The above analysis suggests that a shift in mortality rate and in epidemiology occurred after the 1920s. Based on statistical analysis, one important feature of the transition was that infectious disease and digestive problems gradually lost their

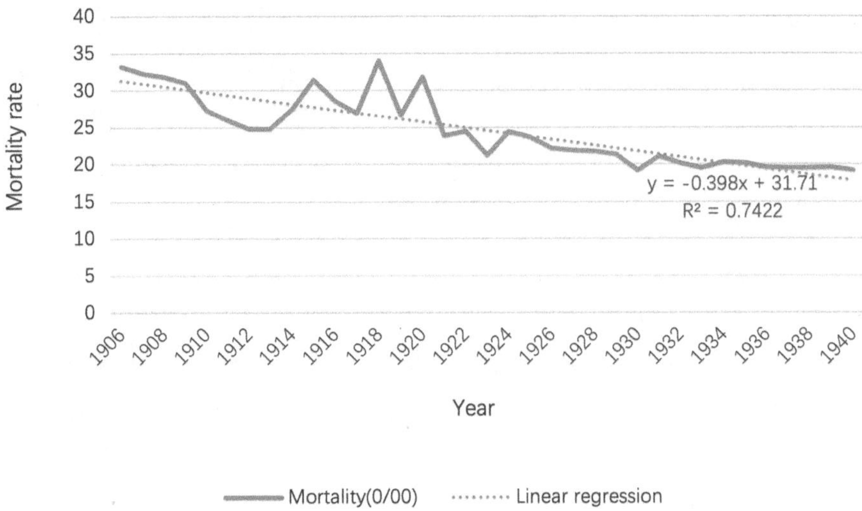

Figure 1.1 Changes of Mortality Rate in Taiwan (1906–1942)

Source: Taiwansheng wushiyinianlai tongjitiyao (Taipei: Taiwanshen xiengzheng zhangquang gongshu, 1946): 326–327.

Note: A semi-log regression of mortality rate can be calculated ln Y(t)=3.4796–0.0166t shows the declines in mortality rates were average 1.6% annually.

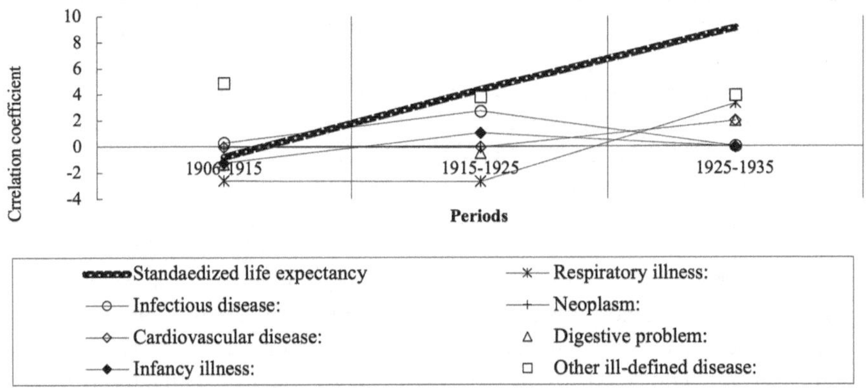

Figure 1.2 The Changing Pattern of Health Transition

Note: The *Y* axis shows the scale of correlation coefficients of certain diseases (e.g., respiratory illness, infectious disease, neoplasm) to the difference of life expectancy between two years (e.g., 1906 vs. 1915).

importance in determining the life expectancy. Moreover, in the 1930s, Taiwan entered its second stage of building a public health system with overwhelming quarantine control and epidemic precaution. Restrictive quarantine and the public's compliance jointly contributed to a health transition with better life expectancy that encompassed a broader range of the life cycle, a multiplicity of diseases with various causes, and less effective political and technological interventions.

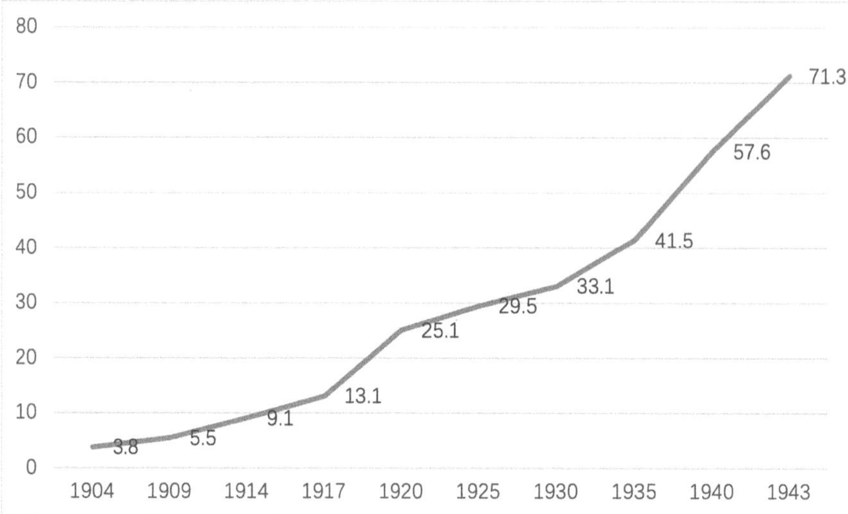

Figure 1.3 Taiwanese School Enrollment Rates (%)

Source: Taiwansheng xinzhezanquankongshu tojishi (Bureau of Statistics, Chief Executive Office, Taiwan Province) ed., *Taiwansheng wushiyinianlai tongjitiyao* (The 51-year Statistical Summary of Taiwan Province), p. 1241.

Since the second stage of the 1930s, the adoption of certain quarantine measure could be internalized to healthy behaviors and current social norms, which affiliated to the promotion of epidemic precaution.

Based on analyses on trends, the health condition in colonial Taiwan after the 1930s obviously improved. However, progress in medical technologies and treatments were not the only reasons for such fast improvement. The Taiwanese school enrollment rates also revealed a sharp increase after the 1920s (Figure 1.3), which indicated more Taiwanese students could receive health education and knowledge of epidemic prevention. The central focus of this chapter is the changing motives of quarantine activities in Taiwan. Such a focus is particularly pertinent because at least an educational theory implies that the adoption related to discipline and order has contributed to a significant behavior formation in certain conditions (Noguera, 2003). Taiwan could be one of them. Generally speaking, as the quarantine control externally reduced the risk of transmitting infectious diseases, the higher school enrollment rates also could be considered to have internally promoted the self-awareness of epidemic precaution in daily life in colonial Taiwan since the 1920s.

Policing Health for Quarantine Control

Armed resistance of the Taiwanese and an unhealthy environment were the two main obstacles that disturbed the colonial government during the early stage of the occupation. To solve frequent health threats, the colonial government launched the public health reforms aimed to reduce epidemic dangers in the 1900s and declared their victory to eliminate major epidemics in late 1920s. Goto Shinpei, the Chief Deputy of Civil Affairs (*Minsei chokan*), and the Consultant of Hygiene (*Eisei komon*) Takagi Tomoe were two main figures for designing public health policies in colonial Taiwan (Tsurumi, 1965; Nagaki, 1989). Among all the public health policies, the sanitary police and constant surveillance systems were two essential tools that not only kept the quarantine functional for the government but also inculcated modern health behaviors to Taiwanese society.

Cholera kept impacting Taiwanese society before the 1920s. Epidemic cholera sporadically occurred between 1908 and 1920. After the medical professionals well knew its pathology and epidemiology, the sanitary police force continuously maintained the same quarantine control as in the early occupation but gradually shifted their focus to the sanitary education of the Taiwanese public. A newspaper columnist echoed such an assertation in 1919, "We [the Japanese] must teach them [the Taiwanese] and improve their hygiene thought. We must inject them with the knowledge of suitable methods of hygiene."[3] As an official slogan revealed later, "community practices meant to protect the community or cure the ill were, in other words, to blamed for the spread of the disease" in the 1920s.[4] The colonial government commonly blames the spread of cholera and other enteric diseases to Taiwanese ignorance of modern health behaviors.[5] It was obviously that since the 1920s, addition to maintain the functions of quarantine controls, the colonial government also paid attention to policing colonized Taiwanese of concepts and disciplines of epidemic precaution by modifying their behaviors and life styles.

The colonial authorities in Taiwan believed that epidemics were caused by filthy environments and unsanitary living styles. As the water-born cholera and typhoid could be linked to filthy environments, animal-transmitted diseases like bubonic plague might be the result of unsanitary behaviors or living styles. Without a reliable conclusion of the bubonic plague in Hong Kong in 1897, Kato Takashi, Director of the Hygiene Section of the Police Department, already expressed much pessimistic feeling to quarantine the spread in Taiwan, because of what he considered to be many Taiwanese filthy and unsanitary behaviors and living habits (Kato, 1897; Liu, 2008). With such an attitude and concerns, the quarantine measures for dealing with the outbreaks remained in line with old laws, focused on isolation of patients, port quarantines, and home searches for infectees (Naoto, 1902).[6] All the measurements and enforcements were heavily relied on a police force. Quarantine laws were, therefore, the fundamental legal base for the police to isolate suspects before the pathogens was caught. Beyond the quarantine control, the sanitary police force also carried the full responsibility for surveillance and disciplining Taiwanese to prevent epidemics.

To fulfill the mission of surveillance and disciplining, the sanitary police department could assign technicians and additional policemen to infected areas, quarantine stations at ports, control traffic and travel for rigid quarantine, and certainly conduct sanitary surveys. Victims and suspects of infection were searched out in house-to-house inspections and then forcibly sent to quarantine hospitals or isolation wards (Chen, 1984). To successfully extend the power over each head of a Taiwanese household, colonial sanitary police infrastructure was integrated with traditional local pao-chia (*hoko* in Japanese) system to form a self-policing structure for searching out the suspects of infection (Fan, 1994). The colonial police were not only responsible for quarantine control during the epidemic periods but also performed functions relating to sanitation and public health, such as draining gutters, inspecting food, and administering quarantine in ports and cities to prevent the recurrence of an epidemic (Chin, 1998; Chiang, 2009). A poster of the police's multiple roles to assist colonial rule from an exhibition in 1926 vividly showed the overwhelming power of the colonial police force in Taiwan. They carried multiple functions from quarantine control to epidemic precaution and education (Figure 1.4).

In addition to the police force, George Barclay attributes health improvements to the medical investment, public health interventions, and educational campaigns undertaken by the Japanese authorities (Barclay, 2015). As the number of medical graduates grew after the mid-1920s, private medical professionals including physicians, nurses, and midwives also deserve some of the credit. By 1930, nearly 300 private physicians were recruited by the colonial government to serve the duty

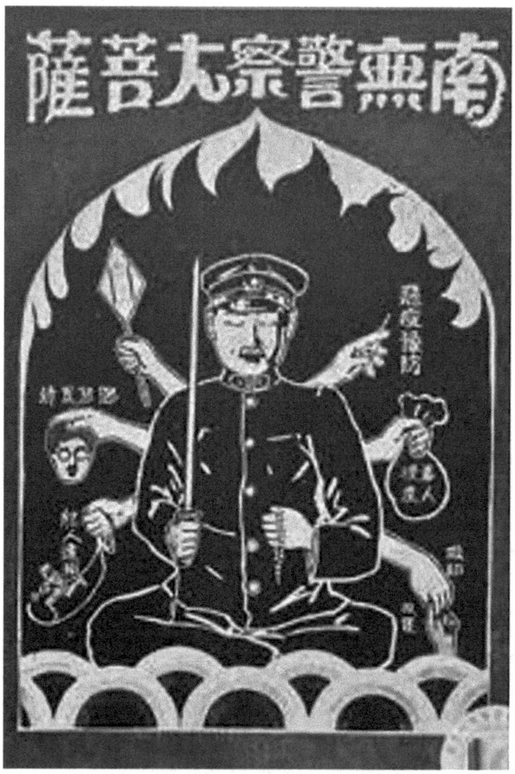

Figure 1.4 Poster "Nanmu 'Police' Daibodhisattva" in 1926

Source: Zhuang Yongming, *Taiwan Shijihuiwei: Shidai gongying* (Tasting Taiwan Eras: Lights and shadows of years) (Taipei: Yunliu, 2011), p. 17.

of public physician (Lo, 2002). Private practitioners and public physicians jointly worked for quarantine control under governmental guidelines and as agents to promote modern public health to local communities (Suzuki, 2005).[7] As the medical doctor was a male-dominated occupation in colonial Taiwan, female health workers, such as midwives and nurses, were essential to bring concepts and guidelines of epidemic precaution to Taiwanese families through the wives and daughters. Increasing numbers of midwives in Taiwan successfully reduced the infant mortality rate (Wu, 1997). The newborns and children were the most vulnerable victims to various infectious diseases such as "diarrhea germs" (Kato, 1998). However, the female health workers did not have legal rights to enforce quarantine control but rather educated the patients to adopt modern public health behaviors. In general, Taiwanese medical practitioners in colonial Taiwan were sensitive to the progress of medical knowledge and current treatments while they constantly played the role of social leaders in communities. Therefore, sometimes paired with the police force, these private medical practitioners were probably impactful in enforcing colonial public health policies in local society.

It is worth noting that the quarantine policy in colonial Taiwan between the 1920s and 1930s did not fully comply with current international mainstream of public health, probably in Japan either. During the 1920s and 1930s in East Asia, the policy practice of colonial medicine gradually shifted from "enclavist" approaches (serving colonial regimes and armies) to "public health" approaches (emphasizing prevention and treatment of contagions facing all societies) (Peckham and Pomfret, 2013). Despite receiving the benefit of a modern public health infrastructure, colonial Taiwan retained the early concept of quarantine control based on the philosophy of disciplining and preaching so-called ignorant colonized population about the "enlightenment and civilization" of modern sanitary behaviors. The improving life expectancy and changing pattern of death of causes were part of the benefit but also illuminated the procedure of adopting of modern public health, which eventually rooted in colonized society. In such a procedure, governmental agents such as the sanitary police, the public physician and private medical practitioners jointly contributed to complete the mission under governmental guidance. However, the roles of female public health workers remained unclear for transforming essential quarantine guidelines and concepts to socio-cultural norms in Taiwanese daily life.

As for the case of colonial Taiwan, there was significant segregation between filthy colonized/Taiwanese and sanitary colonialist/Japanese. In the eyes of Japanese sanitary policemen, colonized Taiwanese could only be disciplined and recognized by the desire to *exploit* their labor, but there was also a competing desire to exclude the colonized from all facets of modern health behaviors due to their ignorance about modernity of modern public health. Quarantine control could be the most convenient means to isolate the infectee while constantly disciplining the public could lower the risk of infection. Over time some strategies of quarantine controls could prove to be untenable, either because they were morally indefensible, or for practical reasons difficult to sustain. To keep the public health condition improving, some disciplines of quarantine controls should, therefore, be voluntarily transferred to regular sanitary behaviors, norms, and customs. In Taiwan, such a process could begin in the 1930s when the school enrollment rates significantly increased and female caregivers ubiquitously appeared in Taiwanese households. An even more significant phenomenon than above finally occurred in Taiwan during the 1960s, namely the early Cold War period.

Self-Discipling Epidemic Precaution in Post-World War II Taiwan

Scholarship on the history of medicine in Taiwan generally considers the period between 1945 and 1949 as either the beginning or the end of an era. This perspective is also applied to the understanding of the quarantine practices in Taiwan. While the public health activities were most commonly associated with the colonial influences in Japan-ruled Taiwan, public health infrastructure as well as quarantine controls in post-World War II Taiwan soon adopted certain aspects of American medicine from the retrocession to the retreat of Republican China in 1949. This resulted in the creation of a unique hybrid model of medical service in contemporary Taiwan (Liu, 2017). Under this transformation, the quarantine control of the colonial legacy of a policing system remained in daily sanitary practices and eventually became integrated into social customs, while the impacts were further boosted by advanced American-influenced medicine and its quarantine criteria and technologies carried out through various foreign aid agencies.

The Relapsing Epidemics to Keep Colonial Quarantine Control Functional

At the end of World War II, Taiwan was returned to China and soon became integrated into China's administrative structure. As far as epidemics were concerned, the island not only underwent changes in the organization of health agencies but also was very much affected by the spread of diseases from the mainland (Chen, 2000). In 1945, the Taiwanese government had reorganized the colonial hygienic model by removing quarantine activities from the police department and placing them in a new Bureau of Sanitation (Weishengju) (Su, 2004). The change did not, however, fundamentally change the core ideology of quarantine control. Various communicable diseases that had been under control in the colonial period reappeared and caused high mortality among the infected population in the early stage of the Taiwan Retrocession (Zhung, 1998). Undoubtedly, post-war Taiwan urgently needed new public health resources and administrative skills to fill the vacuum caused by the withdrawal of the Japanese in August 1945.

The retreat of the Republic of China to Taiwan in 1949 not only caused a sudden demographic surge (see Figure 1.5) but also increased risks of recurrence of several epidemics and endemic diseases. The reconstruction of public health infrastructure, including the capability of quarantine control, was urgently needed to save lives and ensure the political future of the Nationalist Party in Taiwan. The annual growth rate of population in Taiwan reached 2.5% in 1925 and remained around that level throughout the remainder prior to the peak of the Pacific War (1941–1945). Although the actual damage to Taiwanese population was unknown due to the wartime restriction of death registration and incomplete investigation,

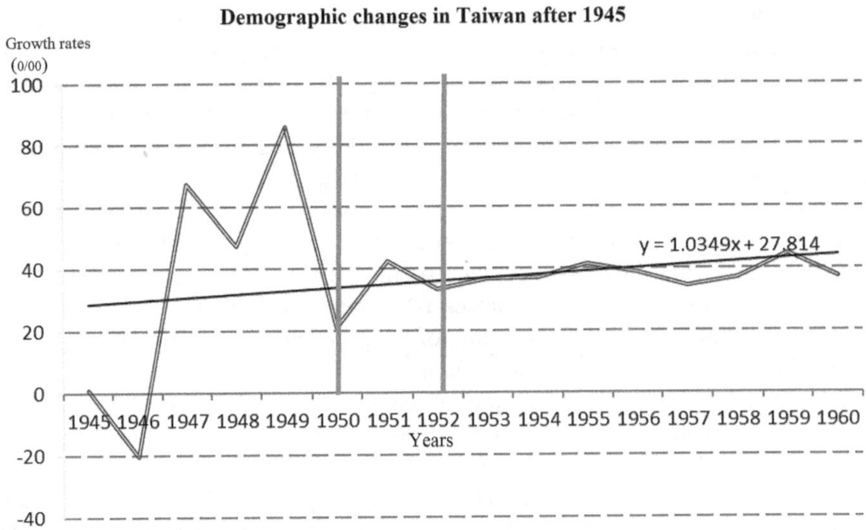

Figure 1.5 The Trend of Demographic Growth Rate in Post–World War II Taiwan

Sources: Statistics are collected from Angus Maddison, "Historical Statistics of the World Economy: 1–2008 AD," http://www.ggdc.net/maddison/ (2021/12/20 accessed). The equation already removed the impact of migration of mainlanders to population growth in Taiwan.

the severe loss of life could also be estimated by post-World War II data (see Figure 1.5). Immediately after World War II the growth rate shot up, reaching a peak of 8.7% in 1949. This large but short-lived increase was due to the heavy migration from the mainland following the exodus of the Nationalists. Even with the surge of mainlanders' migration, throughout the 1950s growth rates remained high, generally well above 3%, until the 1960s when a decline set in.[8] Historically speaking, two effects were commonly counted to explain the population growth: the net migration and the natural increase. The later could be an indicator to evaluate the demographic impacts of public health improvements.

In-migration was again very heavy immediately following World War II, and some slight gains were recorded during the 1950s. However, it was insufficient to offset the fact that natural increase has been and continues to be the main source of population growth in Taiwan (Chang, 1966). According to the statistics above, Taiwan enjoyed an average 6 per thousand population growth rate, while the island suffered the peak setback during the 1950s when rates in excess of 35 per thousand were experienced over several years. Deducting the impacts of migration in the early stage, after World War II, mortality declined even more rapidly between 1947 and 1960 when the death rate fell from 18 to 7 per thousand, or by 78% in a scant 13 years (Bogue, 1969).[9] It is interesting to note that the downward trend has continued since 1961 but the rate of decline has slowed down considerably. The declined mortality trend in the colonial period could have partially contributed to successful quarantine control while the similar situation in post-war Taiwan would have had more complicated reasons.

Mortality levels are of course influenced by the age composition of a population. Probably because sanitary self-discipline was forming since the 1930s, along with the increase of female caregivers, as might be expected, mortality declines have been relatively uniform for all ages for a certain period in the late colonial period. After World War II, from 1949 to the 1960s death rates continued to decline for all ages, but now the biggest declines in the death rates occurred among the pre-school children; the infant death rate also showed a more rapid decline. As mentioned previously, the infant and children mortality were crucial to determine the improving situation of epidemic control in households. The improvement in these mortality rates usually indicates a "younging" effect on overall population age composition (e.g., the age structure of the population in 1968 was as follows: under 15 years—39%, 15–64 years—59%, and 65 years and over—2%),[10] and the increasing awareness of epidemic precaution along with better maternal and child health. Both could be linked to some self-disciplined social customs and personal hygienic behaviors (Preston, 1996).

Figure 1.6 clearly illuminates that immediately after World War II, the crude death rates (CDR) decreased steadily and rapidly, while the crude birth rate (CBR)

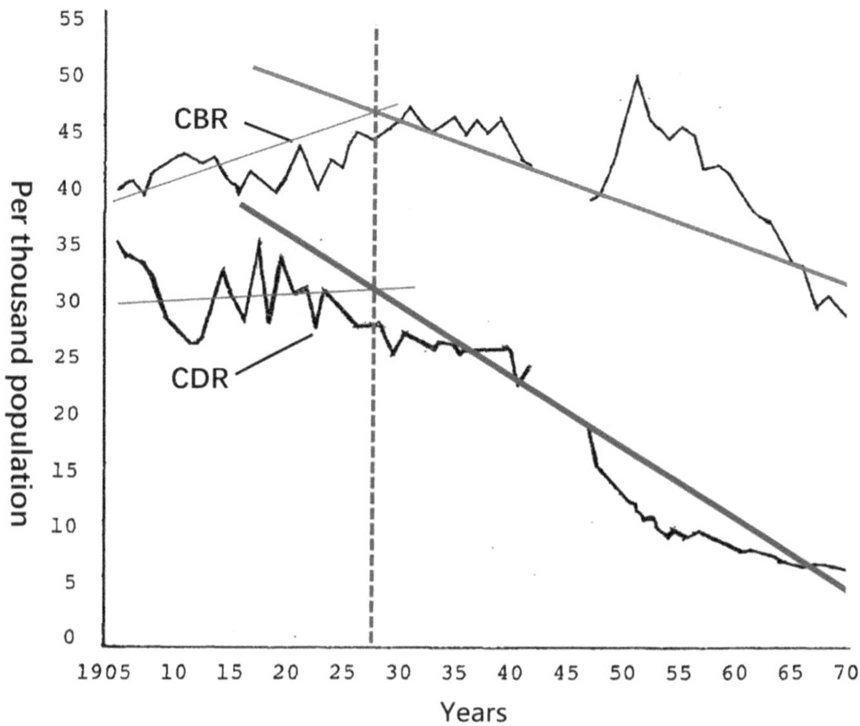

Figure 1.6 The Changing Gape between CBR and CDR, 1905–1970

Source: Statistics are collected from Angus Maddison, "Historical Statistics of the World Economy: 1–2008 AD," http://www.ggdc.net/maddison/ (2021/12/20 accessed).

rose to a peak in the early 1950s. This produced a very substantial increase in the rate of population growth, or what is called the post-war "baby boom." Unlike the children and adult mortalities that both improved after the 1930s in colonial Taiwan, the children mortality in early post-war era showed much improvement. This illuminates that the focus of epidemic control could shift from public sectors, such as the police force and public health agents, to private caregivers in the family. A closer examination of the rate trends depicted in Figure 1.6 further reveals that, from 1946 onward, the mortality decline has been steady and fairly rapid, but fertility has followed two distinct trends. First, beginning in 1946, the birth rate experienced a substantial increase, reaching a peak of 49 per thousand during the period of 1951–1952. One important contributor to this increased fertility is the changing age structure; the number of women of ages 20–24 years increased rapidly during this period. This observation suggests (1) that the conditions that affect mortality also influence fertility, but mortality is more sensitive to them, and (2) that there is feedback between mortality and fertility with either mortality or fertility change requiring an adjustment from the other. Generally speaking, Taiwanese females had a better chance to access knowledge and support of epidemic precaution. To this status, quarantine controls could only be supplemental when certain epidemics broke out.

Changes in the mode of healthcare services and related education quickly opened the way for keeping Taiwanese population growing, away from the threat of epidemics and endemic diseases. These changes influenced both a rise in fertility and a drop in mortality, and produced an initial widening of the birth-death gap (see Figure 1.6). To illustrate, mortality decline may increase the proportion of women entering the childbearing age, and then increase the birth rates. High birth rates with decreasing infant mortality could be because of better epidemic precautions and controls (Creanga and others, 2015). The control of epidemic disease is a most important contributor to mortality decline. However, it is something that can be done by relatively simple public health measures such as better maternal education, nursing, and midwives (World Population Conference, 1974). Additionally, the policing criteria of sanitary behaviors by the guidance of a police force was shortly kept before 1960s, might be later internalized to daily life in Taiwanese society via increasing the population of educated females and wives (Chen, 2014). Population thus increased because fertility behaviors were enmeshed in a web of institutionalized relationships. Not until the social structure takes on a new public health character of epidemic precaution and self-disciplined sanitary habits does a new vital equilibrium emerge (Taeuber, 1952; Hawley, 1973). In the process of societal development, social and cultural norms changed to favor epidemic precaution for diseases control. Rates of infant fertility as well as general mortality also improved.

Considering the severe war damage and sudden population pressure in 1949, the socio-economic development would not be the sole reason to explain the fast demographic growth. The decline in mortality in post-war Taiwan was brought about by three main factors: imported medical aids and public health measures, good health awareness, and where it was reinforced by the force of appreciation to modern criteria of sanitation and quarantine since the colonial period. This was a consequence of man's improved mastery over nature, both in terms of social awareness and public organization to reach the goals of quarantine (Chamberlain, 1970). In fact, the rapid population increase in post-war Taiwan was caused by the dramatic reduction of the death rate made possible by public health measures, successful epidemic precautions, and collective efforts to control rather than by any single efforts to quarantine or isolate infections before the 1960s.

From Policing Health to Self-Discipline of Epidemic Precaution

Under Japanese rule, colonial modernization programs were implemented in a number of areas, such as agricultural production, economic development, and public health. Of particular relevance is the fact that the Japanese administration established and maintained an unusual form of modernity within the colonial situation. Furthermore, since the end of World War II, the island was under the influence of a developmental program initiated by the Nationalist government and the American assistance program. This new political configuration facilitated a move toward recovering some colonial schemes but, this time, was under American guidance and selection (Ekbladh, 2011). It would be essential to note that the economic recovery of post-war Taiwan did not immediately launch until after 1952 when American aid came. Moreover, the expected effects of economic reconstruction in post-war Taiwan took time to unveil, only showing clear signs after the 1960s (Wu, 1988).[11] Therefore, the increase in population before the 1960s implies that, as the existed sanitary policing system remained, changes in voluntarily sanitary habits and the increasing awareness of epidemic precaution greatly helped to control many diseases before the sufficient American aid arrived.

The motives to re-establish a public health system in post-World War II Taiwan in fact is twofold. One is the immediate emergency of recurring epidemics due to long-term war damage. The other one is the goal to resume the public health modernization that had been interrupted by the Sino-Japanese war between 1941 and 1945. American sources on the medical aid given in the 1950s and 1960s included public agencies such as Economic Cooperation Administration, private foundations such as the Rockefeller Foundation, the Population Council, and American Bureau for Medical Advancement in China (ABMAC) as well as the General Headquarters (GHQ) in Tokyo, and universities, such as Princeton and the University of Michigan. Foreign assistance also brought new forms of quarantine criteria and strategies and also introduced the latest concepts and education to promote epidemic precaution and medical prevention for the purposes to control infectious diseases. The results have been nothing short of astounding (Yang, 2008). However, in the 1950s, the core ideologies of top-down administration and authoritarianism resumed under the new belief on "advanced" American medicine.

As for quarantine control, a strategy practiced since the colonial period, it became a mission of recovery and maintenance based on policing health when the Nationalist government transferred control from the police jurisdiction to a new sanitary administration system. Matters related to sanitation and public health were taken over by the first Provincial Sanitary Bureau (Wei-sheng Ju) between 1945 and

1947, and then later at the provincial level by Provincial Sanitary Sector . Both civil institutes were in charge of sanitary affairs while the police force became merely auxiliary to public health works.

Having carried out the mission of recovery, the new public health system under American guidance turned attention to building public health stations in villages and at the township level and establishing a Sanitary Administration (Wei-sheng Yuan) at the prefectural level, which was responsible for supervising the local stations' routine works (Chen, 1954). Without immediately sufficient numbers of medical doctors per population, however, public health nurses and midwives often filled up the functions of health care for the communities and their families.[12] Unlike male ob/gy doctors, midwives in Taiwan had unique opportunities to assist delivery in pregnant women's room and brought medical support and public health education on the emotional base of sisterhood. In short, the Nationalist government transplanted an American-influenced public health infrastructure from Mainland China to the Island of Taiwan. However, due to the difficulty of immediately increasing medical practitioners, who were then mainly the male doctors, female healthcare workers were the majority personnel at these public health stations who provided health care to their communities. It is worth noting that, to complete the mission of recovery, administrative re-construction and re-organization of epidemic control systems could be crippled without insufficient medical powers. Educated females quickly filled the gaps of health care since they were traditionally caregivers in the Taiwanese family and now had received better training in nursing and midwifery.

Like the situation in early colonization, the emergency of epidemic crises always ignited public demand of quarantine control run by the government in Taiwan and people voluntarily rendered personal freedom and privacy in exchange. The most serious vulnerability that Taiwan suffered in these early post-war years was the deterioration in these systems of quarantine control and a weakened sanitary police system. It was through these holes in the quarantine control that bubonic plague, cholera, and smallpox returned to Taiwan along with the population influx from the mainland. It is interesting to note that, however, before Taiwan was returned to China in August 1945, the Nationalist government had already decided to keep their local administration in Taiwan so as to secure the social stability (Chen, 2000). The October 1944 "Draft Outline for the Takeover of Taiwan," which the Taiwan Investigation Committee in Chongching submitted to Chiang Kai-shek,[13] suggested the following policy:

> The laws and decrees from the period of Japanese occupation will all be provisionally valid, except those that oppress and restrain the people, or those that conflict with the Three Peoples' Principles or the laws and decrees of the Republic (Kirby and others, 2001). This is seen as a practical need, and will gradually be revised … in local administration … we will provisionally continue the baojia (*hoko*) system. In each locality, we will take over those governmental and public bodies (including every branch of administration, …, sanitary, waterworks, police, …) and according to Republican laws and decrees, and either dismantle suspend, reorganize, or retain them.[14]

Under the same design, the colonial sanitary police system was saved by the Nationalist government without noticing how severe the war had damaged it.

In the first issue in January 1946 of the *Taiwan Police*, the official magazine of the new Taiwan Provincial Police Training Academy quoted Governor Chen Yi's statements on the high status of the Japanese police in colonial Taiwan. Chen Yi believed that although the Japanese police constantly "enslaved" Taiwanese, they really handled a wide range of duties, spanning "administration, education, hygiene, the economy, etc." He thus claimed that "the things that the police had to do should continue to be done as before" (Chen, 1946). To fulfill such a request, without surprise, the new government continued the training program for police in sanitation and disease prevention, "Sanitary Police Personnel Training" began in June 1946. The training topics widely covered sanitary administration, acute contagious diseases, chronic contagious diseases, port quarantine, restrictions on food and drink, environmental hygiene, malaria prevention, factory hygiene, female hygiene, and school hygiene (Wicentowski, 2007).[15] It was clear that the colonial police system's role to supervise health surveillance and quarantine control was kept on at certain stages while the function of epidemic prevention later transferred, on the surface at least, to the newly established Sanitary Bureau. Such a configuration did not significantly change until the 1960s, even when the local politics went through various crises. However, the importance of female health workers eventually rose in significance while the power of the male sanitary policemen declined.

Chin Hsien-Yu once interpreted the administrative change from male police-led sanitation to female nurse-staffed public health stations as "the feminization of the medical system" and so a key feature of the new public health infrastructure after 1947 (Chin, 1998). The coordination between the male police and the Taiwanese leaders of the *hoko* system meant that the top-down quarantine control was undoubtedly based on the underlying patriarchy, a form of colonial authoritarianism. Since the 1930s, Taiwanese females began to participate, however, in public health works and diseases prevention but they only worked in private roles. In 1951, the Taiwan Provincial Government started to abolish various sanitary functions of the Police Department and remove powers of quarantine inspection and control to the other public health sectors.[16] During the 1950s, nursing and midwifery became dominantly female occupations. In addition to the establishment of a nursing school and department in National Taiwan University, the Provincial Government also gave permission to establish privately funded nursing and midwifery schools. The nursing and midwifery education was, therefore, flourishing (Yeh, 2014). Fu-Ying Vocational High of Nursing and Midwifery in Kaohsiung in 1958 was the first of this kind, and thereby represented a long trend of fast growth of private nursing and midwifery education in Taiwan for decades (Tsay and others, 2006). Chin thus argued, "in general, there was considerable continuity in medical facilities and public health practices from the Japanese colonial period to the rule of the KMT (Nationalist Party) in the 1950s" (Chin, 1998). A very interesting observation further reveals the continuity of the impact of discipling quarantine awareness in the adoption of such consciousness in post-war Taiwanese society. Such a transformation from male police to female public health nurses had vital impacts to the adoption of modern public health as well as of quarantine-control thought and behaviors among local Taiwanese. The public health nurses who also had qualified midwifery training and were based on each public health station after the 1950s brought the female professionals to service the island-wide public health system. They had roles like agents in people's homes by governmental appointment (Li and Zhang, 1975). The famous Taiwanese doctor Du Ts'ung-ming once stated, "since only healthy mothers can give birth to healthy babies, healthy mothers are the key to reproducing the population. Thus, women ought to obey principles of women's hygiene (for our country)" (Du, 1955). With the widespread distribution of public health stations in the 1960s, these stations played a role as a hub to link advanced medical service in the cities and community needs of health services. Thus, the female nurses and midwives in each station eventually had much opportunity to educate local families, replace the sanitary police of the colonial period, and keep similar public health functions ongoing (Chen, 1988; Guo, 1991; Zhang, 2009).

Around the 1950s onward, female health workers such as public health nurses and midwives staffed every health station. Moreover, health stations were often located in the midst of other governmental institutions and so were usually surrounded by symbols of governance like the police station, party headquarters, the courthouse, and the building of the armed forces. Between 1968 and 1973, the Taiwanese government undertook the most extensive expansion on record of the public junior high school system in Taiwan, and as the statistics show, the female school enrollment rate increased. This also directly contributed to the efficient reallocation of females in the Taiwan economy and their family well-being. Prior to the 1970s, while the female school enrollment rate increased, according to the statistics of Figures 1.5 and 1.6, the demographic growth, an indicator of public health improvement, already appeared for nearly two decades (Tsai and others, 2009). It has been a long and deeper tradition that the female was the major caregiver to the family in Taiwan (Zeng, 1998). The Ordinance on Education of 1919 stated that the purpose of the common school was to "(take) care of the development of the health, give moral instruction, impart common knowledge and skills, engender national characteristics, and spread the national language" (Chen, 2006). Probably because Taiwanese family members often intervened in medical decisions, Taiwanese females could not have chance to receive proper education, they were always required to take care of family and search all available or alternative resources, despite the fact that they largely could not have a chance to receive proper education. It also served as an important reason for women to have used more TCM services than men for regular meal preparation (Tsai, 2005; Chuan and others, 2012). Undoubtedly, the public health nurses and midwives during the 1950s and 1960s replaced the top-down discipline of sanitary police, and so provided new ways to educate Taiwanese females in the public health concepts and practices to self-discipline of family health behaviors for the purpose of epidemic precaution (Figure 1.7).

Generally, staffs at health stations were charged with providing medical treatment, controlling communicable diseases, compiling statistics, directing child-rearing and maternal care, making house-to- house visits, distributing public health

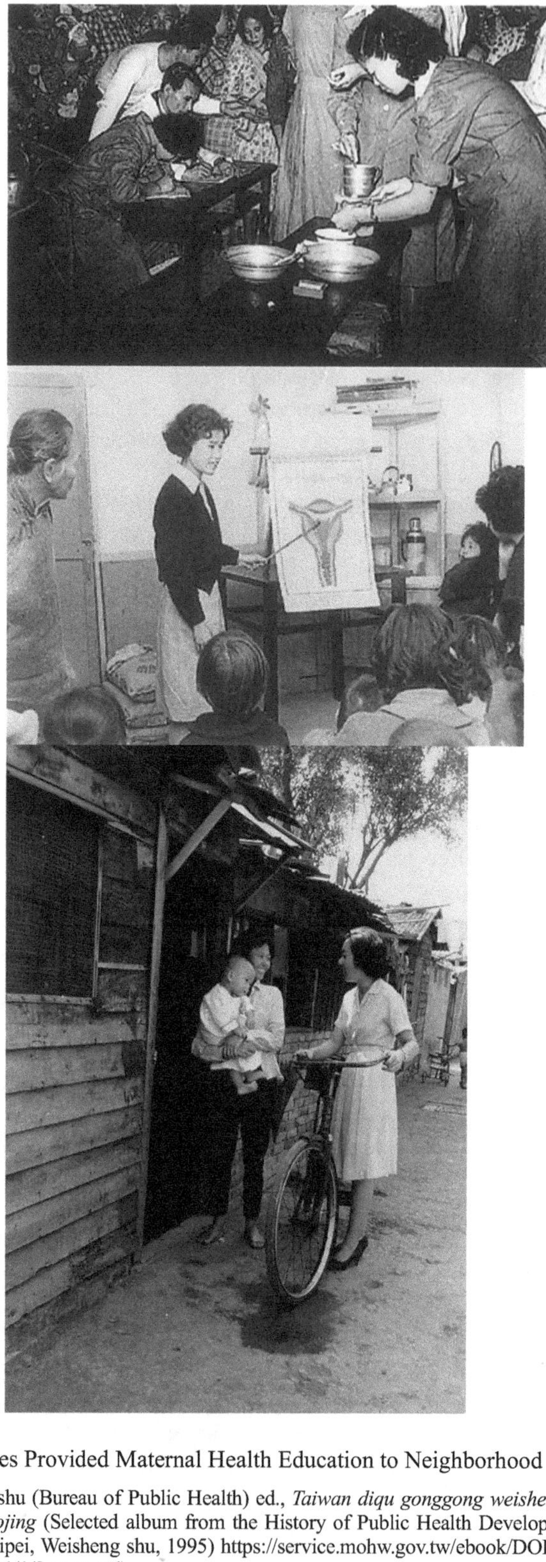

Figure 1.7 Nurses Provided Maternal Health Education to Neighborhood Families

Source: Weisheng shu (Bureau of Public Health) ed., *Taiwan diqu gonggong weisheng fazhan shi zhaopian xuanji (2) baojing* (Selected album from the History of Public Health Development in Taiwan (2) Health Works), (Taipei, Weisheng shu, 1995) https://service.mohw.gov.tw/ebook/DOPL/photo2/chapter3/Welcome.html (2021/1/8 accessed).

information, and helping to administer school hygiene (Yen, 1950). Before the female school enrollment rate accelerated in the 1970s, since they already handled health issues in the family, Taiwanese females received education about the modern hygiene concepts and knowledge of epidemic precaution from these female workers in public health stations. And the nurse-midwifery professionals have provided essential assistance to both expectant women and their family in Taiwan, it is worth pointing out that their contribution to women and family health before the 1960s was significant (Liang and Wu, 2013). By having these female professionals, the top-down function of sanitary police before 1950 was eventually replaced by bottom-up health education to females and their families to maintain the awareness of epidemic precaution. According to the regular services and the roles they played, female nurses, and midwives not only replaced the functions of the colonial sanitary police but also featured the rise of educated women and the penetration of the health surveillance and diseases control to each household.

The rise of female power in the public health field indicates that the stage from self-discipline to adoption of modern diseases control could started at this moment as they contributed to internalized hygienic consciousness and integrated public health behaviors in daily family life. The latest researches on developing countries showed that because education increases consciousness about important health issues, it is also considered to be an important element for improving health outcomes within lesser developed communities. This is possibly the situation of Taiwan in the 1950s. Keats found that female schooling had a positive impact on child health, using Uganda's free primary education program of 1997 as a case study. McAlister and Baskett surveyed 148 countries and observed that female education had the greatest effect on maternal mortality. Anlimachie and Avoada cited the rural education program in Ghana, which had improved the social and health well-being of the citizens. All studies indicated that a higher female education rate increases life expectancy and decreases the adult mortality rate because education creates and enhances awareness and consciousness among females to consume nutritious food, to maintain a healthy life for themselves and for their children. Moreover, the educated female can acquire better health-related information to stay healthy and lead a safe life. As for Taiwan in the early recession period, the replacement of sanitary police by female nurses and midwives enhanced the above effects within a continuously disciplined society from the colonial period to the present.

Insight and Discussion

In 1972, microbiologists Macfarlane Burnet and David White predicted that "the future of infectious diseases … will be very dull" and "there was always a risk of some wholly unexpected emergence of a new and dangerous infectious disease." From Legionnaires' disease first discovered in the 1970s to AIDS, Ebola, the severe acute respiratory syndrome (SARS), and COVID-19, infectious diseases continue to affect world populations (Fong and Law, 2020). COVID-19 the latest pandemic of new infectious disease has mocked modern public health and medical science worldwide.

Facing the COVID-19 pandemic, Taiwan demonstrated resilience at the initial stage of epidemic prevention and effectively slowed down its spread. Based on the analysis of social media and online information, Chih-Yu Chin, Chang-Pan Liu, and Cheng-Lung Wang concluded that the fear of the loss of control best explains why panic behavior occurred among the public. When confronting the highly infectious COVID-19, public epidemic awareness is vital. While fear is an inevitable result when an emerging infectious disease occurs, on the one hand, the strategies to convert social resistance into assistance with quarantine policies further enhanced the strong image of governance (Chin and others, 2021).[17] However, on the other hand, studies in this volume to determine the proportion of individuals who voluntarily reduced interaction with their family members, friends, and colleagues or classmates to avoid coronavirus infection in Taiwan and other surrounding countries since 2019 showed self-discipline and so could be the real reason to voluntarily follow the guideline of quarantine policies and prevent the spread of the COVID-19 pandemic in Taiwan during the pandemic years of 2020–2023. The study by Wei-Po Chou et al. revealed that despite strict social distancing measures not being implemented in Taiwan, more than one-third of respondents voluntarily reduced their interaction with friends and colleagues or classmates (Chou and others, 2020). This study again confirmed that the general public in Taiwan was self-disciplined and voluntarily adopted preventive strategies before the governmental guidelines were issued.

More research has been done on gender difference to deal with the epidemic crisis. Yating Chuang and John Chung-En Liu evaluated mask-wearing behaviors in response to COVID-19 based on 12,208 observations in February 2020 in Taiwan. They find that, compared to men, women are 16% more likely to wear masks as a way to protect themselves during the pandemic. The protective behaviors, however, decrease significantly when people are with others. The gender difference in mask-wearing has dropped the most when people are with a mixed-gender group (Chuang and Liu, 2020). A phenomenon much differed from Wei-Po Chou and colleagues' conclusion. Jointly considering their studies, peer dynamics and potential heritage of adopting awareness of self-quarantine moves should be taken into consideration. This recent Covid experience could echo the above review on Taiwan's history of discipling modern public health under the awareness of quarantine from governance to social consciousness.

"Diseases have no political boundaries" is the widely used expression for advocating social cooperation in quarantine control. The unequal status between colonialist and colonized first brought a top-down administration of quarantine control to Taiwan. The externally applied force to discipline Taiwanese was later adopted by educated youth, especially the females who could play well both the social and domestic roles. The replacement of sanitary police by female public health workers in 1950s Taiwan further accelerated the process to internalize the external guidance of quarantine control as behavior of self-discipline and, finally, adoption. This underlined the colonial legacy behind the contemporary example of Taiwan's anti-COVID-19 scenario.

Charles Rosenberg argues for the importance of identifying similarities between pandemics, especially in the ways that societies inquire into the origin of an outbreak, the ways they demand urgent state intervention (Rosenberg, 1989), and the ways in which collective responsibility can be a framework for communal support. These insights should inspire societies to consider why various strategies are adopted in different contexts and stages of history. While all societies demand a political response, the response to pandemics varies from restrictive quarantine without concern for human rights to ignoring public health warnings and preventative actions. All these responses have repeatedly appeared in the past. Pandemics eventually resolve by a process, as Rosenberg put it, that "starts at a moment in time, proceeds on a stage limited in space and duration, follows a plotline of increasing revelatory tension, moves to a crisis of individual and collective character, then drifts toward closure."[18] The similar drama was playing out with COVID-19—first in China and then in many countries worldwide including Taiwan. History can be a resource to provide inspiration and understanding for controlling pandemics under different social contexts or time spans and is just as essential as the natural sciences are for generating quarantine strategies and treatments. The end of the pandemic depends on a combination of the life cycle of the virus and earnest human efforts at self-disciple and mutual cooperation.

Notes

1 Davidson (1903, p. 364); *Taiwan chiseki shi* (Administrative Achievements in Taiwan) in *Chinese Local Gazetteers, Taiwan Region*, no. 184 (1937) (Taipei: Fuwen, 1985 reprinted), p. 29.
2 *Taiwansheng wushiyinianlai tongjitiyao* (Taipei: Taiwanshen xiengzheng zhangquang gongshu, 1946): 326–327.
3 "Kikenw o shiranu hontojin(Islanders who do not know the danger)," *Taiwan nichinichi shimpo*, August 2, 1919, p. 7.
4 *Taiwan sotokufu keimu kyoku* 1922, pp. 32–33.
5 For example, *Taiwan nichinichi shimpo*, a governmental-own newspaper was pointing to Taiwanese as the source of the spread of infection. "Koeki zokuhatsu: Naichijin ni mo nigikan (Cholera continues: Japanese are also suspected of having it)," *Taiwan nichinichi shimpo*, August 2, 1919, p. 7.
6 After Ogata Masanori successfully conducted his experiment in Taipei in 1897, a policy of catching rates was shortly issued. However, resistance rose from local police force due to "people are indifferent to catching rats." See "Bubonic plague trends and measures for prevention" (Pesuto byo sei narabi ni yobo jo shisetsu tsuho no ken) from Tainan district head Yamagata Naoto to Taiwan Governor-General Chief of Civil Affairs Goto Shimpei, 15 May 1902. *Taiwan sotokufu kobun ruisan* vol. 4678 document no. 1, file dated 1 June 1902, pp. 36–48.
7 Diarrhea was proved the major killer to Taiwanese infants and children by medical doctors and public health surveys. Tetsuzo (2005, pp. 25–213).
8 The number was calculated from numbers taken from governmental publications *Statistical Abstract of Taiwan Province 1962* and *Statistical Abstract of the Republic of China 1973*, while missing number were estimated and inserted from Angus Maddison, "Historical Statistics of the World Economy:1-2008 AD," http://www.ggdc.net/maddison/ (2021/12/20 accessed).

9 The estimation was taken from the numbers of *Taiwan Demographic Fact Book*, 1972. However, infant mortality numbers of 1947–1948 was missing in official reports. The number was therefore taken from the estimation from Bogue (1969).
10 Percentages were only roughly counted from the numbers of *Taiwan Demographic Fact Book*, 1972.
11 Such assertion was made on the argument of Wu (1988, p. 145–52); and "Coordination of MSA/JCRR Policies and Programs," February 19, 1952, Council for International Economic Cooperation and Development (CIECD) archive 36-15-006-001, Institute of Modern History of Academia Sinica.
12 The ration between medical doctors and female health workers were roughly 1 to 21 in the 1950s. Numbers are calculated from *1994 nian weisheng tongji (kongwo tongji)* (Sanitary statistics of 1994 (statistics of public sectors), Table 43; http://www.doh.gov.tw/CHT2006/DM/DM2_2.aspx?now_fod_list_no=10219&class_no=440&level_no=2 (2022/12/01 accessed).
13 "*Taiwan jieguan jihua gangyao caoan* (Draft Outline for the Takeover of Taiwan)," reprinted in Kirby et al. (2001, pp. 107–121).
14 "*Taiwan jieguan jihua gangyao caoan*," p. 108.
15 Taiwan Provincial Government Archives, file 037.3 2, p. 4. The citation was extracted from Joseph Charles Wicentowski, "Policing Health in Modem Taiwan, 1895–1949," PhD dissertation, The Department of History, Harvard University, 2007, p. 166.
16 "Taiwan shengzhefu daidian (Telegram from Taiwan Provincial Government)," *Taiwan shengzhefu gongbao* (Report of Taiwan Provincial Government) no. 54 (autumn, 1951): 648–652.
17 Chin C-Y, Liu C-P, Wang C-L (2021), Evolving public behavior and attitudes towards COVID-19 and face masks in Taiwan: A social media study. PLoS ONE 16(5): e0251845. (https://doi.org/10.1371/journal.pone.0251845, 2021/1/16 accessed).
18 Rosenberg (1989, p. 2).

References

Barclay, George W., 2015, Colonial Development and Population in Taiwan: Princeton, NJ: Princeton University Press.

Bogue, D. J., 1969, The Principles of Demography: John Wiley and Sons, New York.

Chamberlain, Neil W., 1970, Beyond Malthus; Population and Power: Englewood , NJ: Prentice-Hall.

Chang, I-Shing, 1966, The Economic Aspect of Population Problem in Taiwan: The Cultural Foundation of Chia-Hsing Cement Co., Taipei.

Chen, Chi-chan, 1954, Sanitary Administration in China: Taipei Public Health Journal, Taipei.

Chen, Ching-chih, 1984, Police and Community Control Systems in the Empire, *in* Myers, Ramon H. and Peattie, Mark R. eds., The Japanese Colonial Empire, 1895–1945: Princeton, NJ: Princeton University Press, p. 213–239.

Chen, Kung-pei, 1988, Preventive Medicine Foundation Public Health Studies: Main Stream, Taipei.

Chen, Peifeng, 2006, "Doku" No Doshoimu: Rizhishi Qi Taiwan De Yuyanzhengce, Jindaihuayuren Tong (The Different Intentions behind the Semblance of "Douka (Assimilation)": The Language Policy, Modernization and Identity in Taiwan during the Japan-Ruling Period): Maitian chuban, Taipei.

Chen, Shufang, 2000, Zhanhou Zhi Yi: Taiwan De Gonggong Weisheng Wenti Yu Jianzhi 1945–1954 (The Post-WWII Plague: The Questions and Establishment of Public Health in Taiwan 1945–1954): Daoxiang, Taipei.

Chen, Yi, 1946, Opening Statement: Taiwan Jingcha (Taiwan Police), v. 1, n. 1, p. 9.
Chen, Yinshuan, 2014, Kaihuayushixiade Rizhishiqi Taiwan Nutzijiaoyuzhengze: Yi Zhanghuagaonu Welli (Taiwanese Female Education Policy under the Concept of Civilization in Japan-ruled Period: A Case Studies of Zhanghua Female Highschool): Yishu yu wenhua lunhen (A View of Art and Culture), n. 4, p. 91–107.
Chiang, Yu-Lin, 2009, Nanwu Jingcha Dapusa: Rizhishiqi Taipeizho Jingchaweisheng Zhanlanhuizhong De Jingchaxingxiang ("Buddha Police": The Image of the Police in the "Taipei Police & Hygiene Exhibition" during the Japanese Colonial Governance): Chengda faxuepinglun (Chengchi Law Review), n. 112, p. 1–44.
Chin, Hsien-yu, 1998, Colonial Medical Police and Postcolonial Medical Surveillance Systems in Taiwan, 1895–1950s: Osiris, v. 13, p. 326–338.
Chou, Wei-Po, et al., 2020, Voluntary Reduction of Social Interaction during The COVID-19 Pandemic in Taiwan: Related Factors and Association with Perceived Social Support: International Journal of Environmental Research and Public Health, v. 17, no. 21, p. 8039.
Chuang, Y. T., and Liu, C. E., 2020, Who Wears a Mask? Gender Differences in Risk Behaviors in the COVID-19 Early Days in Taiwan: Economics Bulletin, v. 40, n. 4, p. 2619–2627.
Creanga, Andreea A., et al., 2015, Pregnancy-Related Mortality in the United States, 2006–2010: Obstetrics & Gynecology, v. 125, n. 1, p. 5–12.
Davidson, James Wheeler, 1903, The Island of Formosa. Past and Present: Oxford University Press, Oxford.
Du, Ts'ung-ming, 1955, Memories: Lung-wen, Taipei.
Ekbladh, David, 2011, The Great American Mission: Modernization and the Construction of an American World Order: Princeton University Press, Ithaca.
Fan, Yanqiu, 1994, Riju Shiqi Taiwan Zhi Gonggong Weisheng: Yi Fangyi W Ei Zhongxin Zhi Yanjiu, 1895–1920 (Public health in Taiwan during the period of the Japanese occupation: a study focusing on the prevention of epidemics).
Fong, Ben Y. F., and Law, Vincent T. S., 2020, COVID-19 – A Tale of Two Cities: Seattle and Vancouver: Asia Pacific Journal of Health Management, v. 15, n. 3, p. 1.
Guo, Jinping, 1991, Gedi Weisheng Suo Jiqng You Chuntian (All public health stations will have sprint again): Lianhe bao (United Daily News), A6, 1.5.
Hawley, Amos H., 1973, Ecology and Population: Science, n. 179, p. 1196–1201.
Janetta, Ann, 1987, Epidemics and Mortality in Early Modem Japan: Princeton University Press, Princeton.
Kato, Shigeo, 1998, Kindaii Toshiakima to Koshoeisei Jōron: Ten Plus One--Special issue: Tokyo Studies, n. 12.
Kato, Takashi, 1897, Introduction (1896-10-20), *in* Taiwan sotokufu minsei kyoku eisei ka ed., Meiji Nijukyu Nen "Pesu To" Byoryuko Kiji (A Record of the Outbreak of "pesto" in Meiji 29 (1896)): Taiwan sotokufu minsei kyoku eisei ka, Taipei.
Kirby, William C., et al., ed., 2001, State and Economy in Republican China: A Handbook For Scholars, V. 2: Harvard University Asia Center: Distributed by Harvard University Press.
Lamley, Harry, 1970, The 1895 War of Resistance, *in* Leonard Gordon ed., Taiwan: Studies in Chinese Local History: Columbia University Press, New York & London.
Lamley, Harry, 1973, Short-lived Republic and War, 1895: Taiwan's Resistance Against the Japanese, *in* Taiwan in Modern Times: New York: St. John's University Press, p. 241–316.
Li, Yu-hua, and Zhang, Xi-ling, 1975, Xuanze Wo Suo Xingqu De Huli Gongzuo (Choosing a nursing job that interests me): Luxing (Green apricot), n. 26, p. 173–174.

Liang, Hwey-Fang, and Wu, Kuang-Ming, 2013, Muying Zhaohu De Tuishou-Yi Koushu Lishi Yanjiu Fa Tanjiu Zhanhou De Chanpo Shengya (1921–1989) (Playing an Active Role in Maternal-Infant Care: Using Oral History to Explore a Midwife's Career in Postwar Taiwan (1921–1989)): Huli Ji Jiankang Zhaohu Yanjiu (Journal of Nursing and Healthcare Research), v. 9, n. 3, p. 237–247.

Liu, Shiyung, 2008, The Ripples of Rivalry: The Spread of Modern Medicine from Japan to its Colonies: East Asian Science, Technology and Society: An International Journal, v. 2, n. 1, p. 47–71.

Liu, Shiyung, 2017, Transforming Medical Paradigms in 1950s Taiwan: East Asian Science, Technology and Society: An International Journal, v. 11, n. 4, p. 477–497.

Lo, Ming-Cheng M., 2002, Doctors Within Borders: Profession, Ethnicity and Modernity in Colonial Taiwan: University of California Press, Berkeley, CA.

Nagaki, Daizō, 1989, Kitazato Shibasaburō To Sono Ichimon (Kitazato Shibasaburō and his followers): Keiō Tsūshin, Tokyo.

Noguera, Pedro A., 2003, Schools, Prisons, and Social Implications of Punishment: Rethinking Disciplinary Practices: Theory Into Practice, v. 42, n. 4, p. 341–350.

Peckham, Robert and Pomfret, David M. eds., 2013, Imperial Contagions: Medicine, Hygiene, and Cultures of Planning in Asia: Hong Kong University Press, Hong Kong.

Preston, Samuel H., 1996, Population Studies of Mortality: Population Studies, v. 50, p. 525–536.

Preston, Samuel H., Keyfitz, Nathan, and Schoen, Robert, 1972, Causes of Death Life Tables for National Population: Seminar Press, New York.

Rosenberg, Charles, 1989, What Is an Epidemic? AIDS in historical perspective: Daedulus, v. 118, n. 2, p. 1–17.

Shiomi, Syunzi, 1940, The Synopsis of Wei-Sheng-Chu: Taiwan Executive Yuan, Taipei.

Siler, William, 1979, A Competing-Risk Model for Animal Mortality: Ecology, n. 60(4), p. 750–757.

Su, Yaochong, ed., 2004, Zuiho De Taiwan Zongdufu: 1944–1946 Zhongzan Zhiliaoji (The Last Government of Taiwan General-Governor: The Post-war Archive Collection, 1944–1946): Chenxing, Taizhong.

Suzuki, Tetsuzo, 2005, Taiwan Sotokufu No Eisei Seisaku To Taiwan Koi (The Sanitary Policy of the Taiwan Governor-General and Taiwan Public Physicians): Chukyo Daigaku Daigakuinsei Hogaku Kenkyu Ronshu, n. 25, p. 25–213.

Taeuber, Irene B., 1952, The Future of Transitional Areas, *in* Paul Hatt ed., World Population and Future Resource: American Book Co., New York.

Takekoshi, Yosaburo, 1907, Japanese Rule in Formosa: Longman, Green, London.

Tsai, D. F. -C., 2005, The Bioethical Principles and Confucius' Moral Philosophy: Journal of Medical Ethics, v. 31, n. 3, p. 159–163.

Tsai, W. J., et al., 2009, Does Educational Expansion Encourage Female Workforce Participation? A Study of the 1968 Reform in Taiwan: Economics of Education Review, v. 28, n. 6, p. 750–758.

Tsay, Shwu-Feng, Wu, C. H., Chen, Yiong-Hish, and Tai, Michael, 2006, Cong Hulishi Tantao Taiwan De Huli Fazhan Mailuo (An Examination of the Nursing Development in Taiwan-A Historical Perspective): Taiwan Yixuerenwen Qikan (Formosan Journal of Medical Humanity), v. 7, n. 1&2, p. 91–112.

Tsurumi, Yūsuke, 1965, Gotō Shinpei: Tokyo: Keisō Shobō.

Tu, Jow-ching, 1985, On Long-term Mortality Trends in Taiwan, 1906–1980: Journal of Chinese Sociology, no. 9, p. 145–164.

Wicentowski, Joseph Charles, 2007, Policing Health in Modern Taiwan, 1895–1949: Ph.D. dissertation, Harvard University.
World Population Conference, 1974, U. N. Population Change and Economic and Social Development (E/CONF.60/4): United Nations, New York.
Wu, Chialing, 1997, Women, Medicine and Power: The Social Transformation of Childbirth in Taiwan: Ph.D. dissertation. Department of Sociology, University of Illinois at Urbana-Champaign.
Wu, Tsong-Min, 1988, Meiyuan yu Taiwan de Jinjifazhan (American aids and economic development in Taiwan): Taiwan Shehui Yanju Jikan (Taiwan: A Radical Quarterly in Social Studies), v. 1, n. 1, p. 145–152.
Yang, Tsui-Hua, 2008, Meiyuan Dui Taiwande Weishengjihua Yu Yiliaotizhi Zhi Xingsu (U.S. Aid in the Formation of Health Planning and the Medical System in Taiwan): Zhongyang Yanjiuyuan Jindaishi Yanjiusuo Jikan (Bulletin of the Institute of Modern History, Academia Sicina), n. 62, p. 91–139.
Yeh, Mei-Chang, 2014, Shiji Huimo-Taiwan Huli Zhuanye De Yanbian Yu Fazhan (Centennial retrospective on the evolution and development of nursing education in Taiwan): Huli Zazhi (Journal of Nursing), v. 61, n. 4, p. 55–61.
Yen, Ts'un-hui, 1950, The Problems of Public Health on the Local Level: Public Health, v. 9, n. 1, p. 333.
Zeng, Qiumei, 1998, Taiwan Xifuzi Di Shenghuoshiji (The Lives of Sim-pua: The Stories of Taiwanese Daughters-in-Law): Yushan she, Taipei.
Zhang, Qiongrong, 2009, Weisheng Suo Yu Shequ Shuli Guanxi De Lishi Fazhan Fenxi (The Analysis of the Historical Development of Alienation between Public Health Stations and Communities): Master thesis, National Cheng Kung University Graduate Institute of Public Health.
Zhung, Yungming, 1998, Taiwan Yiliaoshih: Yi Taida Yiyune Wei Zhuzho (Taiwan Medical History: Centered on National Taiwan University hospital): Yunliu, Taipei.

2 Policies Tackling the COVID-19 Pandemic

Reflections on Public Health Governance and Public Health Ethics Based on Taiwan's Initial Responses

Ming-Jui Yeh and Yawen Cheng

Introduction

Since early 2020, the COVID-19 pandemic has tremendously impacted public health worldwide. Throughout epidemic development, many factors influence the curves of infection and disease fatalities. These factors include the traits of virus variants, vaccination levels, immunity status of the population, people's disease prevention behaviors, designs and enforcement of public health policies, and the accessibility of post-infection health care.

In Taiwan, like in many other countries, the COVID-19 pandemic has undergone different phases, which were characterized by various epidemic features. At least three phases could be identified in the initial stage. The first phase, marked from the start of the pandemic in January 2020 and up until May 2021, was characterized by very low infection rates and fatality rates despite the rapid spread of the virus around the globe. The second phase started with a rapid outbreak of locally infected cases in mid-May 2021, which was brought under control within two months, followed by another ten months of very low infection and fatality rates up until late April 2022. During the second phase, vaccine shortages were significant policy concerns, but after vaccine supplies were secured through international donations and assistance, vaccination rates quickly caught up, and the epidemic was again kept under control. Finally, the third phase began with a wave of rising infection of less fatal virus variants seen in late April up to late July 2022, subsiding afterward but still evolving.

In this chapter, we focus on policies and strategies undertaken in Taiwan during the first phase. During this phase, Taiwan was expected to be one of the hardest hit countries, given its densely urbanized population and geographical closeness to China. However, to the surprise of many onlookers, Taiwan had effectively contained the spread of the virus for more than 18 months. Taiwan's experiences in the initial phase of pandemic prevention have been widely reported in the media and many academic publications (Cheng, Li and Yang 2020; Lin et al. 2020; Rasmussen 2020; Wang, Ng and Brook 2020). However, a comprehensive overview and analysis of the disease control policies from the perspectives of public health governance and public health ethics are still lacking.

DOI: 10.4324/9781003438380-4

In Chapter 1, Liu examines the impacts of colonial governance in the first half of the 20th century on Taiwan's postwar disease control policies and in the second half of the 20th century while the country was still under tight control by an authoritarian regime. In this chapter, we analyze Taiwan's experiences after democratization, aiming to offer insights into disease control and broader public health policy with an in-depth analysis of the case of Taiwan and discuss the policy actions' repercussions. The purpose of this chapter is to record the early responses as they were under that particular time and space and may serve as a reference for similar scenarios in the future when unknown massive health threats emerge. We start with an overview of the public health governance framework, followed by an overview of disease control governance in Taiwan and major national policies and strategies undertaken during this epidemic phase. We then probe into the structural factors that enabled effective disease control. Finally, we analyze the ethical considerations underlying these policy actions, particularly focusing on the COVID-19 vaccine allocation issue to illustrate the utilitarian nature of most public health efforts. We conclude by pointing out that the ethics of body politic is the ethical mandate that underpins all the state public health policies efforts, as the people's life and health are indeed the sovereign state's primary obligations and the ultimate source of its political legitimacy.

Public Health Governance: Definition and Components

Governance, concerning the relationship between the rulers and the ruled, has been regarded as a significant structural-level social determinant of population health (Solar and Irwin 2010). While "governance" is conceptualized differently, it can be succinctly defined as the process in which authority is conferred on decision-makers and by whom policies are formed and enforced. Correspondingly, the term "public health governance" refers to the process of governance aiming at preventing diseases and promoting population health, in which governments at all levels exercise political power and institutional resources to manage public health affairs (Barbazza and Tello 2014; Carlson et al. 2015).

According to the World Health Organization, elements of good governance include strategic policy frameworks, effective regulations and oversight, coalition building, and accountability (WHO 2010). Among them, accountability is considered essential. It goes beyond the mere responsibility of service delivery, involving how decision-makers respond to the needs of citizens, how policy actions are made transparent to stakeholders and the public, and how decision-makers are held responsible for their actions and policy consequences. In short, it concerns on whose behalf a state is legitimate to rule. The government systems of checks and balances should be established and well-functioning to ensure accountability. Besides, freedom and mechanisms should be provided to stakeholders and all citizens to voice their concerns and influence political decision-making processes. Accountability, therefore, is fundamental to democracy.

Good governance is even more crucial in times of crisis, such as the COVID-19 pandemic. Drawing upon the public health governance framework, we examine policy actions undertaken in Taiwan in the first 18 months to respond to the COVID-19 pandemic. Specifically, this study aims to investigate what infrastructures and preconditions prepared a democratic polity to encounter the epidemic and what societal and political factors have contributed to the swift and effective infection containment. In addition, while some disease control policies have been criticized as infringing civil liberties such as privacy and bodily autonomy, we examine how the state had balanced among different ethical considerations amid the battle against pandemics.

Policy Framework of Disease Control in Taiwan

In Taiwan, the legal and administrative framework of disease control was strengthened as the result of the hard hit by the Severe Acute Respiratory Syndrome (SARS) epidemic in 2003, which led to 73 deaths, of which many were healthcare workers. At that time, and still, until now, Taiwan was blocked from international collaboration networks, thus having limited access to timely epidemic information and virus genome sequence needed for effective testing. In response to this arduous experience, the Centers for Disease Control (CDC), the administration in charge of prevention, surveillance, investigation, and control of communicable diseases under the supervision of the Ministry of Health and Welfare (MOHW), has made tremendous efforts ever since to improve its disease control capacity, by strengthening the regulatory power of the Communicable Disease Control Act (CDC Act), expanding healthcare infrastructure, and increasing professional competence of epidemic control personnel.

In 2005, the MOHW completed a full-scale proposal for the preparedness for the influenza pandemic, in which two areas were emphasized: one regarding the preparation and reserve of needed materials and the other regarding workforce deployment and mobilization. The Disease Control Medical Network (CDCMN) was set up, and designated hospitals were chosen for the provisions of isolation and medical treatment of patients infected with highly contagious and fatal diseases. The operation of the network has been modified throughout the years in response to consecutive epidemics, including the 2005 avian flu epidemic and the 2009 H1N1 influenza pandemic (Ko et al. 2017). Since 2005, the CDC also started recruiting and training Public Health Doctors, who have formed the backbone of the task force in charge of responding to outbreaks. There were 24 public health doctors working at the CDC in 2020. In 2008, the Central Epidemics Command Center (CECC) was written into the CDC Act. Once an epidemic occurs, it is given the highest national authority and has the power to integrate information and coordinate every ministry (see more details in the Discussion section). Besides, according to mandates of the CDC Act, authorities at all levels shall keep a safety stockpile of materials for disease control (2019). Physicians and managers of medical facilities who fail to report a suspected communicable disease within due time are subjected to high penalties, and unauthorized releases of information regarding the epidemic would be monitored and, if deemed unauthentic, censored.

Before the outbreak of the COVID-19 pandemic, there were 21 hospitals being designated as isolation hospitals for communicable diseases in Taiwan. These hospitals would be used exclusively to handle patients, leaving other facilities to operate normally. There were more than 1,100 negative-pressure rooms; the number is higher than in other countries. Accessibility to high-quality masks, gowns, other protection gears, and ventilators has been ensured, as stipulated in the CDC Act.

In addition to these disease control policies, Taiwan also has a universal publicly funded health system, the acclaimed National Health Insurance (NHI), which is a compulsory single-payer social insurance, providing universal coverage of healthcare services to all citizens and residents legally residing in Taiwan (Cheng 2015). The significance of the NHI in tackling the COVID-19 outbreak is twofold. It secures affordable and accessible health services for suspected patients, including virus tests and curative care. Its information technology (IT) infrastructures also allow the rapid identification and tracking of travel and potential exposure history of all citizens.

In sum, the policy framework of disease control is highly centralized and is equipped with reliable legal power, and disease control mechanisms are overseen by trained personnel in Taiwan. The CDC monitors communicable diseases and tackles endemics in ordinary times, and the temporarily established CECC takes charge of policies and measures during epidemics. The well-established NHI is the precondition for effective health services provision and IT applications. The democratic culture and social participation are the preconditions for effective supervision for those in power to make accountable decisions. With these understandings of the basic features of public health governance, we present major policy actions tackling the COVID-19 epidemic.

Effective Policies in Response to the COVID-19 Epidemic

The Establishment of the Central Epidemics Command Center (CECC)

On December 31, 2019, the local health authority of Wuhan issued a notice regarding a mysterious clustering of severe pneumonia cases. On the same day, Taiwan's CDC, upon receiving information through the informal channel, called up an inter-ministerial meeting and started onboard quarantine of all direct flights coming from Wuhan. Border control measures at two international airports began to be implemented. On January 20, in response to the growing severity of the epidemic in China and surrounding regions, Taiwan's CDC enacted the CECC, with the Minister of MOHW as the chief commander and high-rank officials from other ministries as the core members.

Besides, an expert advisory panel was set up, consisting of specialists in different disciplines, including infectious diseases, clinical medicine, epidemiology, medical laboratory science and nursing. In addition, as the members of the advisory panel were external experts with rich field experiences, they would not be bonded with the bureaucratic internal evaluation and could hence make more independent and professional policy recommendations. The centralized command system of CECC helps to effectively mobilize government funds, military personnel, and medical resources for disease control actions.

Board Control, Travel Restriction, Quarantine, and Epidemic Investigation

Since the very beginning of the pandemic, strict border control has been implemented at the two international airports. Health checkups were performed, and entering passengers with suspicious COVID-19-related symptoms were subjected to compulsory viral testing. Soon after the pandemic worsened in many countries in March 2020, the CECC banned all travelers without citizenship or legal residency status from entering Taiwan. Exceptions were allowed only for individuals who obtain entry permission for emergency or humanitarian reasons or on approved business. As the epidemic subsided around June 2020, travel restrictions were eased. However, they were tightened again in mid-May 2021 in response to the surge of infection. Nevertheless, throughout the first 18 months, all entering passengers were subjected to 14-day home quarantine. Regulations concerning local transportation, quarantine hotels, and viral testing are imposed and strictly enforced. In addition, in-depth epidemiologic investigations were carried out for all the confirmed cases to trace the source of infection. Their contacts were identified and subjected to compulsory self-quarantine.

With the coercion power given by the CDC Act, a robust command system led by the CECC, and a sound public health system, the investigating, contact tracing, and quarantining policies have been implemented relatively effectively.

The plausibility of these approaches could be attributed to three major factors. One is Taiwan's natural environment of being an island state. Accompanying the second factor, an effective law enforcement and health administration team, most of the potential infected cases could be identified, and their contacts could be traced. The third factor is the people's active participation throughout the process. There were of course some people who were less willing to cooperate with the government. Still, the majority of Taiwanese citizens respected the ruling of the government and recognized their own role and responsibility in the social cooperation in tackling the COVID-19 pandemic.

Masking, Social Distancing, and Gathering Restriction Policies

During the first 18 months of the pandemic, masking was required in the public transportation systems and in closed spaces, and social distancing policies were practiced while businesses, shops, restaurants, schools, and recreation facilities remained open throughout the period. It was not until May 2021, when the CECC raised the epidemic alert to level three to respond to the rising cases, that all people were mandated to wear a mask all the time when going out, and all leisure and entertainment venues, sports competition venues, exhibition venues, and educational facilities were closed, and most social activities and gatherings were banned.

Intensive Use of Information Technology (IT)

It is worth mentioning that in Taiwan, IT has been intensively applied in disease control measures since the beginning of the pandemic. For example, in early February 2020, the CECC tracked down the digital footprints of passengers of a recreation cruise and used public warning cell broadcast services to warn people who had been in contact with infected persons. Since February 2020, the government has used the NHI card for facial mask rationing and tracking people with higher risks, such as healthcare providers and people returning from other countries.

Soon after the outbreak in May 2021, a different digital system was developed under the leadership of the digital councilor of the Executive Yuan, Audrey Tang. The system asked people to send phone text messages to the number "1922" so their contact histories could be tracked. Owners of shops were also required to post QR codes at the entrance so that people entering their venues can scan sent through their smartphones and send messages free of charge to the system. The government obliged people who have contacted the infected individuals to compulsory 14-day home quarantine. Meanwhile, an App called "Taiwan social distance" was also developed and recommended by the CECC. People who voluntarily installed this app on their smartphones would be notified once they contacted the infected ones that day. With the assistance of digital technology, people's contact histories can be traced effectively. Councilor Tang also helped develop the COVID-19 vaccine reservation system that people could register for vaccine injection via either Internet, smartphone, or machines in convenience stores. In short, the government of Taiwan has applied IT intensively, which contributes to the success of effective pandemic control.

It is also worth mentioning that Taiwan's healthcare system is funded through the National Health Insurance (NHI), a compulsory single-payer social insurance, providing universal coverage of healthcare services to all citizens and residents legally residing in Taiwan. The NHI secures affordable and accessible health services, including virus tests and curative care. It also has advanced IT infrastructures that allow the rapid identification and tracking of travel and potential exposure of all citizens and legal residents.

Vaccination Policies and Vaccine Politics

Vaccination has been recognized as an effective way of COVID-19 pandemic control. However, for many countries which lack vaccine manufacturing capacity, vaccine shortage has been a national security concern. To guarantee the nation's security, starting in mid-2020, the government of Taiwan has tried to procure vaccines from international producers via direct purchase and through the COVAX (COVID-19 Vaccines Global Access) program; however, such efforts encountered political interference from China. Nevertheless, Taiwan still managed to secure 1.02 million doses of vaccines by the early April, 2021 through the COVAX program. However, before the outbreak in May 2021, Taiwanese people, including many healthcare providers, lacked the motivation to receive the vaccine. It was not until the outbreak started on May 14 that vaccine shortage became a public concern.

Policies for Social and Economic Assistance

In response to the economic damage done by COVID-19, the government has issued a series of bailout policies for workers and companies since early 2020, which include extending loan payments, cutting interest rates, providing income compensation, and living allowance. Because the spread of the virus has been contained, the impacts on economic activities and people's daily life are not as severe as in many other countries. In May 2021, the government expanded the coverage of relief packages to cover the unemployed, self-employed, and those who have experienced income loss, people who lack social insurance, those who have insufficient savings for family expenses, and those without other compensations. Besides offering financial support, the government also provided jobs with a maximum wage.

Public Communication

To keep the public informed, the CECC held press conferences on a daily basis, and press releases were put online throughout the period. At these press meetings, the commanding team, led by Minister Chen and consisting of medical experts and top governmental officials, updated the epidemic status, explained regulations and measures, and answered questions raised by the media. All these press conferences are broadcast live on mass media and social media. The willingness of the CECC to communicate with the public, respond to public concerns, and make information open and transparent is evident. These efforts have helped improve social trust and enhance compliance.

Structural Factors Enabling Effective Disease Control Policies

We could reasonably infer that the effective decisions were made on the ground of a responsive, accountable, and transparent democratic administration with active participation and supervision from the society. Below we further extend our analysis of the unique features of Taiwan's experiences.

Centralized Leadership and Professionalism of the CECC

First of all, while some countries might have adopted similar policies, one important difference in Taiwan's case is that during the first 18 months, many policies were adopted one step ahead of the possible turning point of the epidemic. Furthermore, the authority and centralized power enjoyed by the CECC are the results of previous experiences tackling SARS and other epidemics. Legal bases for policies were established by the legislative branch, and epidemic drills were exercised by the executive branch of the government in ordinary times.

The leadership of the CECC and CDC plays a vital role in tackling COVID-19. Policies such as personal hygiene, preventive measures in education and business settings, detecting and isolating suspected and confirmed cases, expropriation of mask manufacturers, and the whole mask rationing system, all require effective collaborations and partnerships between the public and private sectors. Furthermore, the role of the expert advisory panel in the CECC should also be emphasized, as it offers independent professional opinions (as against the political sector and the bureaucracy) within the formal institution and makes policy recommendations that are not otherwise viable from the civil society organizations primarily consist of lay persons.

The decisions made by the CECC were possible only with the overall state capacity. It consists of well-established public health infrastructures such as equitable and affordable access to good quality health care secured by the NHI, relatively dispersed healthcare providers in most of the regions, well-trained and sufficient healthcare professionals, and the civil service team in public health administrations. In addition, the state's capacity is strengthened by Taiwan's strong IT and data science background. The government databases are well instituted and could be interlinked, and the CECC has fully taken advantage of its IT capacity to contain the possibility of infection. Furthermore, the private sector is vigorous and innovative in improvising useful strategies and collaborating with the government to address the epidemic.

In sum, while the CECC enjoys strong political support that sustains its leadership and authority in policy implementation, it also respects and provides enough space for professional inputs in disease control policy formation.

Democracy and Political Accountability

The authority of the CECC relies on the overall social trust toward the current political party in office. Social trust, in response, is maintained by the responsiveness and openness of government. For instance, the CECC holds press conferences on a daily basis, functioning as the single authoritative source of epidemic status updates and disease control-related regulations and policies. The ways the CDC handles this crisis have boosted and reinforced social trust, including quick response, openness, willingness to communicate with the public, and quickly adjusted to social responses.

Civil society organizations and mass media have the capacity to supervise and monitor the legitimacy and legality of the government's policies and measures, questioning when deficiencies are found. It enhances the positive feedback loop between the social concerns and the government's in-time responses, urging the government to maintain its transparency, responsiveness, and accountability.

Political factors, as always, play an essential role in public health policymaking. The CECC and the CDC are backed with full support from the political branch. The premier of the Executive Yuan and other members of the ruling party have helped coordinate and support health affairs since the establishment of the CECC. One thing worth noting is that the ruling party has just won a major victory in the general election of the president and the legislators on January 11, 2020. The election results, in an indirect sense, might have granted the ruling party enough confidence in making decisions for disease control that might appear unnecessary or over-reacted in the first place. With social cohesiveness, social trust, and citizen cooperation—after the competitive and seemingly splitting election, the society quickly comes together to fight against the threat. Effective disease control could be seen as a legacy of democratization in Taiwan.

While many countries have seen rising trends in anti-establishments and social polarization in many aspects, the case in Taiwan shows that an accountable government could boost social trust in institutions, making citizens stand together despite their differences to engage with the common dangers. A stronger democracy might be the key to the maladies of populism in the face of a pandemic.

Lastly, due to the experience of China's persistent attempts to exclude Taiwan from participating in the global community, the Taiwan government, and arguably a majority of Taiwanese citizens, maintains a suspicious attitude toward the validity of any information provided and statements made by the Chinese government (Lien 2020), as well as the international organizations influenced by China's political agenda—in this particular case, the WHO (Buranyi 2020). The development of the COVID-19 pandemic in the first quarter in 2020 has shown that this suspicion and the deploy-in-advance decisions based on it have contributed to the early prevention. It also indicates that models of global health collaborations that are more effective, scientific, transparent, and accountable, either revisions based on the current WHO framework or other alternatives, might be needed (Yeh, Liao and Serrano 2019). The complicated geopolitics in East Asia is one thing, but from the current evidence, we maintain that a democratic, transparent, and accountable decision-making framework is beneficial, if not necessary, for infectious disease prevention and global health collaborations.

Civil Society and Social Participation

The vibrant civil society and broad social participation feature in COVID-19 control. In the case of mask rationing, the cooperation of convenience stores and NHI-contracted pharmacies was the key to the whole mask rationing and distribution process. Despite being burdened with heavy workloads, convenience store workers and pharmacists were not paid or compensated for their extra time and services. The Taiwan Pharmacist Association was vital in negotiating with the government and persuading fellow pharmacists.

One unique socio-culture feature in Taiwan, and arguably in Japan and South Korea, is the general habit of mask-wearing. Solid evidence concerning the effectiveness of mask-wearing among the general public in reducing infection risk is debatable, but such a collective hygienic practice, combined with a sufficient supply of masks, helps to remove the stigma associated with mask-wearing, thus may significantly reduce the risk of spreading the virus from the sick and the asymptomatic-infected.

The general public was also mobilized. Many precautionary measures were possible with the voluntary compliance and participation of ordinary citizens. Through public participation in mask-wearing and mask rationing, maintaining personal hygiene, measuring body temperature at the entry of every public space building, and kindly reminding each other of these healthy behaviors, disease prevention has become the prevalent mindset. Each of the measures might have its effect in tackling COVID-19, but the combination of them as a "disease prevention performance" participated by the people together might exert a synergistic effect greater than the simple aggregation of these measures.

One might draw on the Asian Values or the prevalent Confucianism social ethics in East Asia to explain people's appearing compliance and even voluntary adherence to the government's guidance, and in many cases coercion, in disease prevention. We, however, suggest that it is rather better explained by the overall vigor of civil society. In the practices of democracy and looking after each other, particularly under China's external threats in the global arena, Taiwanese society has developed a durable and resilient preparedness in rapid response to any political and social challenges and is ready to take action accordingly. This assertion is of course subject to further empirical investigation.

Ethical and Legal Considerations

The policies summarized in this chapter warrant further investigations and evaluations on their effectiveness in tackling COVID-19 as well as potential ethical issues. For instance, the expropriation of mask factories, the seemly voluntary cooperation of pharmacists and convenience store staff, and the price control of masks are all exercises of the state's strong governing power. While necessary during a public health emergency, these policies should be monitored with caution since they could infringe on personal and commercial liberties. A centralized decision-making process is essential to handling such a public health crisis. However, if kept not checked, such a governing pattern might have the potential to jeopardize democratic principles (Lin, Wu and Wu 2020). The sophisticated use of medical surveillance and data science techniques is another issue to be concerned about to avoid intrusion into personal privacy and potential misuses.

Concerning contextual factors, if the disease prevention performance was overly taken, it might lead to phobic sentiments or even discrimination against certain sub-populations based on their behaviors, living places, occupations, and so forth. For instance, incidents of caregivers' hostile attitudes toward hospital staffs' children were reported. In addition, the public's overwhelmed and voluntary adherence to the information released by the CECC might form a censoring atmosphere that supports the CECC's actions without proper scrutiny and encourages people's moral supervision of each other's healthy/CECC command-abiding behaviors. These issues warrant further attention.

Scholars have also raised concerns about the allocation of medical resources, border control and travel bans, the potential infringement of individual privacy in the utilization of databases and health surveillance, and the legal basis of administrative measures (Lin, Wu and Wu 2020). Despite being grounded on the CDC Act and the Special Act for COVID-19 and supposedly implemented only during the time of emergency, limitations on citizens' liberty and property rights require further scrutiny.

With the public health governance framework, we discuss the effectiveness of policies, measures, and regulations and their structural enabling factors. These together have made the governance of the COVID-19 outbreak in Taiwan relatively controllable, mitigating its health and socio-economic impacts on Taiwanese society in the first phase of the COVID-19 pandemic. Continuing on the discussion on the potential ethical and legal issues, we analyze the ultimate ethical grounds for these public health governance efforts, arguing for the ethics of body politic, which Yeh first proposed in his brief comments on the COVID-19 vaccine allocation policy in Taiwan (Yeh 2021). Below we further elaborate.

In Defense of State Public Health: The Ethics of Body Politic

Despite these potential ethical and legal considerations of effective disease control policies and measures, an unequivocal fact is that Taiwan's public health policy arrangements appeared to work well in the first phase. From the perspective of public health ethics, the state's public health efforts are primarily justified by their effectiveness in preventing health losses and promoting health gains, that is, the utilitarian account that prefers the maximization of population health outcomes. While considerations like individual autonomy, civil rights and liberties, and non-discrimination are equally important, utilitarian thoughts prevail in public health practices, particularly in the face of pandemics when the health losses at stake are enormous.

Besides its somewhat intuitive feature, utilitarian considerations also have deep connectedness with the nature of public health and the very entity that demands public health practices—the state's popular sovereignty or the body politic. As Krieger and Birn have rightly put it, "public health is indeed a public matter, that societal patterns of disease and death, of health and well-being, of bodily integrity and disintegration, intimately reflect the workings of the body politic for good and for ill" (Krieger and Birn 1998, p. 1603). This distinctive feature marks off the ethical considerations in public health compared to those in biomedical and clinical contexts. The utilitarian account of public health ethics asserts that the most ethical decisions are the decisions that could maximize the health of the body politic. This assertion precisely echoes the very ethical mandate of the body politic.

From the perspective of the ethics of body politic, the most ethically preferable decisions to make are the ones that could best secure or enhance a body politic or a sovereign state's sustainability. In a reductionist sense, a state's sustainability could be described as national security or national interests. It requires the self-preservation of the body politic as the primary ethical goal. Furthermore, since what constitutes the body politic is the people, the ethics of body politic would require the preservation of the people's life and health, so as to fulfill its own self-preservation. Therefore, the ethical demand of the utilitarian account and the ethical demand of the ethics of body politic matches perfectly in the context of public health. This, in turn (at least partially), explains why many people tend to have an intuitive recognition of utilitarian considerations. Following this reasoning, the sovereign state's primary obligations and the ultimate source of its political legitimacy is the fulfillment of the ethics of body politic, and that, under pandemics or other public health emergencies, ultimately underpins the state public health interventions in (and from time to time might against) individuals' autonomy, life, and even rights. Below we take the stark contrast between the state actions of vaccine nationalism and the call for vaccine equity as an illustrative example.

The global allocation of COVID-19 vaccines has been considered a major measure against the pandemic. The World Health Organization, its partner COVAX, and many global actors have collaborated and made a huge contribution. Among the global health cooperation process, many have condemned the so-called vaccine nationalism, as some states refused to take part in the great war against COVID-19 and pay for or support vaccine allocation. The term has now been widely adopted in academic literature to refer to the actions that prohibit the export of vaccine products and obstruct the equitable distribution among rich and poor states, and is believed to be harmful to the battle against COVID-19 (Bollyky and Bown 2020; Hassoun 2021; Katz et al. 2021; Lagman 2021; Wagner et al. 2021). While vaccine nationalism is a concise and catchy term, it may have certain labeling effects and may underestimate the state's primary obligations toward its own citizens. The ethics of body politic could be used to properly recognize these obligations and re-consider the issues of global vaccine allocation.

The ethical foundations of the call for equitable vaccine allocation, or the call against vaccine nationalism, could be well observed from the two priority aims for vaccine allocation put forth by the WHO and COVAX's statement. The first is to allocate in ways that could lead to "the best outcome in relation to ending the pandemic" (p. 15), and the second is to allocate vaccines to "those at greatest need, with a focus on those at greatest risk of becoming seriously ill if infected" (WHO 2020, p. 15). The ethical foundation that underpins these aims is the utilitarian account, which demands the maximization of health, social, and economic benefits of all, or minimization of these harms. This demand is supported by the preliminary evidence so far that more equitable distribution across countries is likely to lead to more effective transmission (Wagner et al. 2021). Besides these two priority aims, the overarching principles for COVAX are equity and fairness. Equity requires that "similar cases be treated similarly" (p. 14), and as of fairness, COVAX leaves its interpretations to the public, only suggesting that no matter what view it may be, it "must be explicitly articulated and defended, and then applied in a consistent manner" (p. 14) (WHO 2020). The COVAX continues to claim that these two principles are grounded on the human rights to health.

Both the utilitarianism and the rights-based approach understood here are cosmopolitan accounts, which take all human beings around the globe as roughly the same ethical significance, calculate their utility as the same, and consider their moral status as the same. No one has any privileges or advantages, regardless of nationality, social or economic status, or other factors. National borders are ethically irrelevant in these cosmopolitan accounts. States' difference in the obligations of helping others only lies in a practical sense in that some are affluent or powerful, and others are less affluent or even disadvantaged. The call for equitable vaccine allocation grounds on these cosmopolitan ethical foundations.

However, there's a dimension of vaccine allocation that has been largely neglected, that is, the ethics of body politic. It appears to be an anti-cosmopolitan account at first glance, as for which the national borders matter, and one's nationality and citizenship are ethically significant when considering the principle of resource allocation. This seems to be exactly what vaccine nationalism had been condemned for. But the ethics of body politic merits certain attention, because it relates the ethical foundation of public health policies to the very core of the meaning and purpose of a sovereign state. The sovereign state's power and legitimacy derive from its commitment to protecting the bodily life and political existence of what constitutes its sovereign, that is, the people. In turn, the people would hold the state accountable by demanding and examining whether the state is really committed to this purpose. This is not only the basic logic of democracy but also the ethical underpinnings of those policies that aim to some form of public health and ask for corresponding limits (or, in a sense, sacrifices) on individuals' rights and interests. In other words, policymakers and public health workers could, of course, educate, campaign, and persuade the people to think otherwise, but at the end of the day, the state should secure as many vaccines as possible if the people demand so.

Therefore, while often being labeled as nationalist or populist, the sovereign state actually has a primary obligation toward its citizens, one that precedes any other secondary obligations. Behind these demands is ultimately the popular sovereignty, a notion that a group of people gathering together to establish justice, promote the public health and general welfare, without which true autonomous personal decisions and freedoms are not possible. The criticism of vaccine nationalism may have certain merits, but the state's primary obligation should not be easily dismissed as well.

The cosmopolitan accounts are not necessarily conflictive to the ethics of body politic, as both require some sense of solidarity shared among peoples because, without the willing cooperation of the public, none of the measures tackling COVID-19 would be effective. The cosmopolitans envision a human solidarity, and the nationalists envision local solidarities. A proper recognition and respect for each other might be an opportunity to forge an identity of global citizen (Lagman 2021) and genuine global solidarity (WHO 2020) in the battle against the COVID-19 pandemic.

Conclusion

At the time that the pandemic of unprecedented severity suddenly swept the world, Taiwan managed to contain the transmission of the virus for one and a half years, gaining crucial time to secure its vaccine and pharmaceutical supplies. Drawing on the WHO's notion of good governance, this chapter has briefly summarized the policy framework of disease control in the first phase of the COVID-19 outbreak in Taiwan. It also delineates the structural enabling factors that have contributed to effective policy efforts against COVID-19, including centralized and professional leadership, democratic and accountable political culture, vigorous civil society, and broad social participation. While the measures against the COVID-19 outbreak must be swift and effective, reflections and check and balance mechanisms are necessary for a healthy and solidaristic democracy to sustain through such a public health crisis. In sum, we evaluate that although not without deficits, the overall health governance up until May 2021 could be considered good governance.

The experiences in Taiwan in later stages and comparisons with other countries should be further examined in global collaborations. The bottom line is that we human beings must stand together in solidarity and insist on political accountability, transparency, professional decision-making, and social responsiveness to national and global health governance. The ultimate ethical ground for these health governance efforts is the pursuit of the self-preservation of the political community constituted by the people. We call this the ethics of body politic. The cross-national, universal global solidarity would be possible with the proper recognition of the ethics of body politic, the preservation of each people's health and life, as the ethical mandate that underpins all the effective and valuable public health efforts arranged and implemented with the exercise of state powers. We conclude that the ethics of body politic is the ethical mandate that underpins all the state public health policies efforts, as the people's life and health are indeed the sovereign state's primary obligations and the ultimate source of its political legitimacy.

Acknowledgments

An earlier version of this chapter was published in *Health Security* in Volume 18, Number 6, pp. 1–8, 2020, titled "Policies Tackling the COVID-19 Pandemic: A Sociopolitical Perspective from Taiwan" (DOI: 10.1089/hs.2020.0095). The contents of this chapter were updated with the newer progress of the COVID-19 pandemic and revised with new inputs, especially adding an extended ethical analysis section. The authors thank the publisher Mary Ann Liebert, Inc.'s generous permission to reuse the chapter.

References

Barbazza, Erica, and Juan Tello. 2014. "A review of health governance: definitions, dimensions and tools to govern." *Health Policy* 116(1):1–11.

Bollyky, Thomas J., and Chad P. Bown. 2020. "The tragedy of vaccine nationalism: only cooperation can end the pandemic." *Foreign Affairs* 99:96–108.

Buranyi, Stephen. 2020. "The WHO v coronavirus: why it can't handle the pandemic." *The Guardian.*

Carlson, Valeria, Marita J. Chilton, Liza C. Corso, and Leslie M. Beitsch. 2015. "Defining the functions of public health governance." *American Journal of Public Health* 105(S2):S159–S166.

Cheng, Hao-Yuan, Shu-Ying Li, and Chin-Hui Yang. 2020. "Initial rapid and proactive response for the COVID-19 outbreak – Taiwan's experience." *Journal of the Formosan Medical Association*: 119(4): 771–773.

Cheng, Tsung-Mei. 2015. "Reflections on the 20th anniversary of Taiwan's single-payer National Health Insurance System." *Health Affairs* 34(3):502–510.

"Communicable Disease Control Act." 2009. *Laws & Regulations Database.* Taiwan: Ministry of Justice.

Hassoun, Nicole. 2021. "Against vaccine nationalism." *Journal of Medical Ethics* 47: 773–774.

Katz, Ingrid T, Rebecca Weintraub, Linda-Gail Bekker, and Allan M Brandt. 2021. "From vaccine nationalism to vaccine equity – finding a path forward." *New England Journal of Medicine* 384(14):1281–1283.

Ko, Hai-Yun, Peng Guo, Yi-Chien Chih, Su-Mei Chou, and Chang-Hsun Chen. 2017. "Maintenance and operation of communicable disease control medical network." *Epidemiology Bulletin* 33(11):198–204.

Krieger, Nancy, and Anne-Emanuelle Birn. 1998. "A vision of social justice as the foundation of public health: commemorating 150 years of the spirit of 1848." *American Journal of Public Health* 88(11):1603–1606.

Lagman, James Darwin N. 2021. "Vaccine nationalism: a predicament in ending the COVID-19 pandemic." *Journal of Public Health* 43(2):e375–e376.

Lien, Yi-Ting. 2020. "Why China's COVID-19 disinformation campaign isn't working in Taiwan." *The Diplomat.*

Lin, Cheryl, Wendy E. Braund, John Auerbach, Jih-Haw Chou, Ju-Hsiu Teng, Pikuei Tu, and Jewel Mullen. 2020. "Policy decisions and use of information technology to fight 2019 novel coronavirus disease, Taiwan." *Emerging Infectious Disease* 26(7): 1506–1512.

Lin, Ching-Fu, Chien-Huei Wu, and Chuan-Feng Wu. 2020. "Reimagining the administrative state in times of global health crisis: an anatomy of Taiwan's regulatory actions in response to the COVID-19 pandemic." *European Journal of Risk Regulation* 11(2): 256–272.

Rasmussen, Anders Fogh. 2020. "Taiwan has been shut out of global health discussions. Its participation could have saved lives." *Time.*

Solar, Orielle, and Alec Irwin. 2010. *A conceptual framework for action on the social determinants of health.* Geneva: World Health Organization (Commission on Social Determinants of Health).

Wagner, Caroline E., Chadi M. Saad-Roy, Sinead E. Morris, Rachel E. Baker, Michael J. Mina, Jeremy Farrar, Edward C. Holmes, Oliver G. Pybus, Andrea L. Graham, Ezekiel J. Emanuel, Simon A. Levin, C. Jessica E. Metcalf, and Bryan T. Grenfell. 2021. "Vaccine nationalism and the dynamics and control of SARS-CoV-2." *Science* 373: eabj7364.

Wang, C. Jason, Chun Y. Ng, and Robert H. Brook. 2020. "Response to COVID-19 in Taiwan: big data analytics, new technology, and proactive testing." *JAMA.*

WHO. 2010. *Monitoring the building blocks of health systems: a handbook of indicators and their measurement strategies.* Geneva: World Health Organization.

WHO. 2020. *Fair allocation mechanism for COVID-19 vaccines through the COVAX Facility.* Edited by World Health Organization. Geneva: World Health Organization.

Yeh, Ming-Jui, Wei-Hsiang Liao, and Ray Serrano. 2019. "Protecting universal health coverage in non–United Nations member states: lessons from Taiwan." *American Journal of Public Health* 109(8):1101–1102.

Yeh, Ming-Jui. 2021. "The ethics of vaccine allocation and mandate in the COVID-19 era." *Applied Ethics Review* 71:119–136.

Part 2

Liberal Democracy and Pandemic Management

3 Leveraging the Power of Digital Technology for Coping with the COVID-19 Pandemic in Taiwan

Li-Chi Chen and Ta-Chien Chan

Background

The coronavirus disease 2019 (COVID-19) pandemic overtook the world quickly and unprecedentedly. Taiwan is geographically located close to the pandemic epicenter of Wuhan, China, and human movement between Taiwan and China is very frequent, with nearly 850,000 Taiwanese citizens residing in and 404,000 working in China (Wang, Ng and Brook 2020). The previous SARS epidemic in 2003, the subsequent avian influenza outbreaks in China, and the 2009 flu pandemic caused the Taiwanese government to seriously monitor and prepare containment and control measures for the next pandemic (Yen et al. 2014). The success of controlling the COVID-19 epidemic in Taiwan can be mainly attributed to the legal authority of the government confirmed by legislation and timely public health policy (Yeh and Cheng 2020). Digital technology through established government infrastructure and public-private partnerships has enabled efficient and effective implementation of public health policy.

Since 2020, most countries have launched non-pharmaceutical policies and control efforts to flatten or mitigate the risk of the pandemic (Chung and Chan 2021). Along with these interventions, digital technology can help in many aspects (Whitelaw et al. 2020) including monitoring and surveillance, contact tracing, screening, risk communication, and resource allocation. However, the advance of digital technology alone cannot be directly applied to the disease control. The digital governance was heavily relied on the consolidated legal framework and public health infrastructure as well as the state-society relationships. The liberal democracy and a vibrant civil society paved the foundation of digital governance to coordinate the resources efficiently. Furthermore, the highly trust of digital governance was correlated to the high adherence to policies from the citizens which is also the influential factor.

The legal framework was majorly formed after SARS outbreaks in 2003 which deeply transformed the regulation of the Communicable Disease Control Act on strengthening administrative power, especially during the pandemic, expanding healthcare infrastructure, and increasing the professional competence of epidemic control personnel (Yeh and Cheng 2020; Su 2021). In 2008, the Central Epidemics Command Center (CECC) was written into the Communicable Disease Control

DOI: 10.4324/9781003438380-6

Act. During the COVID-19 epidemic in Taiwan, the CECC is the highest legal authority to make policies, allocate medical resources, and communicate with different agencies and jurisdictions. Therefore, the legitimacy of the policy was recognized by law and authority (Su 2021). The next challenge was to implement and disseminate policies in a timely and accurate manner.

Many public health infrastructures and applications have been established for many years. The introduction of digital technology to COVID-19 control measures has not been overnight. The major core infrastructure was the national health insurance system, with claims to electronically upload medical visits, clinical diagnosis, drug history, treatments, testing results, and radiology imaging in recent years. Since national health insurance (NHI) in Taiwan is a compulsory single-payer social insurance, the coverage rate of NHI among citizens is over 99% (Wu, Majeed and Kuo 2010). This backbone provides a mainstream information pipeline for surveillance and resource allocation. In addition, infectious disease-related information systems, including notifiable infectious disease reporting, contact tracing (such as with an outbreak investigation on measles [Huang et al. 2019]), cell broadcast service (used in dengue fever), and the Disease Control Butler were all ongoing systems for infectious disease control. The scale-up and extension of these functions were adjusted by modifying for the COVID-19 pandemic.

The state-society relationships can increase and facilitate effective emergency response collaboration across organizations (Liu, Wu and McEntire 2021). During the process, the government played an active role with private sector but still kept its autonomy in making their policy (Yen 2020) which could increase the bureaucracy's efficiency to cope with the COVID-19 crisis. The partnerships with private companies, non-governmental organizations (NGOs), and information technology (IT) communities need long-term communication and understanding. Since 2018, Taiwan government agencies initiated many hackathons to increase the private sectors as well as many IT engineers pay attention to how to use government data for good governance and improve the social good. The Disease Control Butler used during the epidemic was one of the successful examples of this collaboration between Taiwan CDC and one company DeepQ since 2017.

The response time to control highly contagious infectious diseases, such as COVID-19, is very short. The major benefits of introducing digital technology to disease control are to enhance efficiency, prioritize resource allocation, promote residents' compliance, and reduce social anxiety from active risk communication. Many digital technologies have been applied to cope with the COVID-19 pandemic in Taiwan.

First, border control and quarantine policies have been used extensively in many countries. For classifying immigrants into different risk groups, ensuring they adhere to the quarantine policy, the entry quarantine system, and the digital fencing system. The linkage between health insurance data and custom data is crucial to reduce the risk of infection domestically in the communities. If there were some infected cases, contact tracing in the early stages and the completeness of the contacted list determined the effectiveness of the quarantine policy. Based on Taiwan's empirical data (Ng et al. 2021), comprehensive contact tracing requires a large amount of resources, but it has shown promising results in slowing down transmission by measuring the effective reproduction number (Rt). In general, we can classify our contact-tracing approach in Taiwan into two types: location-based and person-based. The location-based approach was to issue alerts to persons unspecific to known risk locations. The real name-based 1922 SMS contact-tracing system and cell broadcast service belong to this approach. The person-based approach can trace the digital footprints of infected persons using telecommunication data or notify the possible contact risks anonymously using the Taiwan Social Distancing App.

Digital technology can also help to screen high-risk populations. Infrared temperature checkpoints are installed everywhere in public places, stores, restaurants, or office buildings. During the local COVID-19 outbreaks in May 2021, silent hypoxia among the infected patients, especially for those elderly or people with chronic diseases, was critical for threatening their lives (Wilkerson et al. 2020). Therefore, oximeters with automatic alerts and Wi-Fi reporting functions can help in the early detection of hypoxia symptoms and facilitate early treatment. In addition, artificial intelligence algorithms applied to radiology imaging can help enhance the diagnostic accuracy for patients with atypical pneumonia from SARS-CoV-2 infection (Liu et al. 2020).

Active risk communication through the Disease Control Butler (Lin et al. 2020a) and daily press conferences on YouTube channels were also very important to increase the residents' confidence and decrease the anxiety of misinformation or non-transparent epidemic situations. The Disease Control Butler is an official LINE chatbot providing bi-directional communication between the Taiwan CDC and residents. The daily press conference provided one-way communication to the public every afternoon at 2:00 PM local time. In addition, the crowd alerts computed from either telecommunication data or live traffic cameras are control measures related to social distancing policy. The Ministry of Transportation or local departments issued this information to control the human mobility of attractions.

Limited supply of medical masks and COVID-19 vaccines occurred in February 2020 and May 2021, respectively. The principles to prioritize the supply to the high-risk population are based on the decisions of expert panels. However, the logistics operation to dispatch these resources to the public fairly and in a timely manner is not an easy task. Digital technology plays an important role in scheduling allocation and dynamically balancing the gap between supply and demand.

Taiwan is a well-known ICT manufacturing hub with a high-quality healthcare system and universal health insurance infrastructure. Taking advantage of these strengths, we list the corresponding applications used in Taiwan and describe the purposes and mechanisms of the applications for coping with the COVID-19 epidemic in Taiwan.

Introduction of the Digital Technology Used in Taiwan

We will introduce five types of technology to cover different purposes of epidemic control, including monitoring and surveillance, contact tracing, screening, risk communication, and resource allocation. In Figure 3.1, we depict the timeline for introducing digital technology in Taiwan during the COVID-19 pandemic period.

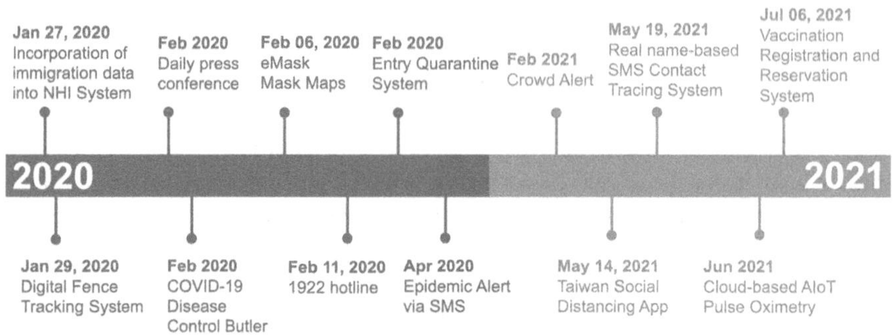

Figure 3.1 Timeline: Applications of digital technology responding to COVID-19 in Taiwan

Monitoring and Surveillance of COVID-19

On December 31, 2019, the World Health Organization (WHO) reported a cluster of pneumonia of unknown etiology in Wuhan City, Hubei Province, China. Simultaneously, the Taiwan CDC began onboard screening for airlines from Wuhan. Since January 25, 2020, Taiwan has restricted foreign passengers from China. Subsequently, travel notice alerts of many areas or countries in the world were elevated from Level 1 to Level 3. Therefore, travelers from these countries were mandatorily requested to quarantine at home for 14 days. Taiwan, merely 81 miles off the coast of mainland China, was initially estimated to be a high-risk country for COVID-19 owing to its geographic proximity and high passenger travel volumes to and from China (Gardner 2020). The border control has been the major policy to reduce the imported COVID-19 risk during 2020–2022 in Taiwan. Owing to the digital technology facilitation of the timely initiation of border control and quarantine policy, Taiwan has one of the lowest incidence and mortality rates of COVID-19 worldwide.

Entry Quarantine System and Digital Fencing Tracking System

During the emergence of the COVID-19 outbreak, one of the most urgent public health tasks was to block the spread of SARS-CoV-2 from the epidemic source region to other regions. The CECC announced travel alerts, based on the criteria including daily newly confirmed and cumulative COVID-19 cases, specific measures taken by local governments, and travel volume between Taiwan and the individual regions/countries (Cheng et al. 2021), raising Wuhan City to Level 3 (Warning) on January 21, 2020. By March 21, 2021, travel notice alerts were raised to Level 3 (Warning) for all countries, and all inbound travelers were subject to a 14-day home quarantine upon arrival in Taiwan.

To attain effective passenger clearance and accelerate inspection procedures electronically, Taiwan's Department of Cyber Security, Executive Yuan, and the Ministry of Health and Welfare jointly developed the Quarantine System for Entry.

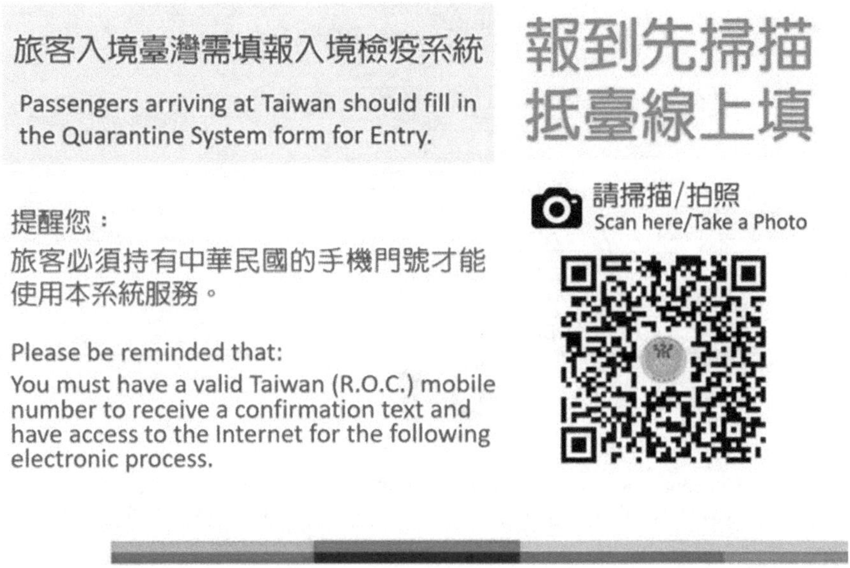
旅客入境臺灣需填報入境檢疫系統
Passengers arriving at Taiwan should fill in the Quarantine System form for Entry.
報到先掃描
抵臺線上填
提醒您：
旅客必須持有中華民國的手機門號才能使用本系統服務。
Please be reminded that:
You must have a valid Taiwan (R.O.C.) mobile number to receive a confirmation text and have access to the Internet for the following electronic process.
請掃描/拍照
Scan here/Take a Photo

Figure 3.2 QR code for the Quarantine System for Entry

The completion of the entire process takes only four simple steps: scanning a QR code at the check-in counter (Figure 3.2), entering health information, receiving health declaration pass via SMS (short message service), and presenting the pass on a mobile phone for faster immigration clearance (Wang, Ng and Brook 2020).

In addition, to utilize mobile phone positioning to track the whereabouts of the quarantined, the Taiwanese government integrated traveler information into the digital fencing tracking system and electronic fence monitoring system by collaborating with the National Immigration Agency and National Communications Commissions. In addition, Taiwan's Department of Cyber Security has cooperated with telecom carriers to track movements using GPS data from the user's mobile phone based on triangulation of base station data. Through the mobile positioning of those in quarantine, if a quarantined individual leaves the designated quarantine area without permission, the system will send an alert message to the individual, health, civil affairs departments, and local police to guarantee full compliance with quarantine rules (MOHW 2020) (Figures 3.3 and 3.4). Violations of related rules will be subject to substantial penalties.

Both the entry quarantine system and digital fencing tracking system were anti-epidemic measures to reduce community transmission. As a means of public health surveillance, facilitating immigration inspection and enforcing home quarantine can isolate possible carriers from the uninfected during the communicable period, thus minimizing the risk of further viral transmission in communities. While digital fencing system is an important tool in ensuring the effectiveness of

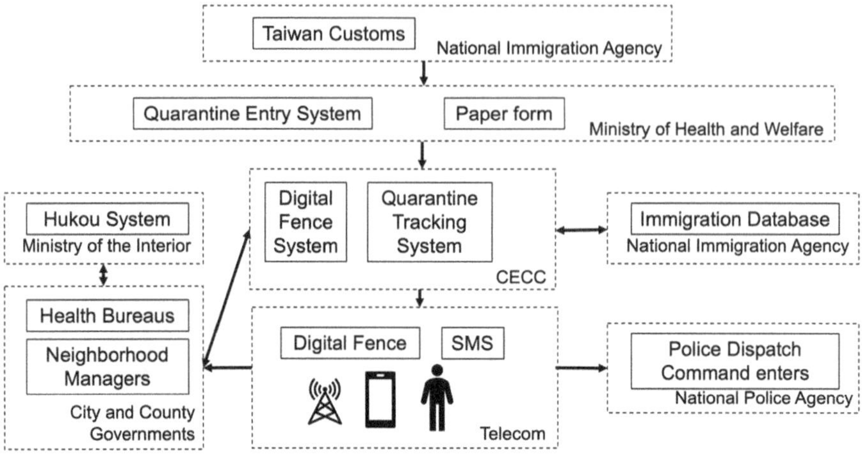

Figure 3.3 Concept Diagram of Digital Fence in Taiwan (Redrawn based on https://blog.schee.info/2020/03/25/digital-fense-system-enacted-in-taiwan-during-pandemics/)

quarantine policies, violations of personal liberties without affirmative authorization by law remain a concern. The legal foundation of digital fencing system needs to be strengthened and regulated to deal with the next pandemic.

Health Insurance Data and Immigration Data

Taiwan has leveraged its single-payer platform to build a comprehensive NHI system which is the backbone of public health surveillance. NHI records, which include travel history, complete health history, underlying health conditions, recent progression of symptoms, treatments, and hospitalization related to respiratory syndrome (Lin et al. 2020b), may help identify high-risk individuals and enhance proactive case findings.

In response to the COVID-19 outbreak for early case detection, the CECC has integrated the immigration and customs database from the National Immigration Agency (NIA) into the NHI MediCloud System, NHI's centralized cloud-based health records, and has provided medical providers access to the complete international travel history of their patients since February 27, 2020. The NHI MediCloud System flagged records of patients with specific travel history to COVID-19 epicenters so that clinicians could be notified in advance (Figure 3.5). Additionally, all confirmed and suspected case contacts reported to the Taiwan CDC were added to the NHI database. As a critical part of the TOCC (Travel, Occupation, Contact, and Cluster history) taken for patient with respiratory or COVID-19-like symptoms, immigration data incorporated into the NHI system generated real-time alerts during a clinical visit based on travel history and clinical symptoms to aid susceptible case identification (Wang, Ng and Brook 2020).

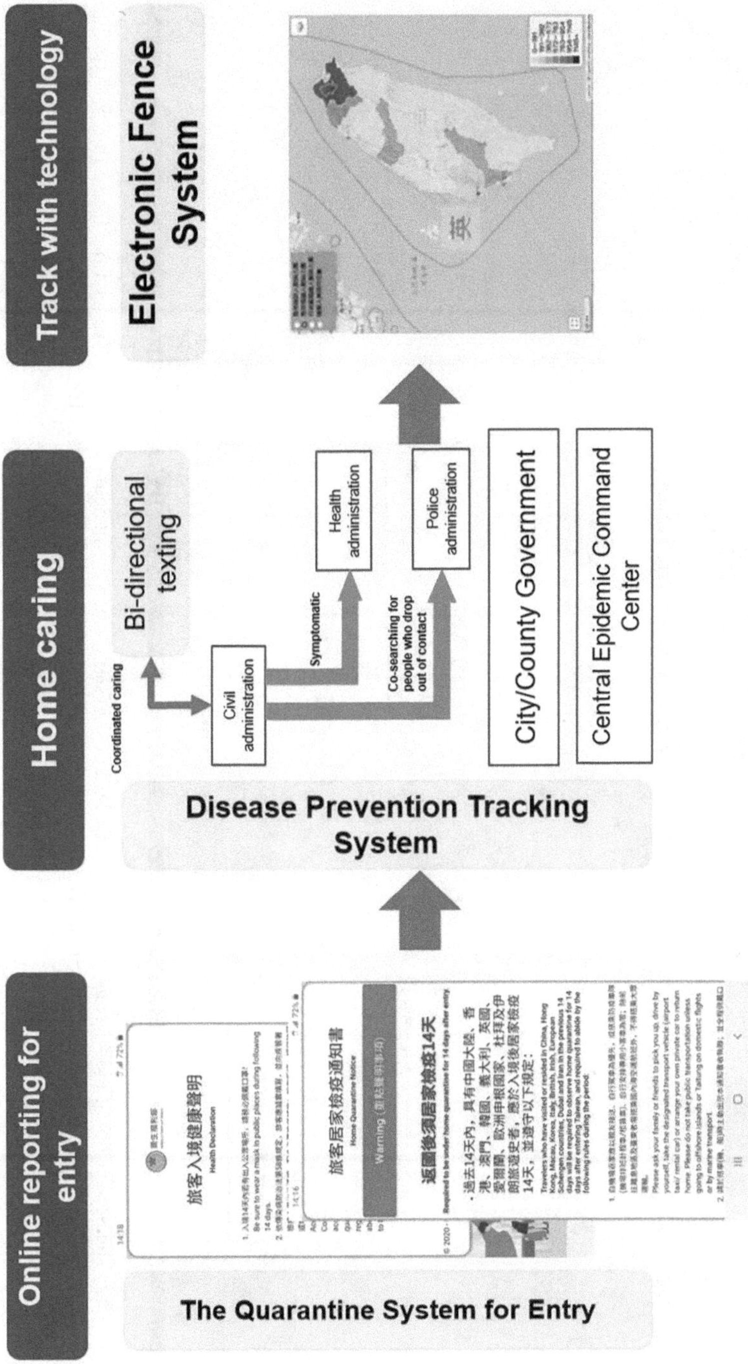

Figure 3.4 Flowchart of Digital Technology Facilitation of Home Quarantine (https://covid19.mohw.gov.tw/en/cp-4775-53739-206.html)

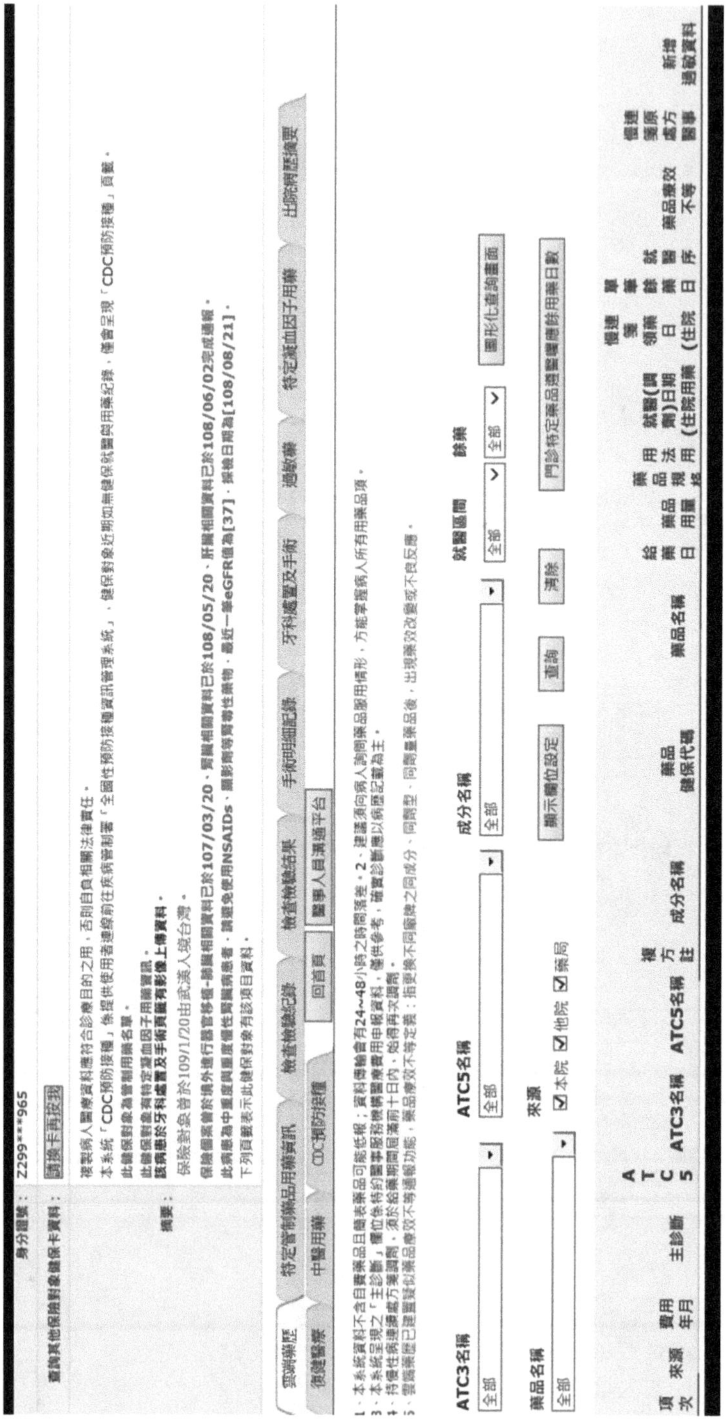

Figure 3.5 The Screenshot of the Alert in the Physician Order Entry System When the Patient Had Travel History from China (https://www.nhi.gov.tw/News_Content.aspx?n=FC05EB85BD57C709&sms=587F1A3D9A03E2AD&s=012016EE70C9A226)

Contact Tracing

Contact tracing, in combination with precautionary quarantine and large-scale testing of contacts, is considered a critical component in mitigating the COVID-19 outbreak (Hellewell et al. 2020). In the face of the pandemic, digital technology deployment utilizes electronic information to identify exposures to infected individuals and high-risk cases. Plus, when it comes to the painstakingly detailed contact-tracing task, digital contact tracing has the potential to tackle the limitations of traditional methods, such as scalability, notification delays, recall errors, and crowd contact in public spaces (Kleinman and Merkel 2020).

Multiple digital contact-tracing strategies have been adopted and can be categorized into location-based and person-based interventions. The former concentrates on identifying locations visited by a contagious person and then tracing down those who were at those locations, while the latter focuses on reaching close contacts, who have been in proximity to a laboratory-confirmed case.

Location-Based Interventions

Real Name-Based SMS Contact-Tracing System

As part of the restrictions of the Level 3 epidemic alert amid the domestic COVID-19 outbreak, all people at public venues must undergo the cumbersome process of either handwriting names and contact information or scanning a QR code and filling out complex forms in case of future contact investigation. In an effort to streamline contact tracing, the Taiwan government, on May 19, 2021, announced a real name-based contact-tracing scheme which utilized QR codes and SMS to simplify the process of providing contact information to the following three steps that can be completed within five seconds:

1 Scan the QR code at stores or public venues with a mobile phone
2 Click on the link that appears
3 In the SMS message box that appears, click “send”

For those with phones that are not equipped with cameras or without an Internet connection, they only need to open the text message function, enter the store code, and send it to the 1922 hotline as the recipient (Figure 3.6).

The user-friendly registration system aims to free people from filling out lengthy forms when they enter stores and public places. The service does not charge mobile phone users or collect personal data. All the information is only used for disease outbreak investigation and will be deleted after 28 days, which is calculated based on two incubation periods.

According to the National Communications Commission, the government has received a cumulative message number of 3,999,666,655 from May 19, 2021, to February 3, 2022, averaging approximately 15 million messages per day (National Communications Commission 2022). The system was canceled on April 27, 2022.

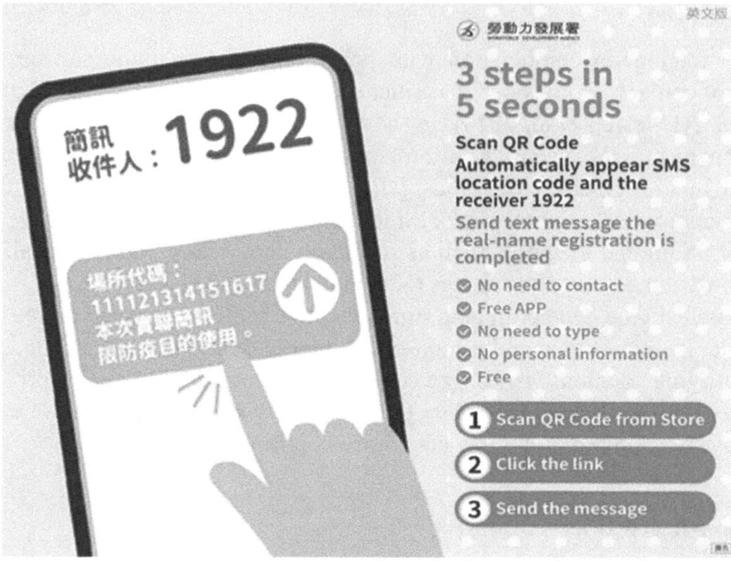

Figure 3.6 Steps to Complete CDC's Real Name Text Message Registration via Cellphone (http://tcmp.cpami.gov.tw/filesys/metro_tc/files/簡訊實聯制-_英文版.pdf)

In January 2022, a high school employee who had worked part time at a steak house in Taoyuan City was identified as a COVID-19 case. Although the employee began to experience symptoms of COVID-19 six days prior, she continued to work, potentially transmitting the virus to many others. Soon after, two migrant workers tested positive after dining at the steak house and had spread the virus to four of their coworkers living in the same dorm in the free trade zone. Thanks to the real name SMS contact-tracing system, close contacts who had dined in the same steak house in that period were quarantined and tested for COVID-19. Nevertheless, there were customers who did not register in the system, which could have generated an undetected transmission chain. Therefore, the CECC attaches great importance to the registration of real name SMS contact-tracing systems when entering public places, especially for restaurants where masks cannot be worn all the time. In addition, when exhaustive details of contact history are required, person-based contact tracing can complement this non-mandatory system.

Epidemic Alert via Short Message Service (SMS)

In response to the local COVID-19 outbreak, the CECC publicized the footprint of confirmed cases and issued epidemic alerts via SMS, which were alert text messages to people visiting specific locations during the same time period as the confirmed cases. For instance, on May 13, 2021, the CECC sent an alert to those who had been near the Wanhua District of Taipei City over the past month in the wake of the local cluster outbreak linked to teahouses in the district. The text message is as follows:

COVID-19 Alert

If you have visited places with a high risk of transmission and experienced any suspected symptoms such as fever, respiratory symptoms, diarrhea, or abnormal sense of smell/taste after April 15, 2021, please seek medical attention at a designated community testing site (Taiwan Centers for Disease Control 2021a) (Figure 3.7).

Likewise, warning messages were sent via SMS responding to the transmission chain regarding Huannan Market in Taipei City and the family cluster involving a pilot of a Taiwanese airline on July 2 and September 4, 2021, respectively.

In addition to the in-depth epidemiologic investigation conducted for all confirmed cases to trace sources of infection, epidemic alert messages indicate potential exposure by the larger unidentifiable public. Furthermore, it notifies affected individuals to self-monitor, voluntarily get tested, and avoid visiting crowded places or using public transportation if they experience any discomfort. For those

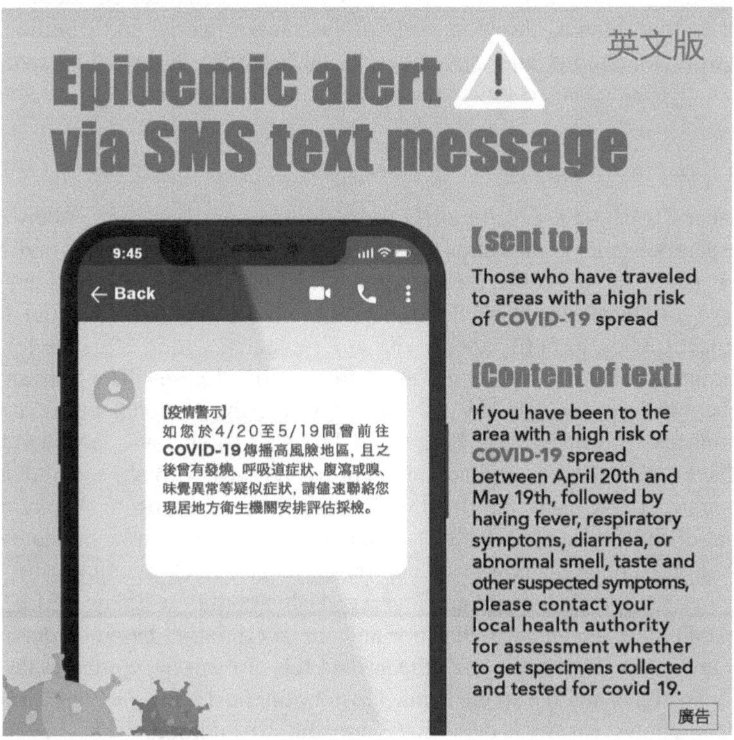

Figure 3.7 The SMS Notification for Those People Have Been to High-Risk Areas (https://fwas.wda.gov.tw/upload/download/c3c091793fc2f477b23b827c80b-c0435b31f8538.jpg)

who seldom watch television, listen to the radio, or are less active on the Internet, this may help heighten public vigilance and compliance with COVID-19 protocols, which complements other contact-tracing measures.

Person-Based Interventions

Cellphone Tracking

The process of contact tracing involves case investigation, contacted case identification, health monitoring, proactive testing, and quarantine of high-risk contacts (Jian et al. 2020). Scalability and timeliness of identification of exposure are pivotal to the process, which can be facilitated by cellphone tracking. Specifically, the interviewing of confirmed cases, which should be completed within 24 hours, includes inquiries about symptoms and clinical course, elicitation of close contacts, and activity history. Hence, the digital footprint of the confirmed case retrieved from telecommunication companies not only expedites contact-tracing efforts but also augments the capacity with the escalation of the epidemic. In collaboration with telecom companies under the governance of the National Communications Commission, the utilization of cellphone geolocation enhances contact-tracing effectiveness and lessens the workloads of case investigators and frontline public health workers. Prompt analysis of the digital footprint, followed by rapid quarantine of close contacts, is key to the prevention of presymptomatic transmission.

Taiwan Social Distancing App

Given that COVID-19 spread mostly through direct or close contact between humans, social distancing measures substantially curtail contacts among individuals, which is necessary to reduce the pace and extent of COVID-19 infection ("flatten the curve") (Thunström et al. 2020). On the other hand, it is essential to carry out contact tracing to notify those with close contact, within 2 meters for a total of 15 minutes or more by definition, with confirmed cases. The Taiwan Social Distance app, co-developed by the Taiwan CDC, the National Information and Communication Security Task Force, and Taiwan AI Labs, was launched to optimize disease surveillance and containment by helping maintain social distancing and keeping at-risk users informed of possible disease exposure (https://covirus.cc/social-distancing-app-intro.html). This is also the example of state-society relationship to create the non-profit app for helping contact tracing.

The Taiwan Social Distance app leveraged Bluetooth Low Energy (BLE) broadcasts to calculate the physical distance and contact duration based on devices carried by app users. The app records the hashed IDs of its users, compares the public list of infected hashed IDs to the contact history on the device, and alerts the user if a high-risk contact history is detected (Figure 3.8). In addition, the hashed IDs were changed every 15 minutes to prevent location tracking or ID information revelation. That is, the decentralized proximity-tracing platform over which anonymous hashed IDs cannot be linked by the government or a third party guarantees anonymity and privacy preservation (Ho et al. 2020). The app helps the public track

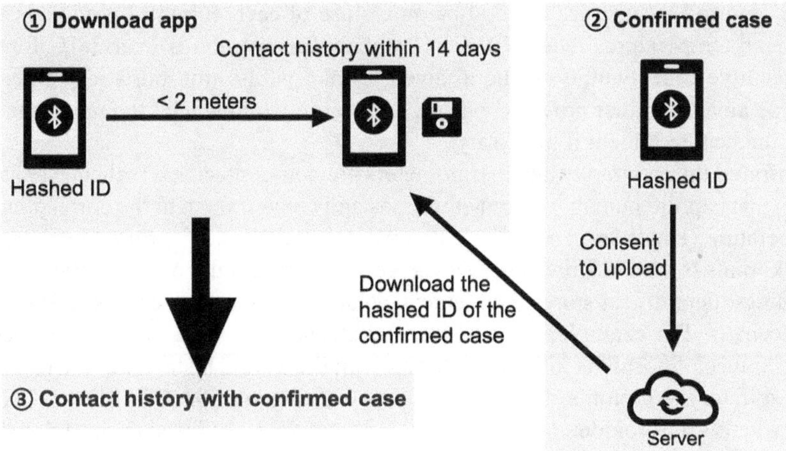

Figure 3.8 Mechanism of Contact Tracing of Taiwan Social Distancing (Redrawn based on https://www.cdc.gov.tw/File/Get/nw1Kx64XF3Yn4WeZzHrvxg)

possible encounters with infected persons in public venues and notifies users to raise their risk awareness and encourage them to get rapid tests in case of infection and subsequent transmission.

Screening

Early screening of infectious diseases is crucial for the identification of infected people, so that they can seek appropriate care and be isolated from healthy individuals. Screening programs for COVID-19 ensure the health and safety of the elderly and immunocompromised individuals to prevent life-threatening infections, and an essential workforce to preserve healthcare capacity. Moreover, accurate and cost-saving screening measures such as testing and hospital beds are imperative for the utilization of limited resources (Neilan et al. 2020). For instance, screening modules, such as AI algorithms, stratify individual risk levels so that those with higher risk can undertake confirmatory laboratory-based tests, polymerase chain reaction (PCR) tests for COVID-19, or quarantine. Hence, adequate screening programs can lead to both the enhanced detection and diagnosis of COVID-19 and the precise distribution of resources.

Infrared Temperature Checkpoints

Fever is the most common clinical presentation in patients infected with SARS-CoV-2 (Siordia 2020), indicating a highly infectious phase. Therefore, the body temperature is a crucial physiological parameter. The detection of febrile individuals intercepts the spread of COVID-19; thus, fever screening has gradually become a ubiquitous screening tool in the disease response. On April 1, 2020, all railway stations, bus transportation stations, airports, and post offices in Taiwan were required to measure the body temperature of each entrant. Individuals with forehead temperatures over 37.5°C or tympanic temperatures over 38°C for two consecutive times would not be allowed to take public transportation, enter the service areas, or other crowded places. They are recommended to stay home and seek medical treatment if necessary.

Infrared thermography and thermometers are non-contact and real-time technologies that capture human infrared emissions and convert them to the corresponding temperature (Khaksari et al. 2021). Extensive installation of infrared temperature checkpoints is seen in Taiwan to mass screen the temperature of the public in office buildings, department stores, convenience stores, restaurants, schools, and recreation centers. For example, infrared thermal checkpoints have been established at the entrance of hospitals in Taiwan. Along with the TOCC history and the presence of respiratory symptoms, fever is a critical warning sign for COVID-19. Febrile individuals are forbidden from hospital entry and are transferred to the emergency department for further evaluation (Hsiao et al. 2020).

With the advent of non-contact technology, this approach facilitates screening programs that minimize the risk of contact with infected individuals. Nonetheless, the measurement of body surface temperature is not a countable surrogate of core body temperature influenced by viral infection (Huizenga et al. 2004). However, in the face of a large-scale epidemic, these measures provide accessible and real-time testing to ameliorate the burden on the healthcare system.

Pulse Oximeter

There are a variety of clinical manifestations of COVID-19 ranging from completely asymptomatic to severe respiratory failure or death. Nevertheless, an atypical clinical picture has been presented in infected patients: the development of severe hypoxemia without proportional signs of respiratory distress, referred to as happy or silent hypoxia (Ottestad, Seim and Mæhlen 2020) which may cause irreversible damage to vital organs if undetected and give rise to rapid deterioration.

By combining the Internet of Things (IoT) technology, which means objects with the ability to transfer data over a network (Hidayat et al. 2020), artificial intelligence, and 5G network technology, a cloud-based oxygen saturation monitoring platform was established to provide healthcare practitioners with real-time information of patients' vital signs without human-to-human interaction (Figure 3.9). SpO_2 (Peripheral oxygen saturation) levels less than 90% trigger an alarm and send warnings to clinicians so that patients requiring medical evaluation and supportive care are recognized in a timely manner. The risk of sudden decompensation decreased accordingly.

In addition, the platform also gives public health agencies access to data that can be utilized by artificial intelligence and deep learning programs to predict healthcare trends and optimize health policies.

Owing to the proliferation of IoT devices and the cloud-IoT paradigm, interconnected wireless platforms facilitate point-of-care testing and real-time monitoring of the growing number of infected patients.

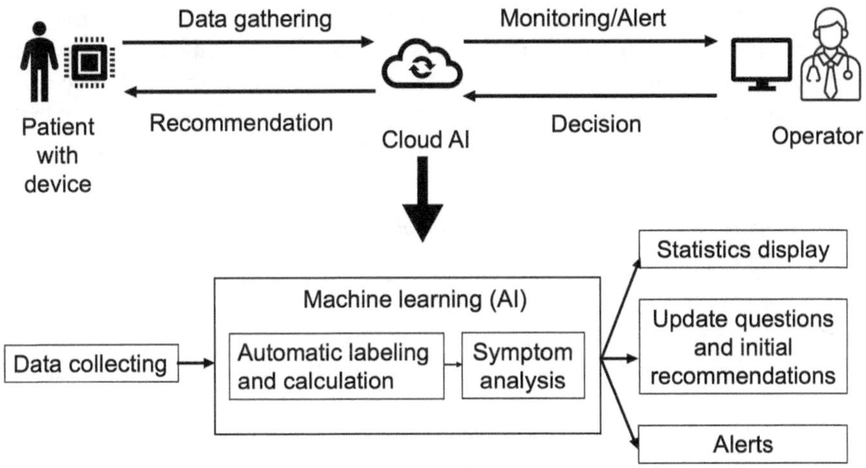

Figure 3.9 Architecture of the Cloud-Based AIoT Platform (Redrawn based on https://www.ncbi.nlm.nih.gov/pmc/articles/PMC8514960/)

Risk Communication

During the unprecedented times caused by COVID-19, effective risk communication is critical for emergency management. As an important component of public health intervention, risk communication focuses on providing timely, accurate, easy-to-understand information and combating misinformation. Taiwan government-guided communication strategies, such as the daily press conference, 1922 hotline, and Disease Control Butler, have contributed to building a two-way communication network, intending to address scientific evidence-based information needs and fight infodemics, which suggests excess information including false or misleading information during a disease outbreak (Eysenbach 2002).

Daily Press Conference through Mass Media and YouTube Channel

Amid the immense level of uncertainty, the Taiwanese government has addressed the challenge of transparent communication. Since January 5, 2020, the CECC has held daily press briefings to update the latest situation of the epidemic, prevention measures, and public health guidelines. Reporting investigation findings of newly confirmed cases and related transmission chains, press conferences educate the public about current policies and guidelines on a daily basis. Such efforts also include announcing border control and quarantine policies, resource allocation, healthcare service capacity, vaccine rollout, and public health education (Su and Han 2020).

Communication is not only top-down but also bottom-up. On the other hand, press conferences also function as conversational and educational platforms to respond to questions and address misinformation and stigma. For example, in

January 2022, domestic COVID-19 cases were linked to Taoyuan International Airport, involving an airport security guard and a taxi driver, which triggered panic and accusation of failing to follow protocols. The CECC used the conference platform to educate the public, encourage all frontline airport workers, and reiterate the importance of following COVID-19 instructions.

Disease Control Butler—Official LINE Chatbot

Joining hands with Line Taiwan Corporation and DeepQ, the healthcare division of HTC Corporation, the CECC developed the Disease Control Butler, an automated chatbot set up for interactive disease communication (Figure 3.10). The Disease Control Butler provides accurate information and fact checks of COVID-19 to dispel fake news and misinformation. Supplemented with artificial intelligence, the chatbot was equipped with a two-way communication system for users to report their health status in a timely manner. As an important part of health monitoring of the quarantined, the LINE bot system allows individuals to report their health status during the 14-day home quarantine, and also sends follow-up messages during the seven-day self-health management after isolation. Moreover, the Taiwan V-Watch System in the chatbot keeps track of users' side effects after vaccination and provides step-by-step instructions if symptoms occur. The Disease Control Butler has been deployed in response to innovative disease containment measures. It merges systems of information dissemination, symptom monitoring, and vaccine registration into one comprehensive platform that aids in fighting infodemics.

1922 Hotline

Complementing other risk communication measures, the toll-free number 1922 served as a helpline offering services on symptom/disease reporting and consultation. The hotline caters for various language-speaking populations, including Mandarin, Taiwanese, English, and Hakka, as well as hearing-impaired populations. It also provides voicemail services for those who do not wish to wait online. Helpline service staff call back as soon as possible (Taiwan Centers for Disease Control 2021b). The disease consultation hotline elevates accessibility owing to its 24-hour service around the globe, which helps shorten the response latency and facilitate risk communication.

Crowd Alerts

The Department of Information and Tourism in Taiwan has launched websites and apps to inform the public of crowd alert levels, indicating the crowdedness of popular tourist destinations. Tourists can browse information before their visits to prevent unnecessary overcrowding during the epidemic period. For instance, in Taipei, crowd alerts of scenic spots, such as Yangmingshan National Park and Maokong, come in three levels: normal flow (green light), slightly crowded (orange light), and overcrowded (red light) (Figure 3.11). The website will also give

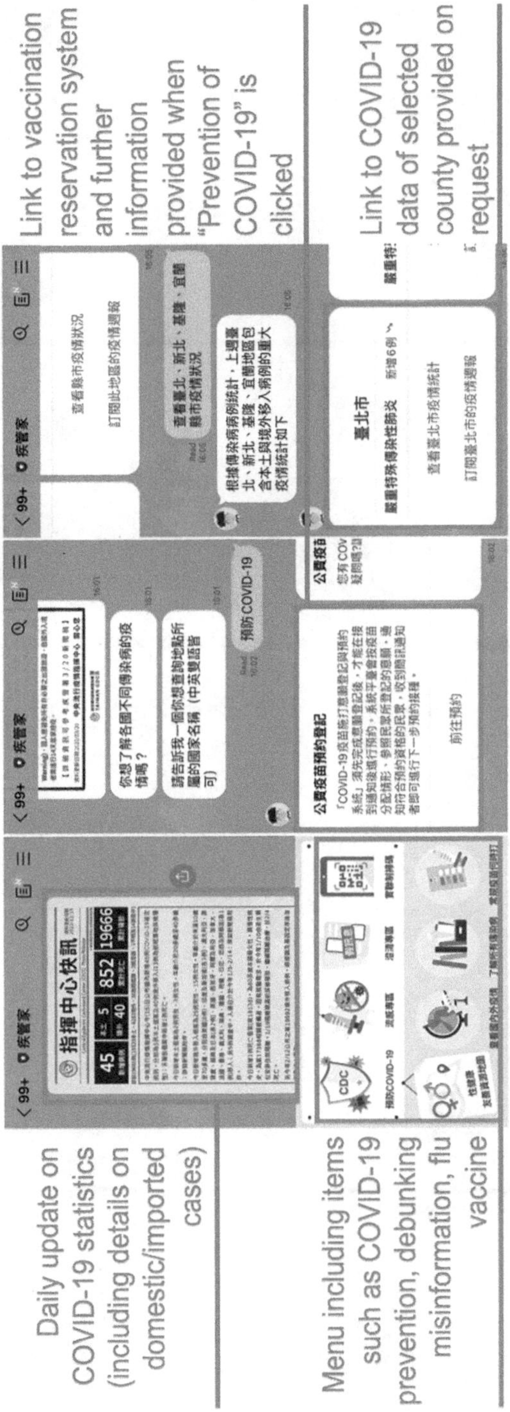

Figure 3.10 The Interfaces of Disease Control Butler

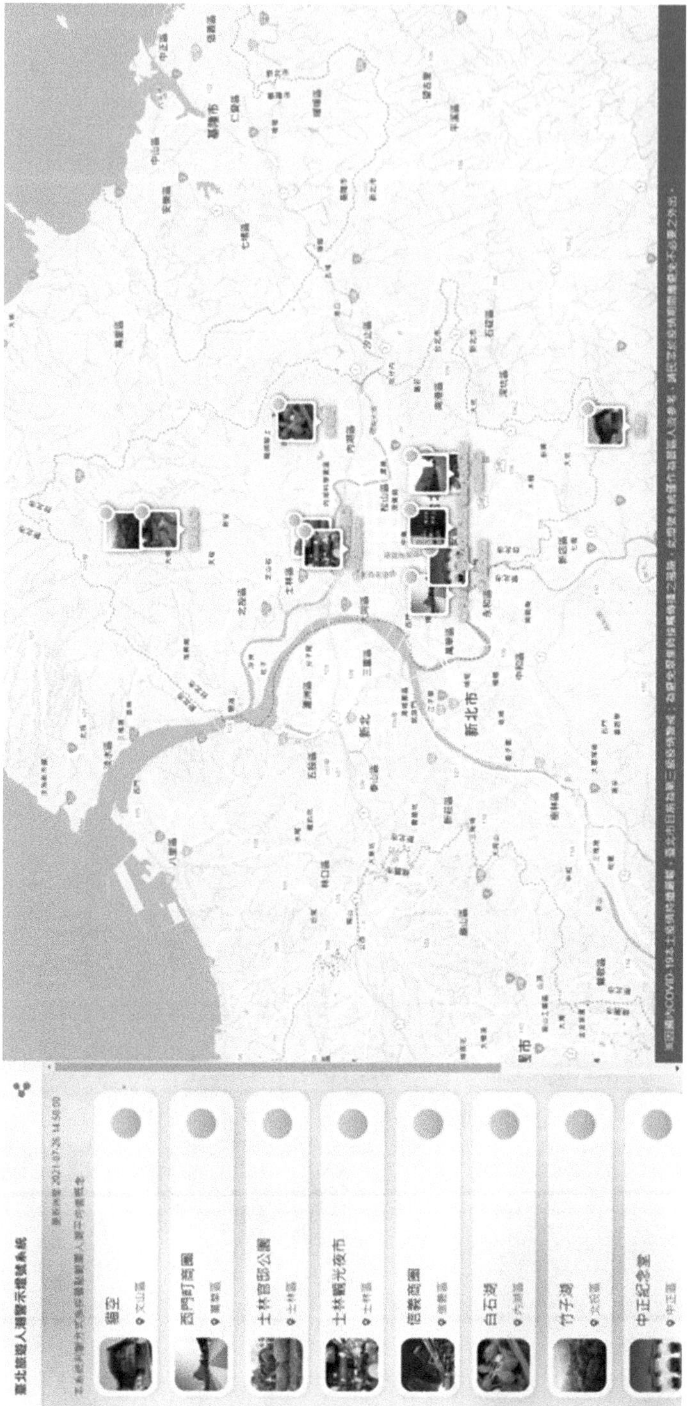

Figure 3.11 Webpage of Taipei Travel Warning Signal System (https://www.travel.taipei/alertofcrowds/#/)

tourists travel instructions that visitors should adhere to the social distancing policy and complete name-based SMS contact tracing.

With crowd warnings or even real-time videos and surrounding traffic conditions for popular tourist attractions, communication efforts regarding risk notification and public health instruction are multifaceted.

Resource Allocation

Mask Supply

Given that the transmission mechanism of SARS-CoV-2 involves a combination of contact, droplet, and airborne modes (Eikenberry et al. 2020), face masks effectively protect against coarse droplets and fine aerosol transmission. The call to wear masks on the general public is critical for curbing the spread of COVID-19. Therefore, the task of adequately supplying and distributing masks is of immense importance.

In anticipation of a demand surge, the Taiwanese government announced an export ban on face masks on January 24, 2020, and then requisitioned domestically made medical and surgical masks and invested to boost production. Furthermore, a name-based rationing system was initiated for the purchase of affordable medical face masks (NTD 4–6 per piece ~ 0.036 USD per piece) on an electronic platform, such as eMask and NHI Express App, or on-site. Under the temporary rationing policy, face masks should be pre-ordered and purchased with the required NHI card registration via the Internet, NHI-contracted pharmacies, and kiosks at convenience stores (Figure 3.12). Every person was permitted to purchase a limited number of

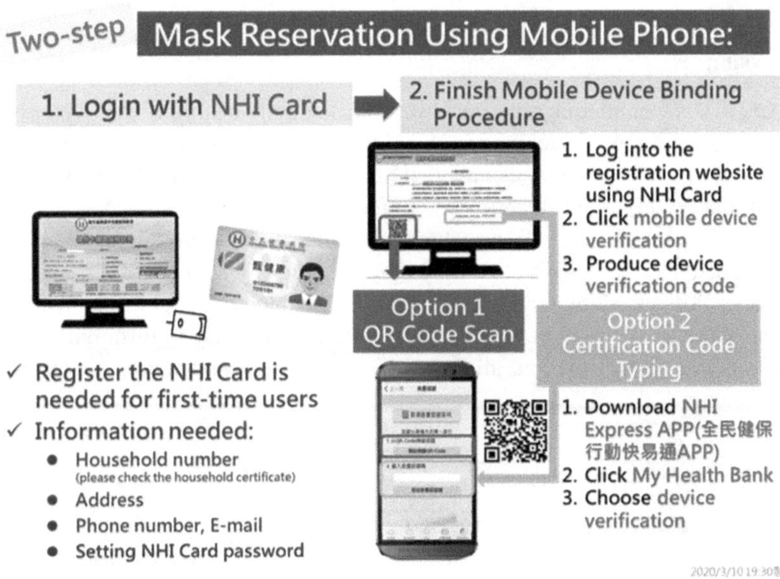

Figure 3.12 Two-Step Mask Reservation Using Mobile Phone

masks within a specific period, for example, three pieces over a seven-day period for adults (five pieces for children) in March 2020. Leveraging the pre-existing NHI system for name-based registration, the rationing system secures mask supply and prevents mask hoarding and price gouging.

To optimize the mask-purchasing procedure, mask maps, which were established by civil collaboration, are websites that locate mask supply points and provide real-time storage. By clearing mask availability near the user, the digital service significantly shortens the waiting queue and enhances convenience.

Vaccination Registration and Reservation System

Effective vaccination is urgently needed to protect humans and diminish the economic and societal impact of COVID-19. To facilitate vaccine rollout, people in Taiwan are able to reserve appointments to obtain a COVID-19 vaccine jab via the vaccination registration and reservation platform. Because a considerable number of vaccine doses in Taiwan were allotted by the COVID-19 Vaccines Global Access (COVAX), it was crucial to ensure effective distribution and equity. The vaccine registration system was linked to the NHI system to ensure the eligibility of registrants. Healthcare personnel, frontline workers with a high risk of contact, and those aged≥65 years were prioritized according to the publicly funded vaccination order. Eligible individuals can book vaccination appointments after registration on a platform via the website (1922.gov.tw, Figure 3.13) or the NHI administration mobile app.

Because of this platform, vaccines can be effectively allocated in order. Reservation-based appointments can also prevent crowds from compromising on social distancing measures.

Discussion

The COVID-19 pandemic remains a worldwide public health threat, even after the increasing coverage of vaccination. Coping with the pandemic not only relied on health system resilience but also needed help from digital technology. In this study, we introduced the digital technology applied in Taiwan to help achieve the goals of epidemic control. The infrastructure of public health informatics, legal support frameworks, and public-private partnerships are the key elements for making these happen in Taiwan. Many countries have also attempted to adopt digital technology to control the COVID-19 pandemic. However, it is not easy to formulate these applications in a short time and allow residents to use these technologies with high compliance.

Public Health Infrastructure

The multifaceted application of digital technologies is vastly attributed to multiple pre-existing infrastructures and regulatory frameworks. Taiwan has a rock-solid public health, medical, and insurance infrastructure with coverage exceeding 99% of the population (Lin et al. 2020b), and this serves as the backbone to fight the

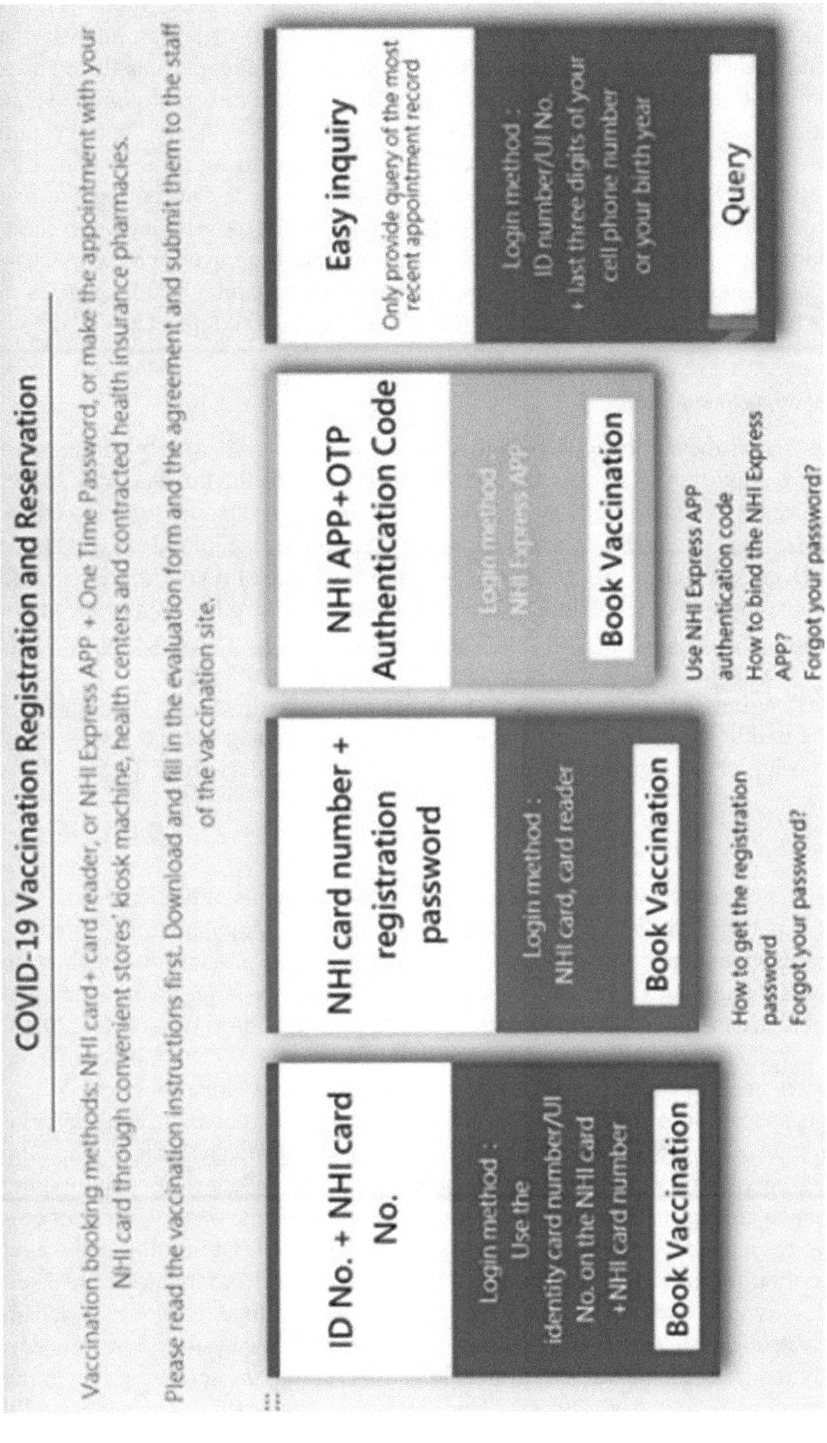

Figure 3.13 The Webpage of the COVID-19 Vaccination Registration and Reservation

outbreak of COVID-19. The Taiwan CDC made innovative use of the NHI database in terms of travel history tracking, name-based mask distribution, and vaccine allocation; therefore, impressively halting community spread, even as the number of confirmed cases surged in most countries. The incorporation of immigration data and medical history enables frontline healthcare providers to query the travel and contact history of patients, which may allow clinicians to assess infection risks and take relevant infection control measures. As for resource distribution, the systems of mask purchase and vaccine registration are linked to NHI cards, recording the purchase of masks and inoculation of the vaccine. Moreover, the comprehensive database of the NHI MediCloud system also allows public health agencies to create big data for analytics and aids in decision-making to combat COVID-19.

State-Society Relationship

In the face of the epidemic, cooperative efforts between civil society and government are important to pioneer better solutions to contain the disease (Yen 2020). For example, the Disease Control Butler, a pre-existing system to fight infectious diseases, was upgraded with a LINE chatbot function for the joint development of HTC DeepQ and the CECC. Mask maps are also successful contributions made by IT communities via the g0v hackthon platform (https://g0v.tw/intl/en/), where attendees apply their expertise to collaboratively come up with solutions to challenges. To recruit a considerable number of IT engineers and generate a great deal of creative innovation for developing applications in a short time is a challenge for the traditional bureaucracy framework. Taking advantage of the state-society relationship, the design of applications can be closer to the needs of the public.

Nationalism and Governmentality

With the governments resorting to conventional instruments of border closure and mask export ban to prioritize the protection of their own population, we witness a resurgent sovereignty and health nationalism in Taiwan. Nationalism, which mean territorial communities known as nations are essential for human flourishing and each nation deserves some autonomy in running its own affairs (Woods et al. 2020), is an entwined and reinforcing processes with globalization. The global pandemic catalyzes the interaction between nationalist thinking and global politics. Policymakers appeal for national solidarity and deploy economy protection and territorial control. The Taiwanese government has utilized social media, such as YouTube and Facebook, and daily press conference to promote messages of solidarity and encourage citizens to work together to fight the virus, which foster a sense of collective responsibility and unity in the face of COVID-19. During the three-level alert period from May 2021 to July 2021, there were localized major outbreaks in Taipei City and New Taipei City of Taiwan for the first time. Health nationalism is reflected in residents' compliance with the soft lockdown policy, which means greatly reducing the movement of people and increasing the screening rate in the communities (Chan et al. 2022). Then, the wave of epidemic was successfully controlled within two months. The government has also taken advantage of the pandemic to showcase Taiwan's technological prowess and demonstrate its capacity to contribute to the global effort to combat the pandemic.

According to Michel Foucault, governmentality is defined as ensemble formed by the institutions, procedures, analyses and reflections, the calculations and tactics that allow the exercise of this very specific albeit complex form of power, which has as its target population, as its principal form of knowledge political economy, and as its essential technical means apparatuses of security (Foucault 1991). The concept of governmentality in the COVID-19 era refers to the justification and legitimation for government actions in response to the disrupted social ecology due to the public health emergency, which forms the foundation of democratic governance in Taiwan. In the debate between human right and governmentality by the public health authorities, elucidation of legal framework and two-way communication are in pressing need. The discussion of the legal clarity and proportionality of health policies, such as border control and digital contact surveillance, should be an ongoing dynamic process and will be the key to reaching universal level of community cohesion and social cooperation.

Legal and Regulatory Framework

During the COVID-19 fight, Taiwan's legal and regulatory framework offers strong legal legitimacy for communicable disease control measures. Equipped with robust legal power, the CECC was established to take charge of centralized and professional leadership (Yeh and Cheng 2020). In addition, the policies of travel restriction, quarantine monitoring, and contact tracing are authorized by the Communicable Disease Control Act and the Special Act on COVID-19 Prevention, Relief, and Restoration. The National Communications Commission clarifies the legal framework that empowers the CECC to enforce disease prevention measures if necessary. Only with transparent and accountable regulations are COVID-19 countermeasures implemented effectively and meticulously by the health authorities in Taiwan.

Regarding database utilization and public surveillance, there are concerns about the potential infringement of individual privacy. For instance, under the digital fence tracking system, personal location is closely tracked by authorities for the purpose of public health security at the expense of individual liberty. Contact tracing via cell phone tracking also suffers from the same issue. Privacy protection mechanisms, such as transparency, proportionality, due process, and expiration (Ching-Fu, Chien-Huei and Chuan-Feng 2020), should not be overlooked to strike a balance between public interest and personal privacy. Although the current approaches to digital technology are well justified and grounded under specific laws, the scope of data linkages, data usage, and tracking of people should be clearly regulated to make sunset clauses in certain situations. Such administrative measures should be implemented only during emergencies and are under further scrutiny so that the public can still keep confidence in the government to prepare for the next pandemic or emergency situations.

Digital Literacy and Accessibility

Digital literacy is the ability to search for information, discern between false and true information, process, condense, produce results, and effectively communicate them (Martínez-Alcalá et al. 2021). In light of the physical constraints and concerns due to COVID-19, it is crucial to proactively explore new options for advancing access to digital tools and resources to support the delivery of important healthcare information. Digital skills and accessibility are of great importance, as the government has already taken several digital measures to contain the epidemic. For example, face mask purchases and vaccine appointments should be reserved via online registration. To facilitate the digital transformation of policy, the government has launched workshops and school curricula to teach the participants hands-on skills so that the gap between technology development and public digital literacy can be shortened, especially among the elderly and socially disadvantaged groups. However, offline manual operation remains a very important approach that can provide fair access opportunities for populations with low digital literacy. In addition, by setting up official channels for some of the most used apps in Taiwan, such as LINE, Facebook, and YouTube, the government can boost the reach and engagement of public health information. In addition to digital literacy, the knowledge to understand the underlying meanings from statistical numbers, such as confirmed cases, severe cases and fatal cases from CECC is also challenging for the public. At the different stages of the epidemic and under different circulating strains of SARS-CoV-2, the linkage between the control policy and the statistics were highly related. The simple and colloquial expression of the statistics can help improve the effectiveness of the risk communication and enhance the policy compliance from the public.

Digital Technology in Taiwan, Japan, South Korea, and Singapore

Regarding non-pharmaceutical policies in the world, there is no gold standard for all countries. Policies need to be adapted by considering the epidemic situation, legal support, and cultural differences for different countries. Here, we selected three kinds of digital technology used in the four democracies in East Asia that have proactively leveraged digital tools to mitigate the negative impacts of COVID-19 on society: social media usage, contact-tracing tools, and tools for quarantine. Comparing the measures taken in Taiwan, Japan, South Korea, and Singapore provides insights into how the public health interventions have been tailored for countries with different cultural, political, and economics factors, as well as the common approaches and potential challenges to inform future policy decisions.

Social Media Usage

Social media platforms play an imperative role in information dissemination, which affects the effectiveness of countermeasures implemented by the public health sector. With more than 90% coverage in Taiwan, LINE has become a ubiquitous platform for news circulation and risk communication. Specifically, the Disease

Control Butler is the official LINE chatbot providing updates on COVID-19 and combating fake news.

In Singapore, WhatsApp, the most widely used message platform worldwide, has been adopted as an official channel for public health information diffusion. The content of the messages included confirmed cases and infection control measures, debunking misinformation, and economic and social support. Studies have shown that subscription to the official WhatsApp channel decreases depression levels. Likewise, increased trust in official WhatsApp messages alleviated anxiety and stress symptoms (Liu and Tong 2020).

Similarly, Korean authorities transmit alert text messages via cellular broadcasting services. The broadcasting approach allows governments to promptly send emergency alerts and publicize guidelines (Heo et al. 2020). With the support of mobile telecom carriers, broadcasting measures act as channels for risk communication and emergency management.

Despite the distinct platforms utilized in different countries, tailored communication strategies are crucial for timely communication and curtailing misinformation. In addition, exposure to officially distributed information can successfully boost psychological resilience and enhance public well-being amidst the uncertainty of COVID-19.

Contact Tracing

Unlike conventional contact tracing, digital mobility data using geospatial technologies from mobile phones or proximity data from Bluetooth (Smith and Mennis 2020) can help identify possible transmission routes and implement precise testing campaigns or quarantine policies. Mobile contact-tracing apps utilize technology to track possible exposure to infection on a large scale.

One study adopted a difference-in-differences framework to examine the effectiveness of voluntary and mandatory mobile contact-tracing apps during the early stages of the COVID-19 outbreak in 2020 (Urbaczewski and Lee 2020). Four countries belonged to the control group (voluntary-based): China, Germany, Italy, and the United States. The other two countries, South Korea and Singapore, belong to the treated group that mandates mobile-tracking apps. The results showed that mandatory mobile tracking significantly reduced new cases per day by 3.3 on average. Although the effect size was not large, a beneficial effect on contact tracing was observed at the early stage. Thus, it is essential for the government to reach a sweet spot that optimally balances compulsory intervention with trade-off assessment and communication.

The feasibility and effectiveness of the COVID-19 contact-tracing app were challenged and doubted owing to its precision, coverage, and privacy concerns. A nationwide cross-sectional study in Japan explored the demographic characteristics of users downloading a contact-tracing app named Japan's voluntary-use contact-confirming application (COCOA) (Ishimaru et al. 2021). Among the 27,036 participants from the online survey, 25.1% had downloaded the app, and workers from public service and information technology were more likely to use the app. However, workers from retail and wholesale, food, and beverages were less likely to use the app. Concerns over the efficacy of voluntary-based contact-tracing apps should be addressed by health authorities. The articulation of consistent and logical evidence-based messages on the value of installing the app to contain the disease. Policy promotion and risk communication were key to incentivizing and emphasizing compliance with such interventions. Moreover, digital literacy and user-friendliness of the app are also key to eliminating technical obstacles to using the app (Lo and Sim 2021).

To address the awareness of possible privacy infringement, governments and health authorities should shed light on privacy-preserving measures and data management. Taiwan Social Distance, the decentralized social distancing app established in Taiwan, elaborates on contact-tracing algorithms and cybersecurity guidelines to reassure users that their anonymous hashed IDs are free from third-party attacks. During the local outbreak period in May 2021, the number of users installing Taiwan Social Distance exceeded 4 million. However, many users have argued about the effectiveness of the app without notifying them of contact with infected cases. The low infection rate, the low installation rate among the general population, and the capability of short-distance detection are all reasons for the rare evidence of good performance.

Quarantine

Home quarantine is effectively reinforced by a comprehensive policy and robust digital fencing system, under which the physical isolation strategy was implemented to mitigate the pandemic. In Taiwan, mobile phone positioning is used to track the whereabouts of quarantined people with its electronic fence monitoring system. The South Korean Self-Quarantine Safety Protection app uses mobile GPS positioning. However, the apps could be cheated by those who left their phones at home, so the authorities developed electronic bracelets to monitor those who had violated self-isolation orders in an effort to improve quarantine compliance. Nevertheless, device-tracking measures are not obligatory, and only the people who consented to wear the band will be monitored (Takefuji 2021). As for Singapore, the multifaceted approaches towards disease control, such as border control implemented prior to its first reported case and strict 14-day mandatory leave of absence for workers returning from China (Yan et al. 2020), have proven to be effective.

With strong initiatives for quarantine strategies and digital technology adoption, Taiwan, South Korea, and Singapore have maintained countries with the lowest per-capita COVID-19 mortality rates worldwide (Zeng, Bernardo and Havins 2020).

Limitation

This study has some limitations. First, the latest utilization rates for each technology are not completely accessible. However, we included the available official data issued by the government. Second, the effectiveness of digital technology in epidemic control is difficult to directly evaluate. Digital technologies are meant to facilitate policy implementation, and the interconnected mechanism of each health policy and digital intervention makes it challenging to quantify the efficacy of every digital application separately. Finally, given that different countries have distinct strategies of digital technology based on their public health policy and law empowerment, Taiwan's experience serves as a modifiable reference for public health response mechanisms instead of an absolute gold standard.

Conclusion

In conclusion, timely public health policies with digital technology can help conduct precise epidemic control, allocate medical resources efficiently, and implement direct risk communication to the public. Meanwhile, it is critical for governments to strike a balance between the reinforcement of health nationalism and the commitment to civil liberties and democratic values. Fortunately, Taiwan stands on the well-based legal authority, health informatics networks, and public-private collaboration to cope with the COVID-19 pandemic in Taiwan. The digital technology of COVID-19 is not a generalized application to all counties. The adaptation process to fit in the context of bureaucracy, legal framework, digital society, public health awareness, and social-cultural differences in each country is an important step in deciding which applications might be appropriate for controlling the pandemic locally. In the race to contain the variants of SARS-CoV-2 globally, the integration of digital technology into pandemic policy and response has remained a critical issue of public health.

References

Chan, T. C., C. C. Chou, Y. C. Chu, J. H. Tang, L. C. Chen, H. H. Lin, K. J. Chen, and R. C. Chen. 2022. "Effectiveness of controlling COVID-19 epidemic by implementing soft lockdown policy and extensive community screening in Taiwan." *Scientific Reports* 12(1):12053.

Cheng, Hao-Yuan, Yu-Neng Chueh, Chiu-Mei Chen, Shu-Wan Jian, Shu-Kuan Lai, and Ding-Ping Liu. 2021. "Taiwan's COVID-19 response: Timely case detection and quarantine, January to June 2020." *Journal of the Formosan Medical Association* 120(6):1400–1404.

Ching-Fu, Lin, Wu Chien-Huei, and Wu Chuan-Feng. 2020. "Reimagining the administrative state in times of global health crisis: An anatomy of Taiwan's regulatory actions in response to the COVID-19 pandemic." *European Journal of Risk Regulation* 11(2):256–272.

Chung, P. C., and T. C. Chan. 2021. "Impact of physical distancing policy on reducing transmission of SARS-CoV-2 globally: Perspective from government's response and residents' compliance." *Plos One* 16(8):e0255873, 1–17.

Eikenberry, Steffen E., Marina Mancuso, Enahoro Iboi, Tin Phan, Keenan Eikenberry, Yang Kuang, Eric Kostelich, and Abba B. Gumel. 2020. "To mask or not to mask: Modeling the potential for face mask use by the general public to curtail the COVID-19 pandemic." *Infectious Disease Modelling* 5:293–308.

Eysenbach, Gunther. 2002. "Infodemiology: The epidemiology of (mis) information." *The American journal of medicine* 113(9):763–765.

Foucault, Michel. 1991. *The Foucault effect: Studies in governmentality*: Chicago: University of Chicago Press.

Gardner, Lauren. 2020. "Update January 31: Modeling the spreading risk of 2019-nCoV." January 31.

Hellewell, Joel, Sam Abbott, Amy Gimma, Nikos I Bosse, Christopher I Jarvis, Timothy W Russell, James D Munday, Adam J Kucharski, W John Edmunds, and Fiona Sun. 2020. "Feasibility of controlling COVID-19 outbreaks by isolation of cases and contacts." *The Lancet Global Health* 8(4):e488–e596.

Heo, Kyungmoo, Daejoong Lee, Yongseok Seo, and Hyeseung Choi. 2020. "Searching for digital technologies in containment and mitigation strategies: Experience from South Korea COVID-19." *Annals of Global Health* 86(1):109, 1–10.

Hidayat, Alfin, Vivien Arief Wardhany, Ajie Setyo Nugroho, Sofyan Hakim, Mirtha Jhoswanda, Ika Noer Syamsiana, and Nur Anis Agustina. 2020. "Designing IoT-based independent pulse oximetry kit as an early detection tool for Covid-19 symptoms." Pp. 443–448 in *2020 3rd International Conference on Computer and Informatics Engineering (IC2IE)*: IEEE.

Ho, Yu-Chen, Yi-Hsuan Chen, Shen-Hua Hung, Chien-Hao Huang, Poga Po, Chung-Hsi Chan, Di-Kai Yang, Yi-Chin Tu, Tyng-Luh Liu, and Chi-Tai Fang. 2020. "Social distancing 2.0 with privacy-preserving contact tracing to avoid a second wave of COVID-19." *arXiv preprint arXiv:2006.16611*.

Hsiao, Shih-Huai, Tun-Chieh Chen, Hui-Chin Chien, Chih-Jen Yang, and Yen-Hsu Chen. 2020. "Measurement of body temperature to prevent pandemic COVID-19 in hospitals in Taiwan: Repeated measurement is necessary." *Journal of Hospital Infection* 105(2):360–361.

Huang, H. I., M. C. Tai, K. B. Wu, W. C. Chen, A. S. E. Huang, W. Y. Cheng, M. T. Liu, and W. T. Huang. 2019. "Measles transmission at an international airport – Taiwan, March–April 2018." *International Journal of Infectious Diseases* 86:188–190.

Huizenga, Charlie, Hui Zhang, Edward Arens, and Danni Wang. 2004. "Skin and core temperature response to partial-and whole-body heating and cooling." *Journal of thermal biology* 29(7–8):549–558.

Ishimaru, T., K. Ibayashi, M. Nagata, A. Hino, S. Tateishi, M. Tsuji, A. Ogami, S. Matsuda, Y. Fujino, and CORoNaWork Project. 2021. "Industry and workplace characteristics associated with the downloading of a COVID-19 contact tracing app in Japan: a nation-wide cross-sectional study." *Environmental Health and Preventive Medicine* 26(1):94, 1–7.

Jian, Shu-Wan, Hao-Yuan Cheng, Xiang-Ting Huang, and Ding-Ping Liu. 2020. "Contact tracing with digital assistance in Taiwan's COVID-19 outbreak response." *International Journal of Infectious Diseases* 101:348–352.

Khaksari, Kosar, Thien Nguyen, Brian Y Hill, Timothy Quang, John Perrault, Viswanath Gorti, Ravi Malpani, Emily Blick, Tomas Gonzalez Cano, and Babak Shadgan. 2021. "Review of the efficacy of infrared thermography for screening infectious diseases with applications to COVID-19." *Journal of Medical Imaging* 8(S1):010901.

Kleinman, Robert A., and Colin Merkel. 2020. "Digital contact tracing for COVID-19." *CMAJ* 192(24):E653–E656.

Lin, C., W. E. Braund, J. Auerbach, J. H. Chou, J. H. Teng, P. K. Tu, and J. Mullen. 2020a. "Policy decisions and use of information technology to fight COVID-19, Taiwan." *Emerging Infectious Diseases* 26(7):1506–1512.

Lin, Cheryl, Wendy E Braund, John Auerbach, Jih-Haw Chou, Ju-Hsiu Teng, Pikuei Tu, and Jewel Mullen. 2020b. "Policy decisions and use of information technology to fight coronavirus disease, Taiwan." *Emerging infectious diseases* 26(7):1506.

Liu, J. C. J., and E. M. W. Tong. 2020. "The relation between official WhatsApp-distributed COVID-19 news exposure and psychological symptoms: Cross-sectional survey study." *Journal of Medical Internet Research* 22(9):e22142, 1–19.

Liu, L. Y., W. N. Wu, and D. A. McEntire. 2021. "Six Cs of pandemic emergency management: A case study of Taiwan's initial response to the COVID-19 pandemic." *International Journal of Disaster Risk Reduction* 64:102516, 1–15.

Liu, P. Y., Y. S. Tsai, P. L. Chen, H. P. Tsai, L. W. Hsu, C. S. Wang, N. Y. Lee, M. S. Huang, Y. C. Wu, W. C. Ko, Y. C. Yang, J. H. Chiang, and M. R. Shen. 2020. "Application of an artificial intelligence trilogy to accelerate processing of suspected patients with SARS-CoV-2 at a smart quarantine station: Observational study." *Journal of Medical Internet Research* 22(10):e19878, 1–13

Lo, Bernard, and Ida Sim. 2021. "Ethical framework for assessing manual and digital contact tracing for COVID-19." *Annals of Internal Medicine* 174(3):395–400.

Martínez-Alcalá, Claudia I., Alejandra Rosales-Lagarde, Yonal M. Pérez-Pérez, Jose S. Lopez-Noguerola, María L. Bautista-Díaz, and Raul A. Agis-Juarez. 2021. "The effects of Covid-19 on the digital literacy of the elderly: Norms for digital inclusion." *Frontiers in Education* 6:716025, 1–19.

MOHW (Ministry of Health and Welfare). 2020. "Combined the "Entry Quarantine System" and "Digital Fencing Tracking System" and utilize mobile positioning to monitor movement of individuals." March 18.

National Communications Commission. 2022. "Cumulative message number of 1922 SMS."

Neilan, Anne M., Elena Losina, Audrey C. Bangs, Clare Flanagan, Christopher Panella, G. Ege Eskibozkurt, Amir Mohareb, Emily P. Hyle, Justine A. Scott, and Milton C. Weinstein. 2020. "Clinical impact, costs, and cost-effectiveness of expanded SARS-CoV-2 testing in Massachusetts." *medrxiv*.

Ng, T. C., H. Y. Cheng, H. H. Chang, C. C. Liu, C. C. Yang, S. W. Jian, D. P. Liu, T. Cohen, and H. H. Lin. 2021. "Comparison of estimated effectiveness of case-based and population-based interventions on COVID-19 containment in Taiwan." *JAMA Internal Medicine* 181(7):913–921.

Ottestad, William, Mari Seim, and Jens Otto Mæhlen. 2020. "COVID-19 with silent hypoxemia." *Tidsskrift for Den norske legeforening* 140, 1–4, doi: 10.4045/tidsskr.20.0299.

Siordia, Juan A., Jr. 2020. "Epidemiology and clinical features of COVID-19: A review of current literature." *Journal of Clinical Virology* 127:104357, 1–7.

Smith, C. D., and J. Mennis. 2020. "Incorporating geographic information science and technology in response to the COVID-19 pandemic." *Preventing Chronic Disease* 17:E58, 1–7.

Su, Sheng-Fang, and Yueh-Ying Han. 2020. "How Taiwan, a non-WHO member, takes actions in response to COVID-19." *Journal of global health* 10(1):010380, 1–5.

Su, Y. C. 2021. "Legislative preparedness for the control of pandemics – using Taiwan as an example." *Medico-Legal Journal* 89(1):19–22.

Taiwan Centers for Disease Control. 2021a "CECC to send out alert message in response to indigenous COVID-19 cases in Wanhua District."

Taiwan Centers for Disease Control. 2021b. "Communicable Disease Reporting and Consultation Hotline, 1922, is accessible from everywhere in world and provides 24-hour service."

Takefuji, Yoshiyasu. 2021. "Analysis of digital fences against COVID-19." *Health and Technology* 11(6):1383–1386.

Thunström, Linda, Stephen C Newbold, David Finnoff, Madison Ashworth, and Jason F Shogren. 2020. "The benefits and costs of using social distancing to flatten the curve for COVID-19." *Journal of Benefit-Cost Analysis* 11(2):179–195.

Urbaczewski, A., and Y. J. Lee. 2020. "Information technology and the pandemic: a preliminary multinational analysis of the impact of mobile tracking technology on the COVID-19 contagion control." *European Journal of Information Systems* 29(4):405–414.

Wang, C. Jason, Chun Y. Ng, and Robert H. Brook. 2020. "Response to COVID-19 in Taiwan: big data analytics, new technology, and proactive testing." *JAMA* 323(14):1341–1342.

Whitelaw, S., M. A. Mamas, E. Topol, and H. G. C. Van Spall. 2020. "Applications of digital technology in COVID-19 pandemic planning and response." *Lancet Digit Health* 2(8):e435–e440.

Wilkerson, R. G., J. D. Adler, N. G. Shah, and R. Brown. 2020. "Silent hypoxia: A harbinger of clinical deterioration in patients with COVID-19." *American Journal of Emergency Medicine* 38(10):2243 e5–43 e6.

Woods, Eric Taylor, Robert Schertzer, Liah Greenfeld, Chris Hughes, and Cynthia Miller-Idriss. 2020. "COVID-19, nationalism, and the politics of crisis: A scholarly exchange." *Nations and Nationalism* 26(4):807–825.

Wu, T. Y., A. Majeed, and K. N. Kuo. 2010. "An overview of the healthcare system in Taiwan." *London Journal of Primary Care* 3(2):115–119.

Yan, Yue, Hanshuang Pan, Nian Shao, Yan Xuan, Shufen Wang, Weijia Li, Xingjie Li, Christopher Y Shen, Xu Chen, and Xinyue Luo. 2020. "COVID-19 in Singapore: another story of success." *International Journal of Mathematics for Industry* 12(1):2050001.

Yeh, M. J., and Y. Cheng. 2020. "Policies tackling the COVID-19 pandemic: A sociopolitical perspective from Taiwan." *Health Secure* 18(6):427–434.

Yen, M. Y., A. W. Chiu, J. Schwartz, C. C. King, Y. E. Lin, S. C. Chang, D. Armstrong, and P. R. Hsueh. 2014. "From SARS in 2003 to H1N1 in 2009: Lessons learned from Taiwan in preparation for the next pandemic." *Journal of Hospital Infection* 87(4):185–193.

Yen, W. T. 2020. "Taiwan's COVID-19 management: Developmental state, digital governance, and state-society synergy." *Asian Politics & Policy* 12(3):455–468.

Zeng, Kylie, Stephanie N. Bernardo, and Weldon E. Havins. 2020. "The use of digital tools to mitigate the COVID-19 pandemic: comparative retrospective study of six countries." *JMIR Public Health and Surveillance* 6(4):e24598.

4 Zero-COVID, Digital Pandemic Control Measures and the Making of the Public Health State in Taiwan

Shun-Ling Chen and Yu-Ling Huang

Introduction

Taiwan's COVID-19 response, praised as a success story in the first years of the pandemic, relied on centralization and digital tools. Border controls, strict quarantines, and comprehensive contact tracing, facilitated by various digital technologies and extensive data sharing, were credited for Taiwan's success. While these developments were not unique to Taiwan, concerns about democratic erosion during pandemic control have been raised (Greitens, 2020). Legal scholars raised concerns about the legality and privacy implications of these measures, especially the legality of Taiwan's excessive digital pandemic measures. With limited available empirical data, we further the question about the legality and legitimacy of intrusive digital contact-tracing measures by offering a preliminary evaluation of the effectiveness of these tools. We do so against a theoretical framework we adapted from political economist Mark Neocleous and conceptualize Taiwan's COVID-19 governance as the emergence of a public health state. Taiwan prioritized security, leading to its emergence as a public health state and the normalization of digital tools and extensive data sharing, without adequately evaluating the effectiveness of such measures. Particularly in early 2022, when the population was widely vaccinated and faced the less severe yet highly contagious Omicron variant, Taiwan did not reevaluate the trade-off between civil liberties and security but instead intensified these intrusive measures to uphold its zero-COVID policy.

The COVID-19 crisis in Taiwan can be divided into two phases: the zero-COVID period (January 2020 to April 2022) and the live-with-COVID period (May 2022 to April 2023). This volume discuss Taiwan's adoption of digital measures during the earlier zero-COVID period, when community transmission was extremely rare. This chapter focuses on the second half of that period, when privacy-intrusive digital measures were implemented due to security concerns following a local outbreak in May 2021. At that time, less than 1% of the population was vaccinated. We examine Taiwan's implementation of digital pandemic prevention measures, including the SMS-based contact-tracing system (SMS-CTS), which was the first measure to normalize the regular collection of personal data of the entire population. Our investigation reveals how the public health state culminated during the

DOI: 10.4324/9781003438380-7

Omicron variant outbreak in 2022, indicating that, with the discourse of effective digital governance, the Taiwanese government exerted patriarchal power over its citizens through public health measures. During this period, the public health institutions, entrusted with the power to control the pandemic and restore normalcy, became inherently and inevitably political. Empowered by an unprecedented level of digital monitoring, the public health authority established a new social order during the pandemic. We explain how the alleged liberal values that Taiwan embraces as a digital democracy were suspended or undermined during this period.

Pandemic Governance and the Public Health State

In response to COVID-19, Taiwan exhibits a governance model of "public health state," a concept we altered from Mark Neocleous's "police state." Neocleous views the police as a political technology through which "the state fabricates order, fashions the market, generates new forms of subjectivity and subsumes struggles" (2006: 27). Policing is not only a form of law enforcement but also a form of political administration, through which the state fabricates order in society (2006: 36). While Neocleous acknowledges the public health angles of "security" in a police state (2006: 36), by calling the Taiwan COVID-19 governance model a "public health state," we emphasize the prioritization of public health administration over the functions typically associated with Neocleous's police institution during the pandemic.

Neocleous's police state places a strong emphasis on the prevention of disorder, which represents an extensive form of social control and political administration (2006: 29–30). Stemming from patriarchal concerns to ensure the majority's well-being and economic prosperity, the police state governs with discretionary power (Dubber and Valverde, 2006: 5). Similarly, public health authorities aim for disease prevention and exercise discretionary power. In Taiwan, the zero-COVID approach not only induced a broad definition of "contacts," subjecting relatively more individuals to mandatory testing and quarantine. This policy also justified the widespread use of digital technologies and personal data. As the virus continued to evolve, the public health authorities stressed the need for "agile governance" (Tang, 2021). The Central Emergency Command Center (CECC), the ad hoc institution that was responsible for coordinating pandemic responses, was granted significant flexibility to deviate from standard legal procedures and utilize ambiguous terminologies for COVID-19 measures (Wu, this volume). Composed of medically trained technocrats, the CECC claimed expertise in epidemiology and biomedicine, supported by exclusive access to pandemic data, which bolstered their scientific authority and minimized external challenges.

For Neocleous, the reason that states often fail to treat emergencies as temporary lies in the *raison d'être* of liberal democracies—civil society grants the state *carte blanche* power to subsume political actions and ensure order (2006: 38). Yet, security is a mythic war that often sees no end (2006: 39). Using security as an ideological tool, the state justifies its decision to keep adopting new regulatory measures and fuels the market for security products. "Temporariness" is often a rhetorical device to justify new, sometimes stricter, security measures. In reality, these measures have the potential to permanently and irreversibly alter political techniques (Neocleous, 2008: 67).

In the case of Taiwan, various factors contributed to a sense of urgency that prompted swift action against the "SARS-like disease" at the beginning of 2020. The traumatic memory of SARS, suspicions surrounding China's official statements regarding COVID-19, and concerns about potential isolation from the international community due to exclusion from the WHO all played a role. Consequently, Taiwan's proactive measures encountered minimal opposition, and by February 2020, Congress had passed special legislation granting the CECC a broad and undefined scope to contain the pandemic.[1] Despite having over eight months without community transmission since April 2020, a lingering sense of emergency persisted in early 2021, fueled by observations of how the pandemic unfolded in other parts of the world.

Neocleous argues that the police state is a product of class society, where the state is used by bourgeois civil society to police and control the poor (2006: 25–26). In our current public health state, the initial high-risk groups for COVID-19 were not the poor, but rather people with relative mobility and resources who were able to travel abroad. Nevertheless, when community transmissions exacerbated, the public health state's COVID-19 measures tended to target the lower class. The adult entertainment industry was the only business category ordered to close in 2020 and its business owners were excluded from COVID-19 compensation programs. Among the businesses closed during the May 2021 outbreak, the adult entertainment was also the last permitted to reopen. These targeted measures could be attributed to intimate interactions often involved in this industry. Considering airborne transmission, busy restaurants are not necessarily a less risky environment than adult entertainment businesses, yet the latter category was more frequently inspected for regulation compliance. Unequal enforcement is also evident in the stricter regulations imposed on migrant workers, such as confining them to their dormitories except during working hours (Amnesty International, 2022).

Neocleous argues that the main purpose of law in bourgeois society is to preserve order, not justice. The belief that law is the foundation of justice and can restrain the discretionary powers of executive agents is a liberal myth (2021: 209–210). This myth has caused internal conflicts in liberal democracies during the pandemic. Public health authorities have exercised discretion to implement extensive measures for pandemic control during prolonged states of emergency, which have encroached upon civil liberties. The authorities have disregarded the concerns raised by legal scholars and activists. The majority of the public has been willing to accept these measures without questioning their necessity, effectiveness, and legality, aligning with the primary goal of restoring order in bourgeois society.

Taiwan, as part of its national identity and geopolitical strategy, positions itself as a beacon of liberal democracy in Asia and a hub of global innovation and advanced technology. Taiwan presents itself as a digital democracy, in contrast to China's digital authoritarian regime. While Taiwan's bio-surveillance during the COVID-19 pandemic was not as extensive as China's, it is worth noting that

Taiwan, despite claiming to uphold privacy protection and other liberal values, granted the public health authority significant discretionary power in deploying digital technologies. The extensive collection and processing of personal data continued for an extended period without sufficient evidence of their effectiveness. In the following discussion, we explore how privacy, an emblematic civil liberty, was derogated by digital contact-tracing tools when the public health agenda prioritized security over liberal values in its pursuit of eliminating the threat of COVID-19, particularly during the second half of the Zero-COVID period.

The Potentials and Criticisms of Digital Pandemic Control Tools

Contact-tracing and quarantine measures play pivotal roles in curbing the spread of COVID-19. Many countries, including those known for being more privacy-conscious, turned to digital tools to expedite contact tracing, thus alleviating the need for stringent lockdown measures (Gasser et al., 2020). However, the extensive use of these tools without sufficient scientific evidence raised legal and ethical concerns about privacy and data protection. To address these issues, international public health authorities and data protection agencies, such as the World Health Organization and the European Data Protection Board, released guidelines on using location data and contact-tracing tools, emphasizing privacy protection and public engagement (EDPB, 2020; WHO, 2020).

East Asian countries like China, Hong Kong, South Korea, Singapore, and Taiwan embraced digital measures to control the pandemic. They implemented a diverse range of tools such as interactive maps, contact-tracing mobile apps, geofencing, and interconnected databases (Lin and Hou, 2020). The relatively low number of cases in these countries during spring 2020 led to attributions of their success in containing COVID-19 to these digital tools (Tan, 2021). Authoritarian tendencies in these nations, influenced by their history or current reality, partially explain the limited public resistance to these technologies. Past experiences with SARS or MERS also fostered a collective mindset prioritizing security over civil liberties and privacy. These experiences further shaped institutional arrangements for proactive pandemic responses (Akbari, 2021; Nageshwaran et al., 2021; Liu, 2021).

In March 2020, a widely circulated commentary highlighted Taiwan's effective crisis management during the early weeks of the pandemic, attributing its success to big data and digital technologies (Wang et al., 2020). Taiwan subsequently adopted the term "big data analytics" to encompass its digital strategies, involving the use of real identity and location data, as well as extensive data sharing between public and private entities for enforcing quarantine and conducting contact tracing (Chen et al., 2020; Ma, 2021).

One significant challenge in assessing these tools is the limited number of experts who have both sufficient knowledge about their design and deployment, as well as access to the necessary data for evaluating their effectiveness. Legal scholars raised concerns regarding whether these measures adhere to the principles of privacy protection, namely proportionality, transparency, accountability, and independent oversight (Lin et al., 2020). Experts in epidemiology, such as medical officers at Taiwan Centers for Disease Control, who possessed exclusive access to contact-tracing datasets, were cautious about the accuracy of new digital tools in identifying high-risk contacts, given their familiarity with the strengths and limitations of traditional methods (Cheng et al., 2020; Summers et al., 2020; Ng et al., 2021).

Some experts embraced digital technologies for emergency use without addressing scientific validity or privacy concerns. Chi-Mai Chen, Taiwan's then deputy premier, co-authored an article with public health scholars and technocrats about how Taiwan reacted after cases were reported on the *Diamond Princess* cruise ship. By utilizing cell tower location data from mobile providers, the government identified 627,386 potential contacts and monitored them through the National Health Insurance database for 14 days to check for respiratory symptoms, without their knowledge or consent. In the end, only 67 "contacts" developed symptoms and no confirmed cases were found. Still, the authors concluded that "[a]lthough over 190 contact persons per traveler [from Diamond Princess] might not be realistic, increasing the targeted contact population with no harm was acceptable as a step against COVID-19 spread in this emergency situation" (Chen et al., 2020).

This broad definition of "contacts" and the collection of data without differentiating risk levels gradually influenced the design and implementation of digital contact-tracing measures against COVID-19 in Taiwan. These measures were widely accepted by the general population (Garrett et al., 2021). Starting from May 2021, the SMS-CTS normalized pervasive data collection and extended it to the entire population. This system preventively collects the daily digital traces of the public at large. The SMS-CTS was the sole digital COVID-19 measure for which the authorities consistently (although limited) published usage statistics. Although incomplete, they provide rare clues to assess the effectiveness and necessity of this tool, especially in relation to its potential invasion of privacy.

This chapter utilized three types of research materials. Firstly, we gathered official documents, daily press meetings, and media coverage related to digital COVID-19 control measures, with a focus on contact-tracing tools. Using document analysis, we examined tool design, implementation, targeted social groups, and enrollment methods. Secondly, we analyzed coverage from United Daily (UD) and Liberty Times (LT), two major news presses obtained from Taiwan News Smart Web Database. Thematic analysis was used to categorize newspaper articles (UD = 108 and LT = 105) published between January 2020 and June 2022, capturing public perception of these digital tools.[2] Lastly, we collected SMS-CTS usage data from sms.1922.gov.tw and the Facebook page of the National Communication Commission (NCC).[3] By comparing case numbers of local transmissions and Google mobility data, we investigated how SMS-CTS usage fluctuated and annotated it with important events. The analysis section provides further explanation of our evaluation rationales.

Early Trajectories of Digital Measures in Taiwan

Decisions on Using Mobile Location Data and Registration Data

Following Taiwan's first reported COVID-19 case on January 20, 2020, the government implemented a 14-day home quarantine for individuals entering from Hubei, China. To enforce this measure, temporary cell phones were provided to track their locations using nearby cell towers. Violators faced police tracking, transfer to quarantine facilities, and substantial fines.[4] This enforcement method later became known as the "digital fencing system" or geofence. Deputy Premier Chen, who purportedly proposed the idea, explained that the government had considered using electronic bracelets or anklets, but opted against them due to privacy concerns and the negative associations they carried. The use of widely available cell phones provided a convenient alternative (SET News, 23 March 2020).

An early landmark event is the *Diamond Princess* (DP) incident, where a cruise ship reported confirmed COVID-19 cases shortly after stopping in Taiwan on January 31, 2020. To trace potential contacts with *DP* passengers, the government used various data sources, including CCTV and cell tower data. By using roaming signals that were detected near the harbor when *DP* passengers disembarked, the government was able to determine their locations and issued cell broadcast service (CBS) messages to warn about potential risks. Since CBS messages only reached individuals who were present in those specific areas at the time the messages were sent, the government requested telecom providers to share historical data from relevant cell towers to retroactively identify cell phone numbers that had been in the same cell as *DP* passengers. Consequently, a total of 627,386 people were identified as "contacts" and were warned via retroactive location-based service (RLBS). These individuals were subsequently monitored in the National Health Insurance (NHI) system (Chen et al., 2020). Given that the DP incident garnered significant global attention as an early pandemic horror, the extensive data requests for contact tracing and the use of RLBS went unquestioned and were widely praised as innovative, proactive, and effective approaches to addressing the public health emergency. However, the full extent of data usage in this incident was not initially disclosed to the public. For instance, the fact that a large number of people were monitored in the NHI database was only revealed when the aforementioned paper co-authored by Deputy Premier Chen was published several months later.

The digital fencing system initially enforced quarantine for those returning from abroad and later expanded to close contacts of confirmed cases. RLBS warnings were used in limited instances in 2020 but became more common in spring 2021. These measures established Taiwan's heavy reliance on cell phone and cell tower data for contact tracing. The implementation involved the sharing of data between various public databases, such as immigration and national health insurance, as well as private databases held by telecom companies. This sharing of sensitive personal data, including real identity and location information, formed the basis of these measures. As the police force was responsible for locating individuals who violated quarantine measures, immigration data was shared with the police and made accessible on the police handheld devices. Unlike South Korea, which has clear legislation allowing for broad data use in pandemic control, Taiwan's digital measures were adopted through administrative discretion. The clauses in the Communicable Disease Control Act, which the Taiwan government referred to as its legal authorization, lacked specific details (CECC, 2020). Despite occasional civil liberty concerns, public support for the government's COVID-19 response, including data sharing, was high due to the low local transmission rate.

In a 2020 survey, 75% of respondents agreed that the government should monitor everyone's whereabouts using cellphone GPS data, while 22% disagreed. It is important to note that this survey question does not accurately reflect the actual technology used (cell tower instead of the more accurate GPS) or the target population (contact tracing instead of monitoring everyone). If the technology measures and target population were described more accurately, the acceptance rate may have been even higher (CECC, 2020).[5]

In spring 2020, many countries initiated discussions on incorporating privacy features such as decentralization, voluntary adoption, and anonymity via transient identity into contact-tracing technologies. However, these discussions failed to gain significant traction in Taiwan. The Taiwanese government had already fixed its solutions on centralized and connected databases, which included mobile location data and registration information from mobile providers. Due to the minimal community transmission in 2020, the Taiwan Social Distancing App (TSDA), the localized Bluetooth-based contact-tracing app that prioritized privacy, was only introduced in April 2021. Instead, the government relied on the RLBS system and later incorporated SMS-CTS as its primary contact-tracing aids. Consequently, TSDA played only a marginal role in Taiwan's COVID-19 response.

Mass Data-Sharing and Flagging High Risk Groups in the National Healthcare Database

The government's approach to pandemic control was anchored on a public mindset that during a public health emergency, high-risk groups should make sacrifices for the benefit of society. This, coupled with the government's focus on security, led private entities to adopt strict precautions. During the 2020 spring break, the CECC issued social distancing reminders through CBS in popular destinations. Some entities then used these messages to identify high-risk groups, resulting in schools and companies asking students and employees who received the reminders to stay home for the safety of others (Commercial Times, 6 April 2020). In other cases, employees were asked to take unpaid leave. The CECC did not discourage private entities from implementing these measures. In response to a legislator's inquiry regarding these actions, a senior officer at the Ministry of Health and Welfare (MOHW) stated that they welcomed both public and private entities taking these precautionary measures (CNA, 6 April 2020).

During the pandemic, the CECC flagged higher-risk individuals in the NHI system to protect the healthcare system and alert healthcare providers to take precaution (CNA, 28 January 2020). Data sharing between the National Immigration

Agency and the NHI allowed for marking individuals with recent travel to high-infection regions, expanding from Wuhan to all foreign countries by mid-March 2020. The high-risk group grew to include certain occupations (e.g., health providers, flight attendants, quarantine hotel staff), clusters, and contacts with confirmed cases (United Daily, 29 March 2020). The public health authorities exercised discretion when differentiating between high and low risk. For example, although the infection rate varied significantly across countries in mid-March 2020, the CECC flagged all individuals with recent international travel history.

Public health authorities failed to provide clear standards or scientific explanations for their line-drawing decisions. Furthermore, the categorization of high-risk groups was done with little evaluation of the potential adverse impacts on individuals and society. Individuals flagged as cluster and contact cases were often uninformed and unable to challenge their status, leading to stigmatization and denial of health services. Instances of mass flagging, such as at Taoyuan General Hospital in January 2021 and in Wanhua, Taipei, in May 2021, were only revealed when affected individuals were denied healthcare or access to hospital. A few legislators and human rights NGOs questioned the basis of these flagging decisions. However, these incidents of mass flagging did not receive significant attention, and discussions were limited (Yi Media, 26 May 2021; Liao and Hsu, 2020). The public and media showed little concern about the lack of transparency and scientific evidence, as the overall aim of preserving and securing society was widely accepted.

SMS Contact Tracing and the Normalizing Data Collection of Daily Activities

During the early stages of the zero-COVID period, digital technologies in pandemic control primarily focused on the high-risk group, sparing most Taiwanese from disruption in their daily lives. Measures such as digital fencing and flagging in the NHI system were deemed necessary evils to safeguard the general public. Although the RLBS warning system required access to every individual's cell phone metadata, it was rarely used in the first year of the pandemic due to limited community transmissions. In May 2021, when the first local outbreak occurred, Taiwan introduced the SMS-CTS, an SMS-based guest list system, as a new addition to their digital COVID-prevention toolkit. Unlike previous measures that targeted high-risk groups, the SMS-CTS proactively collected personal identity and location data from all individuals, gradually normalizing the practice of data collection in our daily activities.

The SMS-CTS was launched on May 19, 2021, coinciding with the country's "Level Three Alert" period until July 26, 2021. It allowed locations (business, vehicle, venue, etc.) to obtain a unique ID and QR code for visitors to scan with their cell phones. Visitors could scan the QR code using their cell phones to automatically fill in the location ID and send a text message to the government hotline (1922), with no cost to the sender.[6] This process generated a location visit record (SMS-CTS record) that included the sender's personal identification (via cellphone registration information), the location ID, and a timestamp. These records were kept by the sender's cell phone provider for 28 days. The Executive Yuan conducted a special press conference to introduce the SMS-CTS system and emphasized the need for efficient and effective contact tracing in light of the increasing number of cases (Executive Yuan, 2021). However, the government downplayed privacy concerns and inaccurately claimed that the system would not require users' personal data. Due to the urgency of maintaining order in the public health state, there was no opportunity for public deliberation regarding this new tool. Instead, the government presented the swift development, implementation, and adoption of the SMS-CTS within a three-day timeframe as a testament to their capable, technologically advanced, and proactive governance.

In May 2020, the CECC already advised location operators to keep a voluntary guest list and issued data protection guidelines. By the end of the year, digitized guest lists became common for large events. When the Level Three Alert was issued, the CECC made it mandatory for restaurants and eateries to keep a guest list, even though they were only allowed to offer take-out services. However, this initial mandate did not apply to other types of businesses.[7] This decision seemed puzzling as shopping at grocery stores was not necessarily considered less risky than buying take-out food from restaurants. Nonetheless, many businesses voluntarily adopted guest lists as a gesture of solidarity with public health goals. When adopting the SMS-CTS, the burden of data protection for location operators was eased by the fact that records were stored with cell phone providers. Some business owners even refused to provide hand-written alternatives, leading to occasional disputes. Overall, driven by a sense of urgency and collective pride in maintaining Taiwan's reputation as a COVID-free haven, the SMS-CTS was adopted without much controversy. The aforementioned inconsistency regarding risk levels and mandates went unnoticed, and the presumed efficiency, effectiveness, and necessity of the SMS-CTS were largely unquestioned in the initial weeks.

The initial statistics published on the SMS-CTS in June 2021 raised doubts about its effectiveness and necessity. Out of the 6.19 million SMS sent, contact tracers only requested 303 records, leading some to question whether traditional contact-tracing methods could have been sufficient, considering the decline in local transmissions from hundreds to double-digit figures per day. Despite these doubts, the CECC insisted that the SMS-CTS contributed to the contact-tracing efforts. When Taiwan reduced the alert level after July 27, the requirement for guest lists did not end but expanded to include all types of public locations. Collecting personal data was seen as a necessary compromise to ease other pandemic restrictions and restore a sense of "normalcy" for everyone. The limited number of data requests in the early months might have been attributed by the CECC to logistical issues, suggesting that the mass data collection began before the public health authorities fully understood how to utilize it. However, the CECC did not address the concerns about the effectiveness and necessity of the SMS-CTS and the extensive data collection it entailed.

To address the logistical problems, the CECC developed the Contact-Tracing Assistance Platform (CTAP), providing frontline contact tracers with easy access to SMS-CTS records. From September onward, daily case numbers consistently remained in the single digits. In October 2021, the question of whether the SMS-CTS should be retained sparked public discussions. The CECC promptly responded that the system would remain in place until at least June 2022, arguing that data requests through the SMS-CTS could offer greater precision compared to the RLBS warning system (Broadcasting Corporations of China, 2021). Despite the absence of an actual emergency, the CECC justified the extensive and regular data collection of all residents in the SMS-CTS for precautionary reasons, preparing for potential future outbreaks.

The usage of SMS-CTS (the number of SMS-CTS records) significantly decreased since October 2021, despite expanding mandates and increased community traffic flow (Figure 4.1). In December 2021, with minimal local transmission, daily usage was even lower than during the system's initial week in May. A lab leak in December resulted in the first and only local transmission case in months. Although the CECC listed 479 people as contacts, none tested positive. Since there were no other active contact-tracing cases, it is likely that all CTAP data requests during that time were related to this single incident. The first two days alone saw nearly 240,000 requests.[8] Given the low case numbers, it is difficult to determine the effectiveness of SMS-CTS as a contact-tracing tool. However, the lab leak case sheds light on the significant number of data requests that can arise from a single incident. The lack of protocols from public health authorities leaves uncertainty regarding the scope of data requests, their filtering process, and the effort involved. It remains unclear how many of the 479 contacts could not be identified using traditional contact-tracing methods.

The January 2022 case uptick which began with an Omicron cluster only slightly increased SMS-CTS usage. It should be noted that by this time, more than 70% of the population have received two doses of vaccination. It was the CECC's late January reiteration that restaurants must comply or offer take-out that significantly increased usage, likely due to strengthened enforcement by store owners. In January and February 2022, the CTAP processed over 10 million data requests. While some found the SMS-CTS "useful" for contact tracing, it was unclear if contact tracers could have reached the same individuals without SMS-CTS records. With the multiplication of local cases and the lack of separate contact-tracing statistics for each case, it became impossible to compare the number of identified contacts against the number of CTAP data requests. As public health authorities mandated testing for identified contacts, we investigated the correlation between the increase in the number of reported tests and the CTAP data requests in January and February 2022. Since there were no separate statistics for tests administered for different reasons (e.g., contact tracing, quarantine for inbound travelers, community stations, and institution-based screening), we could only examine how the curve changed from December 2021. Figure 4.2 shows very little correlation between the number of data requests and reported tests. Temporary testing stations set up at institutions (e.g., schools, factories) or neighborhoods when there were confirmed cases often contributed a few thousand tests per day and were likely more significant sources of the reported test increase.

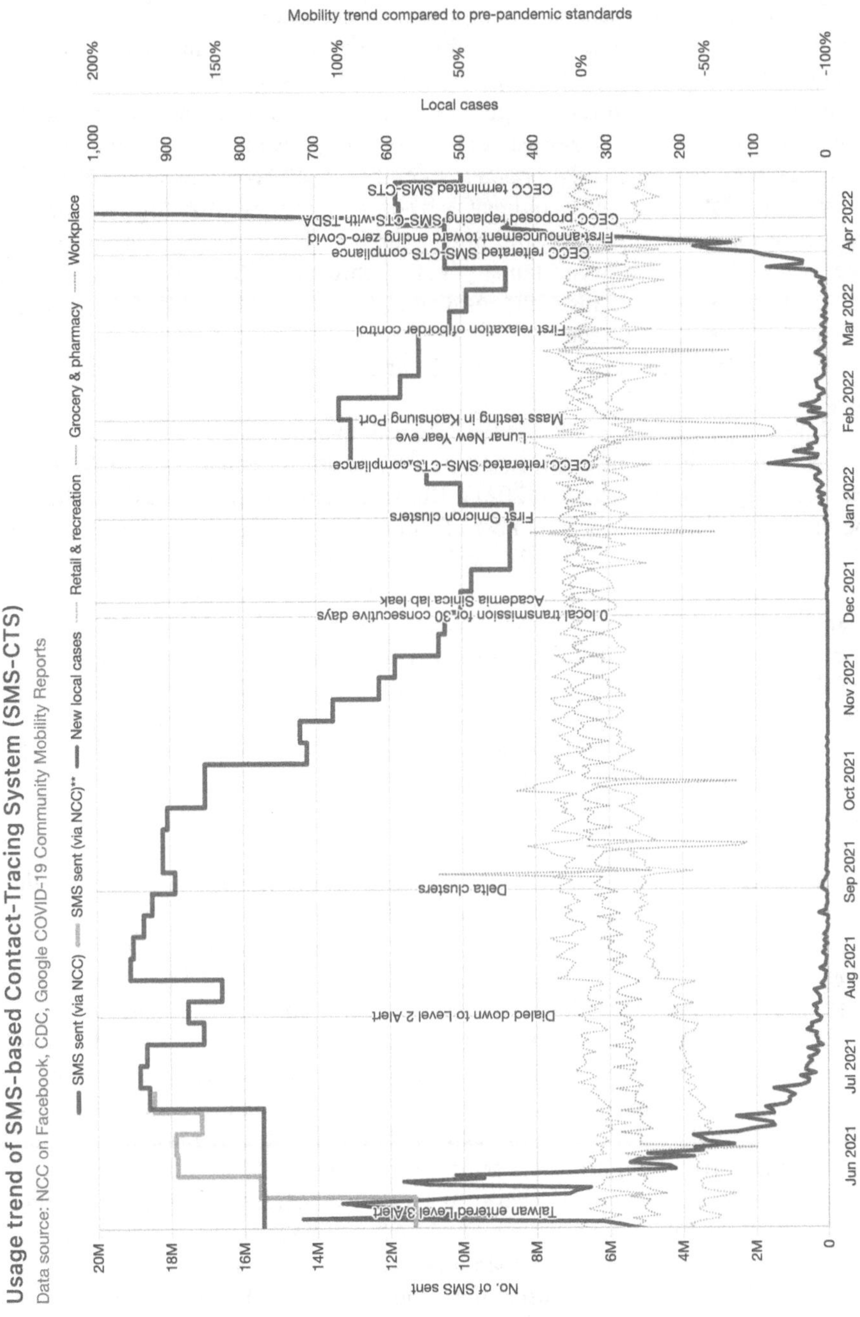

Figure 4.1 Usage Trend of SMS-based Contact-Tracing System

The NCC published the weekly number of SMS-CTS messages sent and the number of messages deleted for having expired the 28-day retention period on its Facebook page (https://www.facebook.com/ncc.gov.tw/).* All reference periods are from May 19 until the day before the report date. We inferred the weekly average by calculating the difference between the total number of sent messages from two consecutive reference periods. Since the first reference period for the total number of sent messages was as long as 40 days, we used the total number of deleted messages of the early reports to infer the weekly average in the first weeks.

We used data from the Google COVID-19 Community Mobility Reports as a reference for the change in traffic flow. (The baseline is the median value from the five-week period between January 3 and February 6, 2020.) We excluded data related to parks, public transit, and residential areas, where the SMS-CTS was usually not required or enforced.

*Some of the reports had a two-week interval because the NCC occasionally skipped reporting.

When the necessity of the SMS-CTS was questioned in October 2021, the CECC argued that it is more precise and thus less intrusive than the RLBS (Broadcasting Corporations of China, 2021). But this claim is unsupported. In the first outbreak in 2022, the highest number of daily CTAP data requests was 660,418 on February 21, followed by 417,968 on February 20. Assuming these data requests were to identify "contacts" of new local cases between February 14 and 20, more than 1 million SMS-CTS records were accessed for a total of 65 cases. During the *DP* incident, to track potential contacts with more than 3,000 roaming signals, 627,386 local cell phones received warning messages. While the SMS-CTS and RLBS function differently and are not directly comparable, the scale of data requests in the SMS-CTS raised concerns regarding privacy protection.[9] It is also important to note that Taiwan did not retire the RLBS warning system after the introduction of the SMS-CTS.

In March 2022, SMS-CTS usage declined again. Despite the case number reaching three digits by the end of the month, the level of usage was only slightly higher than the lowest point recorded in December 2021 when there were almost no cases. CECC's reiteration of the guest list mandate reiteration on April 1 led to a mild usage increase. As the case number continued to spike, the CTAP data requests also grew exponentially with daily requests reaching six or seven digits, peaking at 3,838,724 on April 19. The daily number of reported tests in April ranged between 30,000 and 70,000. Although this increase was not insignificant when compared to January and February, when the number of daily reported tests ranged between 10,000 and 50,000, it was far from exponential, unlike the increase in case numbers and data requests during the same period. This could be partly attributed to insufficient testing capacity. However, as the public health system became strained due to the surge in cases, the volume of CTAP data requests simply overwhelmed the contact tracers' processing capabilities. Consequently, on April 27, 2022, the CECC made the decision to discontinue the SMS-CTS, five weeks ahead of the original schedule (Figure 4.3).

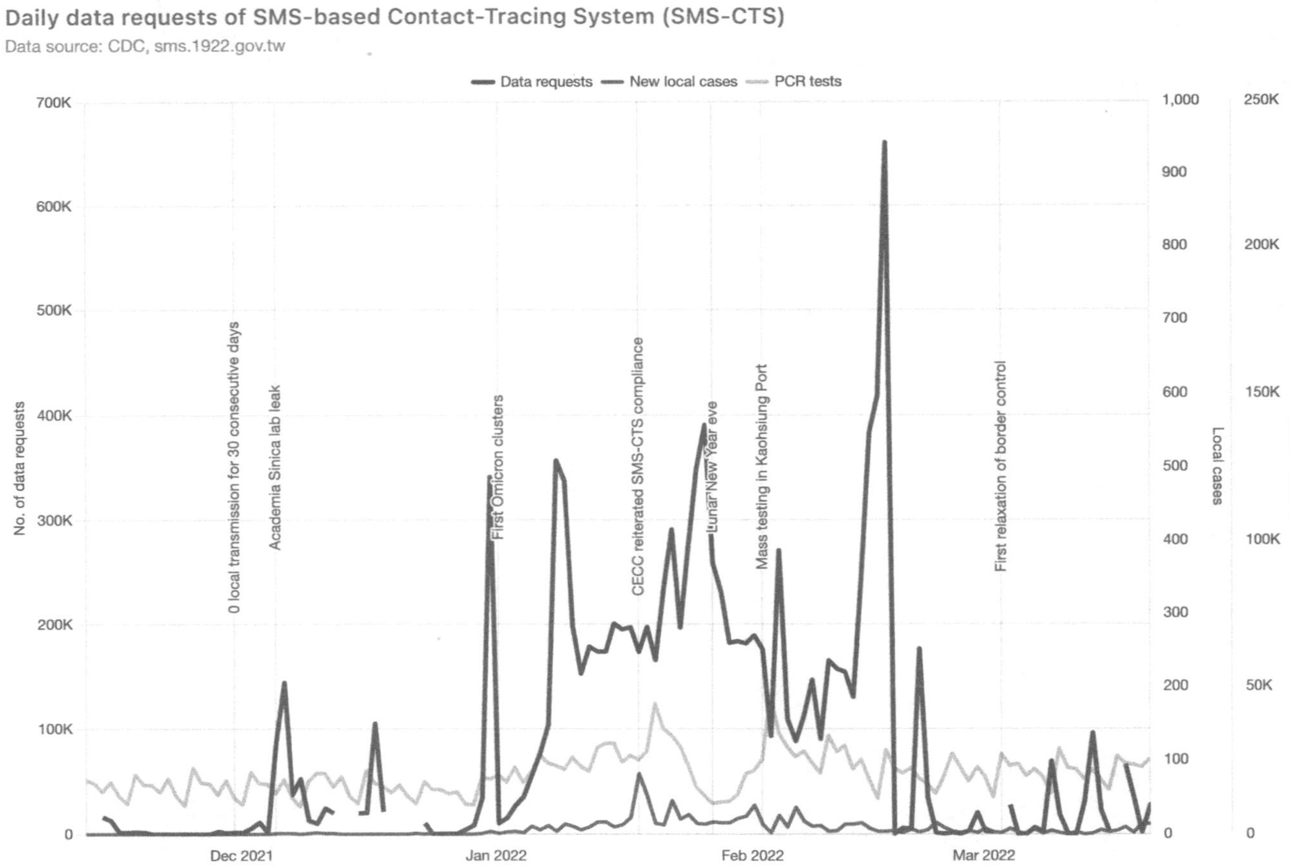

Figure 4.2 Daily Data Request of SMS-based Contact-Tracing System (November 16, 2022–March 25, 2023) sms.1922.gov.tw updated the total number of requests daily. We noticed and began collecting data in mid-November 2021. We inferred the number of requests of a given date with the difference between two consecutive report dates. The website skipped some dates without updating, hence the gaps in the blue line.

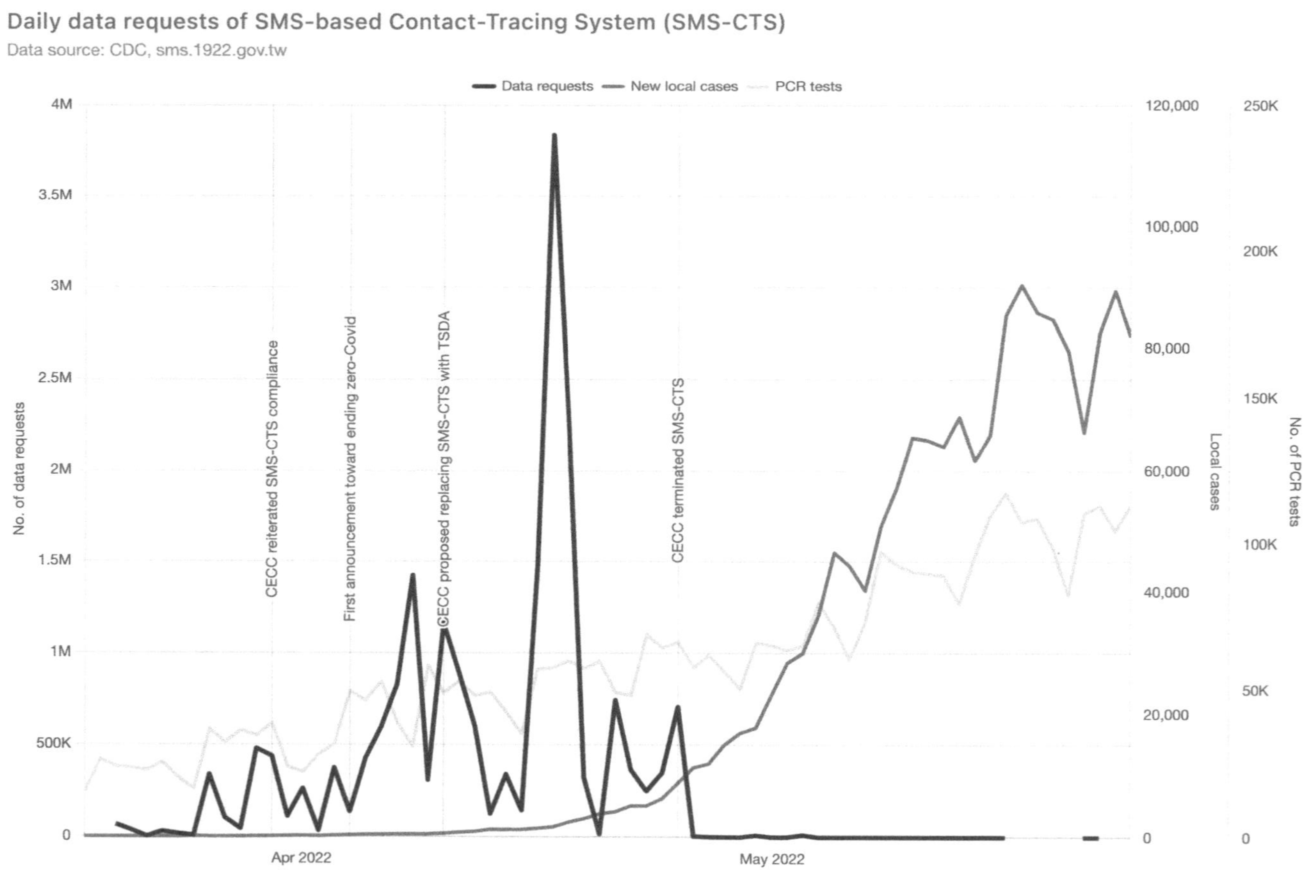

Figure 4.3 Daily Data Request of SMS-Based Contact-Tracing System (March 20–May 26, 2023) sms.1922.gov.tw Provided Daily Updates on the Total Number of Requests. We Noticed and Began Collecting Data in Mid-November 2021. We Inferred the Number of Requests of a Given Date by Calculating the Difference between Two Consecutive Report Dates. The Website Skipped Updating on Certain Dates, Resulting in the Gaps in the Line

Since Spring 2021, the official rhetoric of "precision pandemic control" shifted toward the goal of finding every needle in the haystack.[10] Even in the absence of immediate public health emergencies, privacy became dispensable in pursuit of zero-COVID. While the police faced criticism for using SMS-CTS records for crime investigation, the extensive and unsupported data requests for pandemic control largely went unquestioned.[11] The effectiveness and necessity of the SMS-CTS contact-tracing tool were assumed but never evaluated. From May 19, 2021, to its termination on April 27, 2022, almost 4.8 billion records were sent through SMS-CTS, with nearly 43 million CTAP data requests, approximately 43% of which were made in April alone. Due to limited data availability, we cannot fully address the question of whether the SMS-CTS is effective or necessary. However, our analyses indicate that its effectiveness is questionable, thereby raising doubts about its necessity. Until the CECC was closed in May 2023, the public health authorities failed to provide any evidence-based study justifying the effectiveness or necessity of the SMS-CTS, a system that preemptively collects personal data and individuals' whereabouts. It remains unclear whether the public health authorities ever intended to evaluate the effectiveness or necessity of the SMS-CTS.

Our analysis of newspaper coverage sheds light on various aspects of contact-tracing tools, with a special focus on SMS-CTS. We identified four primary themes that dominate the public discourse on the SMS-CTS: (1) enrollment; (2) dysfunction or destabilization; (3) civil avoidance; and (4) termination. Among the 213 articles analyzed, comprising 108 articles from UD and 105 articles from LT, enrollment emerged as a central theme in the news coverage on the SMS-CTS (N=155, UD-65 and LT-90). These articles provided information on how, when, and where the general population should incorporate the SMS-CTS into their daily activities. A few pieces discussed the potential penalties, as a forceful means of enrollment, imposed on business operators who fail to maintain a guest list. The issue of dysfunction or destabilization of the system is consistently addressed in UD (n=29) but to a lesser extent in LT (n=14). These articles discuss various aspects such as the technical constraints of the system (e.g., Liberty Times, 17 May 2021), the misuse of contact-tracing data by the police (e.g., United Daily, 20 June 2021), and the practical challenges faced by outdoor vendors in adopting the system (e.g., United Daily, 18 October 2021). The third category encompasses instances where individuals rejected, avoided, or bypassed SMS-CTS, highlighted in 16 articles (e.g., Liberty Times, 14 January 2022). For example, many people who bought groceries in the traditional markets pretended to use SMS-CTS to get in (United Daily, 5 June 2021). Considering the magnitude and widespread utilization of SMS-CTS, it is rather astonishing that reports pertaining to its termination are scant (n=10). Discussion about retrospective evaluation of this tool is also absent. Our analysis also revealed that the adoption of the SMS-CTS involved invoking a sense of civic duty and solidarity. Public health authorities used forcible measures like fines or business restrictions for enrollment. LT focused more on articles about the enrollment, while UD highlighted the technical and social shortcomings of the SMS-CTS.

While other countries also faced the need to enroll their populations in digital contact-tracing tools during the pandemic, their domestic media extensively discussed themes such as data governance, the role of IT giants, scientific rigor, voluntariness, and functional efficacy (Amann et al., 2021). These topics were comparatively rare in Taiwan. The public reactions recorded in the news coverage reflected Neocleous's notion that restoring order is the primary concern of bourgeois society. The majority of the public were willing to accept regulatory measures without critically examining their imperative, efficacy, and adherence to legal frameworks.

The Public Health State and the Failed Liberal Promises of Digital Democracy

Taiwan has branded its COVID-19 response as the "Taiwan model," highlighting its transparency and balanced use of digital technology and big data while protecting human rights and privacy (ALDE Party, 2020; Sun, 2020). The government asserted that their tools are in accordance with the principles of adequacy, necessity, and proportionality of privacy law (CDC, 2021). However, the extensive data collection and requests have raised concerns about their necessity. Upon closer examination of the adoption and enforcement of the SMS-CTS, characteristics of a public health state that contradict Taiwan's proclaimed liberal and democratic values as a digital democracy become apparent.

Lack of Public Participation and Deliberation

The SMS-CTS was often touted as the result of collaboration between civic technologists and the government. This claim helped establish Taiwan internationally as a digital democracy and distinguished it from China as an example of digital authoritarianism. Domestically, it allowed the system to gain more trust and induce compliance. While it is true that g0v (gov-zero), a loosely connected group of civic-minded developers and open government/open data enthusiasts, contributed to the design of the tool by organizing discussions on their Slack channel, public participation played only a marginal role. The government made top-down decisions on how to deploy the SMS-CTS, and the public was not consulted when the CTAP was introduced to allow easier data access.

The initial mandate for location registration and its later expansion were decided by the CECC in an "agile governance" fashion. However, this approach led to the CECC violating a basic rule-of-law principle more than once by issuing orders after their alleged effective dates. This hurried roll-out precluded public deliberation. Privacy concerns raised by activists were dismissed by the CECC. Instead, the CECC evaded these questions by dismissing "certain misinformation on Facebook" that claimed the SMS-CTS was a government surveillance tool. They warned that spreading misinformation could lead to jail time and fines. This intentional misinterpretation of legitimate privacy concerns, along with the threatening tone, discouraged criticism and hindered conversation (TAHR, 2021). This attitude reflects Neocleous's account that when security is a priority, a nation would find anything remotely approaching "critical," "thoughtful," or "intellectual" problematic (2008: 135).

Privacy versus the Rhetoric of Security

The government's claim that the SMS-CTS was "free, easy and secure" requires unpacking. There are at least three security concerns: data security, public health security, and national security in pandemic geopolitics. Although national security was not spelt out, it was this notion of security that assisted the public health state in mobilizing the population, involving civic technologists in shaping the SMS-CTS concept, appealing to citizens' sense of solidarity, and countering activists' criticisms regarding the discretionary nature of COVID-19 measures.

As mentioned, to address public health security, the CECC advised location operators to keep guest lists in May 2020. In May 2021, as cases increased, the public health authority expanded its contact-tracing capacity and began mandating guest lists. Many location operators were unequipped or unwilling to bear the burden of providing adequate data protection. The SMS-CTS was initially proposed as a solution but introduced its own data security issues with a more centralized data structure, which became more acute after the CTAP allowed a wider and easier data request process. The public health authority downplayed or disregarded concerns about centralized databases, instead emphasizing that SMS-CTS protected citizens against lurkers flipping through hand-written forms in stores. This implied that ill-intentioned individuals and irresponsible location operators failing to protect customer data were considered the primary threats. Although these are valid privacy concerns, the omission of addressing the database structure and accountability mechanism in this extensive data collection program was a significant oversight. Similarly, the public health authorities dismissed concerns from human rights activists, refusing to acknowledge that a bio-surveillance state itself poses a threat to privacy and civil liberties. Instead, they assumed the role of a caring patriarch seeking to protect their subjects.

The So-called "Gold Standard" for Digital Pandemic Control

Following the introduction of the CTAP to address logistical challenges, the CECC launched the sms.1922.gov.tw website for people to check data requests within the past 28 days. Taiwan's Digital Minister Audrey Tang praised the revised SMS-CTS request system as "the gold standard" and a "milestone for digital epidemic control," noting that allowing people to check the access record is an example of how accountability, a principle of open government, is embodied in the system (Tang, 2021). Although this feature deserves some credit, it had limited impact on the discretionary nature of extensive data collection. During the zero-COVID period, individuals identified as "contacts" faced mandatory 14-day quarantine regardless of negative PCR test results. Since the public health authorities never publicize data requests guidelines or protocols, there is little opportunity to dispute their classification. The revised system's accountability was minimal, as the rationale of the access request it provided did not go beyond "for contact-tracing purposes."

Conclusion

Taiwan prioritized security and embraced digital tools for pandemic control, but this came at the expense of privacy and civil liberties, possibly even "celebrating bio-surveillance" (Schubert, 2021). While Taiwan aimed to establish itself as a digital democracy that successfully contained COVID-19 while upholding liberal values, it compromised even the most fundamental political right in liberal democracies—voting rights—in favor of COVID-19 measures. During the "live-with-COVID" period, which began seven months before the municipal elections in November 2022, no alternative arrangements were made for citizens who tested positive at voting stations. If individuals tested positive and were still within the mandated quarantine period, they were effectively barred from casting their ballots, risking a prohibitive fine for breaking quarantine.

The Taiwan government's COVID-19 responses in 2020 laid the foundation for its pandemic containment efforts. From border control to contact tracing, the public health state has shown a fetish for data, relying on centralized and linked databases to enforce its policies. The SMS-CTS episode is indicative of how Taiwan operated under the rationale of a public health state that prioritized security. The hasty roll-out of the SMS-CTS during the public health emergency not only prevented any public deliberation, but also guaranteed a chaotic data governance structure. The prolonged sense of emergency, despite low local transmissions, led to continued data collection through SMS-CTS, even though its effectiveness was questionable. The public health authorities neglected to address the different risk levels of activities, resulting in unnecessary data collection. Through the SMS-CTS and other digital pandemic control measures, the state employed public health as a political technology to fabricate order (normalizing extensive data collection and sharing for exhaustive contact tracing, differentiated treatment for high-risk groups), shape markets (preference for SMS and telecom providers over other tools and services), generate new forms of subjectivity (monitored high-risk bodies, good citizens, and responsible business operators that pay hyper attention to ensure they would not become the "weak link" in the COVID-19 prevention), and subsume struggle (dismissing critiques as misinformation or as signs of lacking solidary).

Although the excessive daily data collection and access of the SMS-CTS is now history, data sharing between private and public databases for border control and for quarantine persisted in the "live-with-COVID" period. Geofencing and flagging in the NHI database have become normalized as case numbers increased and international travel became more common. While Taiwan ended COVID-19 measures in April 2023, these measures may become institutionalized in the planned revision of the Communicable Disease Prevention Act, following the pattern set by Taiwan's response to SARS. When celebrating Taiwan's early pandemic success as a model for pandemic governance, one should not overlook the civil liberties cost paid under the public health state.

Acknowledgment

We are grateful to Shun-Ling Chen's assistants, Poren Chiang and Cathy Lee, for helping with the collection, analyses, and visualization of the SMS-CTS data.

Notes

1 The special legislation had an initial sunset clause to terminate in June 2021. It was renewed in 2021 and again in 2022.
2 We used TNSW because online news outlets often publish the same stories repeatedly. United Daily (UD) and Liberty Times (LT) are chosen because they represent different political views.
3 The numbers on sms.1922.gov.tw were renewed daily but ephemeral, as they were replaced by the next update. Neither source offers statistics in the open data format. We published both sets of data we collected on GitHub: https://github.com/IIAS-infolaw/sms-registration-data.
4 In 2020, the penalty for a quarantine who refused the traceable cell phone could be as high as 10,000 USD (RTI, 29 January 2020).
5 Question 10 of the survey asked whether one agrees that the government can use cell phone GPS data to monitor everyone's whereabouts. Among the 1,253 respondents, 404 strongly agreed, 541 agreed, 191 disagreed and 85 strongly disagreed (Center for Survey Research, 2020).
6 To fund the system, the NCC expedited a procurement with major mobile providers.
7 The initial mandate applied to certain events, such as religious activities, funerals and weddings, but did not apply to other businesses.
8 Given the contact tracing process can last several days, this number is a rather conservative estimate.
9 The high number of data requests may be partly due to how the SMS-CTS is enforced. For example, shopping centers generally demand customers to check in with the SMS-CTS at the main entrance.
10 In 2020, Taiwan's "precision pandemic control model" used to mean targeted testing, which explains the very low number of total PCR tests until spring 2021.
11 The COVID-19 special legislation did not authorize the CECC to override wiretapping law or other privacy laws that permit government agencies to access personal data beyond the purpose of collection. Nevertheless, prioritizing the public health objective, the CECC demanded that law enforcement excluded such data, *de facto* overruling the wiretapping law.

References

Akbari, A., 2021, Authoritarian Surveillance: A Corona Test: Surveillance & Society, v. 19(1), 98–103, https://doi.org/10.24908/ss.v19i1.14545.

Alliance of Liberals and Democrats for Europe Party (ALDE Party), May 6, 2020, The Taiwan Model Is Something that All the Liberal Democracies Can Learn from, accessed May 25th, 2023, at https://www.aldeparty.eu/the_taiwan_model_is_something_that_all_the_liberal_democracies_can_learn_from_2020.

Amann, J., Sleigh, J., and Vayena, E., 2021, Digital Contact-Tracing during the Covid-19 Pandemic: An Analysis of Newspaper Coverage in Germany, Austria, and Switzerland: PLoS One, v. 16(2), e0246524, https://doi.org/10.1371/journal.pone.0246524.

Amnesty International, 2022, Taiwan 2021, accessed May 25th, 2023, at https://www.amnesty.tw/sites/default/files/news/files/20210112%20ICCPR%2C%20ICESCR%2C%20List%20of%20issues%20of%20Taiwan.pdf.

Broadcasting Corporations of China, Oct. 12, 2021, SMS-CTS Costs 2M NTD/Day, Chen: It Is Useful for Contact Tracing, at https://bccnews.com.tw/archives/59600 [in Mandarin].

Center for Survey Research, 2020, Taiwan Social Image Survey 1st Report of 2020: Academia Sinica, Taipei.

Central Epidemic Command Center, Sep. 9, 2020, Letter to Taiwan Association for Human Rights, at https://www.tahr.org.tw/sites/default/files/u147/yi_qing_zhi_hui_zhong_xin_gong_kai_shu_ju_.pdf [in Mandarin].

Chen, C., Jyan, H., Chien S., Jen, H., Hsu, C., Lee, P., Lee, C., et al., 2020, Containing COVID-19 among 627,386 Persons in Contact with the Diamond Princess Cruise Ship Passengers Who Disembarked in Taiwan: Big Data Analytics: Journal of Medical Internet Research, 22(5), e19540, https://doi.org/10.2196/19540.

Cheng, H., Jian, S., Liu, D., Ng, T. -C., Huang, W. -T., Lin, H. -H., and Taiwan COVID-19 Outbreak Investigation Team, 2020, Contact Tracing Assessment of COVID-19 Transmission Dynamics in Taiwan and Risk at Different Exposure Periods Before and After Symptom Onset: JAMA Internal Medicine, v. 180(9), 1156–1163, https://doi.org/10.1001/jamainternmed.2020.2020.

CNA, Apr. 6, 2020, MOHW Supports Public and Private Organizations to Collect Travel Histories of Spring Break: Central News Agency, at https://www.cna.com.tw/news/ahel/202004060185.aspx [in Mandarin].

CNA, Jan. 28, 2020, NHS Warning Expands to People Returning from Hubei and Close Contacts: Central News Agency, at https://www.cna.com.tw/news/firstnews/202001280126.aspx [in Mandarin].

Commercial Times, Apr. 6, 2020, NCKU Prohibited Students and Faculties with Specific Travel Histories from Entering Campus: Commercial Times, at https://ctee.com.tw/livenews/ch/chinatimes/20200406004168-260405 [in Mandarin].

Dubber, M. D., and Valverde, M., editors, 2006, The New Police Science: The Police Power in Domestic and International Governance: Stanford University Press, Stanford, CA.

European Data Protection Board (EDPB), 2020, Guidelines 04/2020 on the Use of Location Data and Contact Tracing Tools in the Context of the COVID-19 Outbreak, at https://edpb.europa.eu/our-work-tools/our-documents/guidelines/guidelines-042020-use-location-data-and-contact-tracing_en.

Garrett, P. M., Wang, Y., White, J. P., Hsieh, S., Strong, C., Lee, Y., Lewandowsky, S., Dennis, S., and Yang, C., 2021, Young Adults View Smartphone Tracking Technologies for COVID-19 as Acceptable: The Case of Taiwan: International Journal of Environmental Research and Public Health, v. 18(3), 1332, https://doi.org/10.3390/ijerph18031332.

Gasser, U., Ienca, M., Scheibner, J., Sleigh, J., and Vayena, E., 2020, Digital Tools against COVID-19: Taxonomy, Ethical Challenges, and Navigation Aid: The Lancet Digital Health, v. 2(8), e425–e434, https://doi.org/10.1016/S2589-7500(20)30137-0.

Greitens, S., 2020, Surveillance, Security, and Liberal Democracy in the Post-COVID World: International Organization, v. 74(S1), E169–E190, https://doi.org/10.1017/S0020818320000417.

Executive Yuan, 2021, *The Executive Yuan Gazette*, v. 110(78), 375.

Liao, J., and Hsu, S., 2020, The Privacy Concerns about People from Wanhua are Marked in the NHI System: Hsu & Associates, at https://hsu.legal/article/60 [in Mandarin].

Liberty Times, Jan. 14, 2022, Security Guards Shut Down the Elevator as a Man Refused SMS-CTS When Entering the Building, at https://news.ltn.com.tw/news/society/breakingnews/3800976 [in Mandarin].

Liberty Times, May 17, 2021, Passengers Jammed Taipei's SMS-CTS App and Causes Public Discontent, at https://news.ltn.com.tw/news/life/paper/1449130 [in Mandarin]

Lin, C., Wu, C., and Wu, C., 2020, Reimagining the Administrative State in Times of Global Health Crisis: An Anatomy of Taiwan's Regulatory Actions in Response to the COVID-19 Pandemic: European Journal of Risk Regulation, v. 11(2), 256–272, https://doi.org/10.1017/err.2020.25.

Lin, L., and Hou, Z., 2020, Combat COVID-19 with Artificial Intelligence and Big Data: Journal of Travel Medicine, v. 27(5), https://doi.org/10.1093/jtm/taaa080.

Liu, C., 2021, Chinese Public's Support for COVID-19 Surveillance in Relation to the West: Surveillance & Society, v. 19(1), 89–93.

Ma, K. S., 2021, Integrating Travel History via Big Data Analytics under Universal Health-care Framework for Disease Control and Prevention in the COVID-19 Pandemic: Journal of Clinical Epidemiology, v. 130(February), 147–148, https://doi.org/10.1016/j.jclinepi.2020.08.016.

Nageshwaran, G., Harris, R. C., Guerche-Seblain, and C. E., 2021, Review of the Role of Big Data and Digital Technologies in Controlling COVID-19 in Asia: Public health interest vs. privacy: Digital Health, v. 7(January), https://doi.org/10.1177/20552076211002953.

National Communications Commission (NCC), 2021, Statistics of the SMS-based Contact-tracing System, accessed May 25, 2023, at Facebook at https://www.facebook.com/permalink.php?story_fbid=3023169064584095&id=161231844566917l.

Neocleous, M., 2006, Theoretical Foundations of the "New Police Science", *in* Dubber, M. D. and Valverde, M., editors, The New Police Science: The Police Power in Domestic and International Governance: Stanford University Press, Stanford, CA, 17–41.

Neocleous, M., 2008, Critique of Security: Edinburgh University Press, Edinburgh.

Neocleous, M., 2021, A Critical Theory of Police Power: Verso, New York, NY.

Ng, T., Cheng, H., Chang, H., Liu, C., Yang, C., Jian, S., Liu, D., Cohen, T., and Lin, H., 2021, Comparison of Estimated Effectiveness of Case-Based and Population-Based Interventions on COVID-19 Containment in Taiwan: JAMA Internal Medicine, v. 181(7), 913–921, https://doi.org/10.1001/jamainternmed.2021.1644.

RTI, Jan. 29, 2020, CECC: The Home-Quarantine Will Get Punished If They Refuse to Track via Cellphone: Radio Taiwan International, at https://www.rti.org.tw/news/view/id/2049647 [in Mandarin].

Schubert, G., 2021, The Governmentality of Taiwan's Anti-epidemic Politics: Northern England Policy Centre for the Asia Pacific Policy Brief at the University of Central Lancashire (UCLan), v. 2021(1), at https://www.docdroid.net/0rW8vT5/nepcap-2021-01-gunter-schubert-pdf.

SET News, Mar. 23, 2020, Digital Fencing System Inquired by Several Countries; SETN Interviews Proponent Chi-Mai Chen: SET News, at https://www.setn.com/News.aspx?NewsID=712983 [in Mandarin].

Summers, J., Cheng, H., Lin, H., Barnard, L. T., Kvalsvig, A., Wilson, N., and Baker, M. G., 2020, Potential Lessons from the Taiwan and New Zealand Health Responses to the COVID-19 Pandemic: The Lancet Regional Health – Western Pacific, v. 4(November), https://doi.org/10.1016/j.lanwpc.2020.100044.

Sun, J., undated (published on Nov 4, 2020), The Taiwan Model for COVID-19 Prevention (sponsored content): The Boston Globe, at https://sponsored.bostonglobe.com/taipei-economic-and-cultural-office-in-boston-teco-boston/taiwan-model-covid-prevention/.

Taiwan Association for Human Rights (TAHR), May 31, 2021 Who Audits the SMS-CTS? Public Debates Should Not Be Dismissed as Misinformation, Press Release, at https://www.tahr.org.tw/news/2959 [in Mandarin].

Taiwan Centers for Disease Control (CDC), June 29, 2021, The Use of SMS-CTS Data Follows the Principle of Legality, Legitimacy and Necessity: Press Release, at https://www.cdc.gov.tw/Bulletin/Detail/HS0hjvHxAOTCPtNPmDo7Bw?typeid=9 [in Mandarin].

Tan, E., July 13, 2021, South Korea, Singapore and Taiwan Take on Coronavirus, at Medium at https://medium.com/digital-asia-ii/south-korea-singapore-and-taiwan-take-on-coronavirus-7650a40bcde.

Tang, A., Aug. 26, 2021, The Gold Standard: 1922 SMS: CommonWealth Magazine, at https://english.cw.com.tw/article/article.action?id=3065.

United Daily, June 20, 2021, CECC: We Never Passed the SMS-CTS Data to Police, p. front page A2 [in Mandarin].

United Daily, June 5, 2021, Chaos in Covid-19 Prevention Measures and People Hide Away from SMS-CTS, p. front page B1 [in Mandarin].

United Daily, Mar. 29, 2020, Flight Attendants Are Discriminated Against in Health Care, at https://web.archive.org/web/20200330042145/https://health.udn.com/health/story/120950/4451498 [in Mandarin].

United Daily, Oct. 18, 2021, Puzi Night Market is Over-crowded, p, front page B2 [in Mandarin].

Wang, C. J., Ng, C. Y., and Brook, R. H., 2020, Response to COVID-19 in Taiwan: Big Data Analytics, New Technology, and Proactive Testing: JAMA, v. 323(14), 1341–1342, https://doi.org/10.1001/jama.2020.3151.

WHO, 2020, Ethical Considerations to Guide the Use of Digital Proximity Tracking Technologies for COVID-19 Contact Tracing, accessed May 25, 2023, at https://www.who.int/publications/i/item/WHO-2019-nCoV-Ethics_Contact_tracing_apps-2020.1.

Yi Media, May 26, 2021, Internal Documents Show that the CECC Collected the RLBS Receivers in Wanhua and Marked High Risk Groups in the NHI System: Yi Media, at https://yimedia.com.tw/investigate/117647/ [in Mandarin].

5 Digital Pandemic Measures in the Age of COVID-19

Taiwan's Challenges with Regard to Privacy and Personal Data Protection

Chuan-Feng Wu

Introduction

During the COVID-19 pandemic, novel digital technologies have been used in Taiwan to support pandemic investigation needs. Effective digital governance using big data analytics and smart technology is regarded as an important factor in Taiwan's success in containing the pandemic (see Chapter 3). With impressive success battling the novel virus, the government's emergency powers to use these technologies to extensively collect personal data have been generally accepted in Taiwanese society (Garrett and others, 2022).

However, despite digital democracy challenges (discussed in Chapters 4 and 6), privacy experts and human rights advocates have expressed fear that the use of information technology-based surveillance measures and tracking tools (hereinafter "digital COVID-19 measures") may lead to the derogation of privacy and personal data protection (Calvo, Deterding, and Ryan, 2020); thus, it is important to evaluate the pandemic's implications for privacy and personal data protection in Taiwan, and society's response to these privacy challenges. This chapter first investigates the following questions to determine whether Taiwan's digital COVID-19 response policies hold up under the Personal Data Protection Act (PDPA) as well as constitutional scrutiny and the precedents set by the Constitutional Court in terms of the personal data protection principles: (1) Do the digital COVID-19 measures comply with the principles? (2) If the principles are compromised due to the pandemic, has the government provided proper justification establishing the necessity of restricting individuals' privacy right, the evidence-based efficacy of each digital COVID-19 measure, and justification of the trade-off between privacy protection and the pursuit of public health security? The personal data protection principles, including lawfulness, purpose limitation, data minimization, and transparency, are adopted here because they are more specific than general privacy concepts and can provide normative guidance in assessing personal data protection, which is regarded as an essential aspect of privacy, during the pandemic (Tzanou, 2013a, 2013b). Second, in addition to the legal doctrines, this chapter attempts to understand the rationale underlying Taiwanese society's widespread acceptance of the digital COVID-19 measures with only limited privacy intrusion concerns. The question lies with whether or not the boost in social trust in institutions during the pandemic is either due to the difference in the

DOI: 10.4324/9781003438380-8

social perception of privacy between the Taiwanese culture and the Western notion or due to Taiwan's strong democracy.

Digital Measures in Response to COVID-19 in Taiwan

Spurred by the need for public safety during the COVID-19 pandemic, the Taiwan government adopted several digital measures to combat the novel virus. The following are some of the digital approaches to personal data collecting, storing, using, transferring/sharing, or disclosing (hereinafter "personal data processing") and surveillance that the Taiwan government employed in its response to COVID-19.

1 Database linking and sharing: Multiple databases maintained by government agencies and private entities (such as telecommunications operators) were linked. For example, to efficiently monitor travelers from abroad, the National Health Insurance Administration (NHIA) linked their medical database with the immigration database maintained by the National Immigration Agency.[1] Furthermore, the information, accompanied by the patient's career information (such as "flight crew") and contact/cluster history, is marked on their National Health Insurance (NHI) card so that physicians can check a patient's travel history and COVID-19 exposure risk without obtaining their consent.[2] The digital notification system was eventually expanded to include populations who are determined, by the government, to be under high COVID-19 exposure risk.[3]
2 Intellectual digital surveillance fence: The National Communication Commission (NCC) required the telecommunication companies to deploy a digital surveillance system on individuals' mobile phones (self-owned or temporarily provided by the government) to trace their movements in quarantine or during self-health management.[4] If an individual leaves the quarantine site, the digital fence system sends a short message service (SMS) alert to the individual, the related administration, and the local police. Furthermore, the system is connected to the Police Cloud Computing System (M-police),[5] a big data mobile computing platform that combines multiple digital surveillance systems, such as the real-time surveillance camera system, instant photo comparison system (linked to personal ID card, criminal record, and missing persons' report databases),[6] and instant license plate recognition system.[7] By combining the digital fence and the M-police, the government is capable of aggregating and analyzing massive amounts of personal information.
3 SMS contact-tracing system: After requiring individuals to register their real names and contact information when they visit public places, a QR code-based real name registration system, known as the "SMS contact-tracing system", was developed by the government. In this system, facilities such as stores, restaurants, and public institutions are each assigned a QR code with their location information, and individuals are required to scan the QR code and send an SMS message with the QR code to the CDC (1922 hotline).[8] Through the system (and possibly supplemented by surveillance cameras), tracking of patients' daily routes down to the hour is disclosed to the public so that individuals who visit

the same locations simultaneously can be alerted for potential transmission.[9] The SMS messages are stored in the telecommunication companies and should be deleted after 28 days as requested by the NCC.[10]

4 Social distancing app: Taiwan's social distancing app was developed by the CDC and Taiwan AI Labs and first launched in May 2020.[11] The mobile phone app uses Bluetooth technology to sense whether a user has come within two meters of a confirmed COVID-19 case for more than two minutes over the past 14 days.[12] The data collected by the app is encrypted and will not be used to investigate individuals' locations, as disclosed to the public in the technical white paper.[13]

Privacy and Personal Data Protection in Taiwan

Although the privacy right is not enumerated in Taiwan's Constitution, it has been long recognized by the Constitutional Court as an indispensable fundamental right under Article 22 of the Constitution[14] for purposes of preserving human dignity and the integrity of personality, as well as protecting the private sphere of life from intrusion and the self-determination of personal information (Judicial Yuan Interpretation Nos. 585 and 603). In 1995, the notion of privacy, especially the right to information privacy, was adopted in the PDPA, where the personal data protection rules were set out with reference to EU Directive 95/46/ EC (later replaced by the General Data Protection Regulation [GDPR]) to provide more data protections than any previous Taiwanese legislation (Chang, 2014).

To be noted, in theory, privacy and personal data protection are not identical rights (Tzanou, 2013a, 2013b). But the distinction is not clear in Taiwan and in practice these two rights are intertwined in policies and judicial decisions, where personal data protection is analyzed on the basis of privacy and vice versa (Chang, 2014, Liu, Li, and Tu, 2020). For example, the Supreme Administrative Court stated in *Tsai et al. v. NHIA* that the PDPA is a mechanism providing tools and procedures to protect privacy.[15]

It is also worth noticing that the Constitutional Court did not assert that privacy is an absolute right. In Interpretation No. 603, the Court explicitly left open the possibility of the mass collection of personal data, insofar as the collection is subject to the purpose specification and data minimization principles as well as organizational and procedural safeguards (such as the proportionality principle). Similarly, the PDPA allows the government to be exempted from some personal data protection principles if it is necessary for the government to ensure national security or public interest or to perform its statutory duties (PDPA Articles 6(I)(2) and 16(I)(2)). Namely, during the pandemic, the government can justify its processing of personal data derived from the digital COVID-19 measures and restrict the privacy right by raising compelling interests or appealing to statutory duties delineated in the Communicable Disease Control (CDC) Act. It is consistent with the European Data Protection Board's (EDPB) opinions, which stated that the personal data protection rules do not hinder pandemic control because the rules provide legal grounds for personal data processing when it is necessary to protect public health or vital interests (GDPR Articles 6 and 9) or to comply with legal obligations (EDPB, 2020c, WHO, 2020).

However, as criticized by the Constitutional Court in its recent Judgment No. 13 of 2022, personal data protection in Taiwan is still incomprehensive due to the absence of an independent monitoring mechanism, the lack of unambiguous requirements for entities accessing personal data, and the ignorance of the right of informational self-determination.[16] These issues then turned into privacy challenges for the digital COVID-19 measures.

Privacy Impacts of COVID-19: Digital COVID-19 Measures and Personal Data Protection

Although the Constitutional Court and the PDPA have elaborated that the balance between privacy right and public interest shall be subject to the examination of necessity and proportionality, the pandemic has undermined privacy protection standards, that is seemingly robust in normal times, due to the unprecedented magnitude of COVID-19. The digital COVID-19 measures in Taiwan were not properly or strictly scrutinized and remains debatable whether all of them qualify as "necessary measures" that pass scrutiny under the rule of law principles (Lin, Wu, and Wu, 2020, Liu, Li, and Tu, 2020). The ignorance may be caused by the lack of knowledge about the novel virus, fear of the enormous destruction brought about by the pandemic, and the need for a prompt response in a manner that may not allow sufficient time for regular constitutional scrutiny, parliamentary deliberation, or regular administrative procedures (Bastos and de Ruijter, 2019, Knowles, 2014).

However, considering the ongoing and open-ended nature of the privacy restrictions imposed by the digital COVID-19 measures and the fact that mass digital surveillance techniques have become a convenient tool for the government to employ to combat the pandemic, it is unreasonable to avoid a stricter level of review that can serve as a critical check on the exercise of government power in its use of the digital COVID-19 measures. For example, the digital COVID-19 measures were mostly affected through scattered executive orders or administrative gazettes, or worse, unofficial announcements or press releases. It is questionable whether the CECC's vague, broad orders/gazettes and press releases, which grant the government extensive powers that can infringe on an individual's privacy right through the digital COVID-19 measures, ignore statutory formalities required by the legislature and exceed or undermine the delegation that the legislature has entrusted to the administration (Li, 2020a). To prevent the digital COVID-19 measures adopted during this state of emergency from becoming the new normal, a bottom line needs to be clearly drawn (O'Mathúna and Gordijn, 2018).

The bottom line is fairly straightforward: While some exceptional measures may be justified by the legality of emergency, ignoring the existing rule of law and privacy protection safeguards is a dangerous move that may ultimately institutionalize exceptionalism and leave a lasting impact on privacy protection (Farrow, 2021). To address this issue, the PDPA personal data protection principles should be applied as substantive and procedural safeguards to review the justifications of

Taiwan's digital COVID-19 measures and to ensure that the privacy right is not unduly sacrificed or burdened in exchange for health security (Liu, Li, and Tu, 2020, Weng, 2021). For the purposes of this chapter, the following analysis focuses on the principles of lawfulness, purpose limitation, data minimization, and transparency enshrined in the PDPA.

Lawfulness

As regards the lawfulness of personal data processing, it can be carried out either based upon the data subject's consent or some other legitimate basis laid down by law. The lawfulness requirement is used as a structural safeguard to hold administrative agencies legally accountable for the use of data and to enable the democratically accountable legislature to oversee these digital pandemic responses (Bradford, Aboy, and Liddell, 2020).

The potential lawful basis for Taiwan's digital COVID-19 measures can be found in the PDPA because most measures are either necessary for the performance of a task carried out in national security or public interest (PDPA Article 16(I)(2)), for the protection of the data subjects' or others' vital interests (Articles 16(I)(3) and 16(I)(4)), or for the exercise of official authority vested in the administrative agency as a statutory duty (Articles 6(I) and 15(I)(1)). Additionally, the CECC cites the CDC Act as well as the Special Act for Prevention, Relief, and Revitalization Measures for Severe Pneumonia with Novel Pathogens (the COVID-19 Special Act), which authorize the government to impose necessary pandemic control measures, as the lawful basis for the digital COVID-19 measures since these measures are necessary tools to combat COVID-19.

However, simply identifying a legal provision as the lawful basis is insufficient to meet the lawfulness requirement. Whether or not the lawful basis is clear and precise and its application is foreseeable to persons subject to it, as well as the necessity and proportionality of the envisaged measures, need to be assessed (see e.g., GDPR Recital 41) (Kotschy, 2020). The problem here then is that, although the lawfulness requirement can be fulfilled in formality, it is debatable whether the lawful bases applied to the digital COVID-19 measures are substantially justifiable and are not invalid under the void-for-vagueness doctrine (or the principle of clarity) (Larkin, 2021).

The answer is in the negative. ***First***, when the statutory duty/public interest exemptions delineated in the PDPA are applied as the lawful basis for processing personal data, the Taiwan government has failed to explain what specific purpose the government is seeking to achieve through each specific digital COVID-19 measure and whether the measure is necessary and proportionate to the purpose. A lack of proper explanation greatly increases the risk of administrative agencies abusing their authority and misusing personal data for purposes other than pandemic control (Huang and Lo, 2021, Lin, 2020). For this reason, rather than simply repeating the vague legal texts (such as statutory tasks or public interest) set out in the PDPA as the lawful bases, the government should strive to fulfill the lawfulness requirement by further articulating the public health purposes of the proposed digital COVID-19 measures and elaborating on why they are conducive to these purposes. Furthermore, as proposed by the EDPB, in addition to the general personal data protection legislation (the PDPA), specific legislations for implementing individual digital COVID-19 measures are still necessary in order to protect the privacy right by setting out functional requirements for the use of such measures (EDPB, 2020c). Recently the Constitutional Court also concurred with this argument by confirming that the PDPA is a "framework norm", which alone cannot be the lawful basis for the reuse of the government's databases, and therefore specific legislations defining explicit requirements of specific personal data processing need to be adopted as lawful bases.[17]

Some may argue that certain digital COVID-19 measures' purposes are self-evident, for example, the digital fence is set up for the purpose of ensuring the compliance with isolation/quarantine orders and the real name registration system for contact tracing. But the issue here is not about whether or not the policy purposes can be self-evident; it is about whether or not the government can conveniently use the ambiguous statutory duty/public interest claim as a lawful basis to justify its processing of personal data. Namely, even if the policy purposes are self-evident, the interpretation of these purposes may still be arbitrarily expanded by the government when the legitimacy of these measures is based upon vague lawful bases.

Second, the CDC Act and the COVID-19 Special Act, with vague terminology such as "various effective investigations" (CDC Act Article 7) or "other necessary measures" (CDC Act Article 58(I)(4) and COVID-19 Special Act Articles 7 and 8) to control communicable diseases, are also cited by the government as the lawful bases for its digital COVID-19 measures. However, the concepts of "various effective investigations" and "other necessary measures" are overly abstract and generalized and have made it easier for the government to attribute the establishment of almost any kind of digital measure to pandemic response measures (Wu, 2020). The vagueness also literally gives the CECC the power to issue any order it deems "necessary" while affording a person of ordinary intelligence no notice of what personal data will be processed (Larkin, 2021). It is unreasonable to believe that the legislature intended to empower the government to indiscriminately process personal data through any digital measure that the CECC could devise. Therefore, applying the ambiguous terms of the CDC Act and the COVID-19 Special Act as lawful bases for processing personal data should be regarded as invalid under the void-for-vagueness doctrine.

Some have argued that the lawfulness requirement and the void-for-vagueness doctrine need some flexibility in the pandemic because it is impossible for the legislature to foresee all possible digital COVID-19 measures and potential uses of personal data, and to explicitly, expressly codify the proper lawful bases for individual digital measures into law (Cimini, 2005). Additionally, without broad delegation the government cannot well address a rapidly changing pandemic that is uncertain and dynamic in nature. For example, in Judicial Yuan Interpretation No. 702 the Constitutional Court stated that the void-for-vagueness doctrine would not be regarded as violated if the legislature, after weighing the complexity of society, uses general terms in the statutory language as long as the meanings of such terms are not difficult to understand, foreseeable for the people affected, and subject to judicial review.[18] This regulatory flexibility affords the government some space to implement digital COVID-19 measures predicated upon vague lawful bases as necessary during the emergency to contain the spread of the pandemic (Abiri and Guidi, 2021, Chen, 2020).

However, regulatory flexibility is not unlimited (Wurman, 2021). General terms in the statutory language (such as other necessary measures) should not be used as a blank check to unconditionally permit the government's digital processing of personal data during a public health emergency. Proper explanations or additional guidelines should be provided to limit the scope, length, or manner in which the government applies a broad, general legal provision as a lawful basis.

Returning to the lawfulness requirement for the digital COVID-19 measures, it is unlawful to apply ambiguous legal concepts, such as "various effective investigations" and "other necessary measures", as broad legal bases for the digital COVID-19 measures unless rational individuals already have a basis, legal or de facto, for clearly understanding the scope of privacy restrictions imposed by the digital measures, or the administrative agency can provide reasonable interpretation. As an example, Article 7 of the CDC Act, used as the lawful basis for several digital COVID-19 measures,[19] only vaguely stipulates that the government "shall conduct various investigations and effective preventive measures to control communicable diseases" without any typification or exemplification of legitimate bases or normative facts regarding what "investigations" or "measures" may refer to. Additionally, since digital COVID-19 measures are novel tools used to combat the pandemic for the first time, it is, therefore, uncertain whether society can foresee which digital measures fall under the "effective preventive measures" the legislature referred to in this provision. Since Article 7 fails to provide a reasonable person fair notice of the scope of personal data processed and is so standardless that it may authorize the arbitrary exercise of agency discretion, it is not a justifiable lawful basis for the digital COVID-19 measures unless supplement guiding principles are provided (Li, 2020a). Similar issues can also be found in the COVID-19 Special Act Article 7 (Huang, 2020).

In other cases, the government ignores the specific instances provided in the general legal provisions and instead uses vague stipulations to exceed the scope of its powers endowed by the legislature. For example, Article 37(I)(6) of the CDC Act, which authorizes the local government to adopt "other disease control measures", is cited as the lawful basis for the SMS contacting system.[20] However, a review of the specific restricting measures (e.g., regulating schooling, meetings, and traffic volume) stipulated in Article 37(I)(1)–(5) as examples for the vague term "other disease control measures", makes it clear that Article 37(I) is designed to grant the government the power to regulate group activities and to control the number of people in certain facilities, rather than to collect personal data when citizens enter public places. Since the SMS contact-tracing system is irrelevant to achieving the purpose assigned by the legislature in Article 37(I), it is unjustifiable to apply this provision as the lawful basis for personal data processing in the SMS contact-tracing system.

The debate about the vague lawful bases for the digital COVID-19 measures exposes concerns about broadly written statutes where the government's expansive emergency authority to enact restrictions is tethered only to its subjective belief that its actions are reasonable. To iron out the corollary discrepancies such as vague terminology and inappropriate discretion and achieve principled personal data protection goals within the context of public health, it is essential to have proper scrutiny of the lawfulness of the expansive derogations of personal information safeguards resulting from the digital measures (EDPB, 2020c).

Purpose Limitation

To collect personal data, one must have one or more specific, explicit, and legitimate purposes, and the personal data must only be used within the necessary extent of such purposes. That is, to comply with the purpose limitation principle, the government must define up front what the personal data will be used for and limit the processing to only what is necessary to meet that purpose (PDPA Article 5). The purpose limitation principle is vital to privacy during the pandemic because it can guarantee that personal data collected through new and innovative digital technologies is not used for purposes other than curbing COVID-19 to ensure that an emergency power does not creep into matters unrelated to the emergency (Gil, 2021, Newlands and others, 2020).

To satisfy the purpose limitation principle, the personal data processing using the digital COVID-19 measures must fall within the scope of the policy purposes that were disclosed to the public (through privacy notices, terms and conditions, or consent forms) during the time of collection (EDPB, 2020a). Furthermore, not all "purposes" can be encompassed by "specific purposes" (Chang, 2014, Lee, 2013). Policy purpose purposed for digital personal data processing must be based on unambiguous arguments that are comprehensible, foreseeable, and judicially reviewable rather than abstract legal jargon such as "pursuing the public interest" or "maintaining social order" (Lee, 2013). Namely, the policy purpose of personal data processing must be made abundantly clear, and include theoretical and empirical bases, public health monitoring approaches, public health impacts (i.e., reducing disease prevalence, incidence, or mortality, or changing health behaviors), and impacted groups (Article 29 Data Protection Working Party, 2013, EDPB, 2020b). Additionally, the policy purposes of digital measures need to be detailed enough to validate the use of personal data, the choice of digital technology, and the expected results (Li, 2020b).

However, the Taiwan government has neglected to explicitly address the policy purpose of individual digital COVID-19 measures and to evaluate whether the big-data-driven practices of public health surveillance qualify as "necessary measures" on a case-by-case basis. Vague and overbroad claims, such as "pandemic prevention", "reducing disease prevalence", or "to combat COVID-19", have been consistently and indiscriminately used to describe the public health purposes to be achieved through different digital COVID-19 measures. The vagueness results in failures to conduct sound, properly conceived privacy impact assessments, hinders public understanding of and debate over the legitimate purposes of these measures, and allows the government to bypass privacy safeguards with false or ostensible trade-offs between privacy and public health (Chang, 2014).

To cite one instance, after the COVID-19 outbreak in Taipei's Wanhua district, the CECC required the telecom operators to provide the phone numbers and location data (through cell tower triangulation) of all residents in the district as well as those who do not live in but work in the district. The personal information was later sent to the NHIA to add special notations to their NHI cards.[21] According to the CECC's reply to the Taiwan Association for Human Rights, the policy purpose of such pandemic measures is "to prevent the spread of the pandemic" and no notice or consent is required because preventing pandemic spread is the government's statutory task based upon the CDC Act in general.[22] But the policy purpose provided by the CECC is vague and overbroad because it lacks clear boundaries for personal data processing and appears to be overinclusive in collecting the whole community's personal data. Similar vagueness can also be found in the rationale behind imposing the overly strict digital surveillance measures on all residents and workers in Wanhua district, where the CECC simply stated that these people were at high risk of COVID-19 exposure based upon "time, specific areas, confirmed cases, and other factors", without further explanation (or administrative decree/guidance) on how these factors were applied to determine who was at high risk of COVID-19 exposure. The absence of a specific policy purpose then undermines the society's capacity to assess whether the digital measure is proportionate and does not go beyond what is necessary to achieve the claimed purpose, creates ambiguity regarding the boundaries of personal data processing, and makes the protection of privacy vulnerable to the government's emergency powers (EDPB, 2020b, Van der Sloot, 2021).

Some have argued for allowing exceptions to the purpose limitation principle in extreme situations (Rozenshtein, 2020). Admittedly, granting the CECC great delegated powers and extensive discretion in an emergency may be justified because it may not be possible for the legislature to set up *ex-ante* criteria and specific policy purposes due to the uncertainty of the emergency (Lin, Wu, and Wu, 2020). However, proper explanations should be offered as external detection controls. There should still exist appropriate advice provided by the legislature or the administration for society to foresee, to a degree that is reasonable in the circumstances, the consequences that a given digital measure may entail. For example, even where digital technologies are regarded as an efficient tool to combat the pandemic, there have been different measures which require different types and amounts of personal data. Therefore, the government has the obligation to provide proper information regarding the specific purpose of each digital measure so that the society can be capable to evaluate the relationship between the measures and the desired policy purpose, to assess the necessity of the scope of personal data processing, and to choose legitimate digital COVID-19 measures (Li, 2020b).

In conclusion, since the purpose limitation principle may be undermined by the urgency and uncertainty of the pandemic, the broad policy purpose should be interpreted and applied in a supplementary manner in accordance with the CDC

Act, and legal and ethical guidance should be developed to help delineate the scope of an unwarranted, broad authority under the guise of "pandemic prevention" (Dubov and Shoptawb, 2020). Additionally, an *ex-post* review and accountability mechanism should be adopted so that the specific purpose of each digital COVID-19 measure can be periodically evaluated and revalidated (Lin, Wu, and Wu, 2020).

Data Minimization

Data minimization refers to the concept of limiting the processing of personal data to what is necessarily and reasonably related to legitimate purposes. Article 5 of the PDPA stipulates that personal data processing "shall not go beyond the necessary extent of the purposes for which the data was collected, and must be reasonably and justifiably related to such purposes". The Constitutional Court also states that personal data shall be collected by the government only in situations of necessity and relevancy (Judiciary Juan Interpretation No. 603). Under the data minimization principle, the legal and technical design of the digital COVID-19 measures must ensure that only the "narrowest possible set of data elements" are processed, with minimal impairment of privacy and data security, and all data must be kept only for a limited duration and deleted upon termination of the legal authorization (Gil, 2021).

The data minimization requirement should not be arbitrarily compromised during the pandemic in order to avoid personal data abuse and function creep (Bradford, Aboy, and Liddell, 2020, EDPB, 2020b). For instance, the policy purpose of social distancing apps is primarily to provide COVID-19 exposure notifications to at-risk users. To achieve this purpose, proximity data (e.g., proximity/contact data collected via Bluetooth) is sufficient for contact tracing and disease spread prevention (EDPB, 2020b). Since the effective operation of the apps is not reliant on information such as detailed geolocation data and the identities of contacts, processing such information would be a violation of the data minimization requirement.

A clearly and definitively stated policy purpose for personal data processing can serve as the basis for determining the minimum data required to achieve that purpose and measuring whether data minimization has been satisfied (Blauth and Gstrein, 2021). Therefore, the ***first*** challenge Taiwan faces regarding data minimization lies in how to assess the data minimization requirement for the digital COVID-19 measures when their policy purposes are mostly vague and broad. As discussed in Section IV(2), the policy purposes of digital COVID-19 measures are obfuscating in Taiwan's legal framework. The lack of specific policy purposes provides no basis for the society and the court to assess whether the adoption of a less intrusive alternative digital measure, which burdens privacy to a lesser extent with minimum personal data, can still achieve the same purpose. For example, in addition to daily routes, in some cases the COVID-19 patient's gender, age, occupation, workplace, and sometimes address were disclosed online by the CECC.[23] Although the information can be used to identify a specific patient, the CECC argues that revealing the information is necessary to protect the public interest, but without clarifying the specific purpose.[24] It is then difficult for the society to verify the CECC's claim of necessity—whether or not the purpose can be achieved by revealing less information—since the CECC provided no specific purpose of the disclosure of more information than daily routes.

The ***second*** challenge lies in establishing criteria to restrict the categories of personal data that can be collected through the digital COVID-19 measures. For example, in addition to the government-operated SMS contact-tracing system, which requires only the mobile phone number and location data, several private entities also developed their own real name registration systems, some of which collect not only phone number but also name, age, address, and email address, among others (Lin, 2021). Human rights advocates have criticized this practice, noting that the amount of data collected through the systems is beyond necessary and thus violates the data minimization requirement.[25] The government did not respond to the criticism until May 2020 by issuing the Guidance on the Real-Name Registration Measures, which requires the collection of personal data to be subject to the necessity principle, where the systems should collect, process, and store as little data as absolutely necessary to fulfill the specific public health aim.[26]

Third, although the practice of data minimization can lower the risk of function creep, there is no guarantee that the data controller cannot pair the data collected to its queried or autogenerated data.[27] Therefore, whether the digital COVID-19 measures feature data minimization and whether the data controller will be held accountable is a reasonable concern which should be well addressed and monitored by an independent third party (Unger, 2020). But Taiwan's legal framework has neither proper norms and mechanisms nor independent third parties to assess whether the personal data collection of the digital COVID-19 measures meets the data minimization requirement (Weng, 2021). As a result, decisions regarding the scope of personal data processing necessary for pandemic control, which should be evidence-based decisions, then may be subject to political interference, and the value of privacy right may be significantly eroded without a proper supervision mechanism to rule out interference.

Transparency

In terms of transparency, the government should be required to inform the data subjects of how and what personal data is collected, the purposes of data processing and sharing, and the possibility of secondary use of the data (EDPB, 2020c). That is to say, an institutional culture of transparency should be embedded in the digital COVID-19 measures (Gil, 2021). For example, for pandemic prevention measures that involve algorithms (e.g., social distancing apps), the government should make the algorithms (source code) available for public scrutiny and invite independent experts to review them periodically to avoid potential biases and maintain accountability (EDPB, 2020c). The public health authorities also have the obligation to periodically and upon request produce relevant information to administrative and legislative supervisory bodies, and this reporting should be made available to the public (Levy, Chasalow, and Riley, 2021). Transparency is important to the protection of the privacy right when society is asked to accept digital pandemic controls because it can help to enable effective oversight of the digital measures, inform legislative deliberation on extending or terminating the measures, and ensure accountability (Booth and others, 2021)

Additionally, transparency is not a one-dimensional concept: On the one hand, transparency is an organizational phenomenon, where an organization needs to demonstrate transparency by outlining how it processes data; on the other hand, transparency entails the idea of verifiability as well as the notion of explainability and inspectability (Booth and others, 2021). Thus, transparency should not only be regarded as a data protection principle but also an important tool for spurring meaningful discussion about policy goals of digital COVID-19 measures in accordance with personal values and beliefs regarding privacy.

Accordingly, in addition to matters related to personal data processing, the rationales for the policy purposes of digital COVID-19 measures should be publicly available for the widest possible scrutiny regarding how to identify and evaluate the efficacy of the digital COVID-19 measures and how to protect individuals' privacy right under the existing resource and technology development restrictions. Reasonableness must be supported by scientific evidence and explainable rationales, including reasonable construal of rationality and reasonable cost-effectiveness analysis. Failing to be clear about these rationales behind the state's digital pandemic responses hinders individuals and communities from precisely foreseeing what considerations are included in policymaking process, examining the accuracy of the policy evaluation, and rerunning the policy evaluation with alternative assumptions and inputs (Syrett, 2007).

The government argued that the digital COVID-19 measures in Taiwan are implemented with a large degree of transparency. The CECC holds daily public briefings with the affected population to ensure public trust. Regarding the SMS contact-tracing system, citizens can check how many times their personal data collected by the system has been processed by the government in the past 28 days.[28] To convey and transform complicated technical information into concrete disease control measures to the public, the government has also employed both formal and informal channels (such as social media platforms and messaging apps) to facilitate two-way communication between the CECC and the public. Studies have shown that part of Taiwan's success comes down to transparency, and rather than dictating policies to its citizens, the government has involved them in solutions and provided transparency throughout its processes (Chang and Lin, 2021).

Nevertheless, it should be noted that human rights advocates still question the efficacy of daily briefings and argue that they generally consist of top-down announcements without detailed content or reasonings (Lin, Wu, and Wu, 2020). For example, the government has declined to disclose information regarding the operation of the digital fence system due to concerns that citizens may find ways to cheat the system.[29] Namely, the CECC is still reluctant to be totally transparent about the deployment of digital measures and operating mechanisms. Although the scope of information to be disclosed under the transparency principle is debatable, human rights advocates' transparency concerns are not without reason because detailed layer of information with clarity about what is going to happen or has happened with personal data is crucial for the data subjects, especially when the digital COVID-19 response policies involve making ethically contestable decisions about the use of coercive powers (Zanfir-Fortuna, 2020).

From the legal perspective, there are still some challenges regarding the transparency requirement. ***First***, although Article 8 of the PDPA requires the data controller to expressly inform the data subjects of any information relevant to the processing of their personal data, the data controller can be exempted from the duty to inform if "the collection of personal data is necessary for the government agency to perform its statutory duties or the non-government agency to fulfill its statutory obligation" (Article 8(II)(2)). This exemption then is used by the government to avoid its duty to inform. Because the government argues that the lawful basis of the personal data processing that is carried out in the digital COVID-19 measures is the fulfillment of its statutory duties stipulated in the CDC Act (see Section IV(1)), the government then claimed that it is exempted from the duty to inform.[30] Therefore, accessibility to information about personal data processing under the digital COVID-19 measures is obstructed and the transparency requirement may be restricted. Although individuals can still actively exercise their rights, stipulated in Article 3 of the PDPA, to access information related to the processing of their data and the details regarding the operation of the digital measures, in this case the transparency requirement can only be partly addressed by *ex-post* review and accountability mechanisms, which may be prone to hindsight bias (Lin, Wu, and Wu, 2020).

Second, a similar challenge can also be found in the freedom of information act. According to Article 5 of the Freedom of Government Information Law (FOGIL), Article 5 of the Freedom of Government Information Law (FOGIL), the government is required to disclose its information (including the rationales behind the digital COVID-19 measures) upon request. But this open data initiative is restricted in Article 18(I)(3), where government information regarding "the draft for internal use or other preparatory works before the agency makes a decision" is restricted from being made available to the public. For example, whether putting notations on high-risk populations' NHI cards qualifies as an "effective investigation" stipulated in the CDC Act Article 7 (see Section IV(1)) is decided by the CECC based upon the results of internal discussion or expert meetings. However, according to Article 18(I)(3) of the FOGIL, the government is exempted from the duty to disclose the rationales behind the decision because the rationales are considered as the preparatory works. Additionally, although Article 7(I)(10) of the FOGIL requires the government to make the meeting minutes of government agencies available to the public, the disclosed information is limited to the "gist of motions, programs, content of resolutions and list of the members who attend the meeting" (Article 7(III)). These restrictions then hinder the transparency requirement and discourage careful reflection by the government.

Finally, the application of novel digital technologies to combat the pandemic also created new offenses for using personal data (Gunawan and others, 2020). But the scope of information disclosure required by the PDPA and the FOGIL is sufficient to cope with the latest technological developments, resulting in the possible diminishment of the transparency requirement. For example, there is no law in Taiwan requiring the algorithm (source code) of the social distancing apps to be open to the public. But without such information, society's concerns regarding the technical security of the application or background personal data collection then cannot be assuaged (Gunawan and others, 2020). Namely, the transparency requirement should not be limited to the information listed in the PDPA and the FOGIL and needs to be reevaluated during the pandemic. This is important because the digital technologies and amount of personal data used in digital pandemic responses are unprecedented and the emergency power of the government to implement intrusive digital measures is far greater than in normal times.

Social Trust and Privacy Restrictions in the Pandemic

Although there are grave privacy concerns regarding the digital COVID-19 measures from the perspectives of lawfulness, purpose limitation, data minimization, and transparency, Taiwanese society's acceptance of these measures is quite high (Garrett and others, 2022). Admittedly, individuals who feel their safety is threatened are more likely to support privacy-restrictive measures to ensure the public safety (Hetherington and Suhay, 2011). The severe acute respiratory syndrome (SARS) outbreak in 2003 may have further reinforced this attitude and reshaped Taiwanese citizens' relationship with the government in terms of the trade-offs they are being asked to make between privacy and health security. But even considering these two factors, the social attitude toward the potential impacts on privacy caused by the digital COVID-19 measures still remains comparatively positive in Taiwan (Hsieh and others, 2021).

Some find that cultural relevance is a key dimension of the stark contrast between citizens' acceptance of digital pandemic response programs in Asian and Western countries (Huynh, 2020). Although privacy is a universal human need that gives rise to a fundamental human right, it may take on disconcerting forms because the perceived value of privacy is affected by culture and varies considerably in different societies (Whitman, 2004). This cultural difference then is likely to be highlighted or amplified in a society's response to digital COVID-19 measures (Li and others, 2021).

More specifically, unlike European/American societies who view privacy as a human right and reserve their distrust for the government or corporations, Taiwanese society, with its heritage of Confucian thought, Daoism and Buddhism, views individuals as relational beings in society and defines the privacy value through an individual's relationships with other persons, rather than through an isolated quality such as rationality (Ess, 2007). Namely, the conception of privacy in Taiwanese culture, unlike that developed in the modern West around the notion of the autonomous but atomistic self, refers to the collective privacy of the family vis-à-vis the larger society and reflects society's emphasis on the values of the common good and obedience/conformity and the lack of individualism as a cultural trait that are associated with positive attitudes toward government intervention (Chen, Frey, and

Presidente, 2023). The cultural legacy of Taiwanese society is regarded by some as the reason for public acceptance of the stringent digital measures taken by the CECC.[31]

However, in my view, local privacy culture is not the key factor shaping Taiwanese society's willingness to share personal data to control the spread of COVID-19. ***First***, young people in Taiwan are influenced by their exposure to Western notions of individual privacy and generally insist on the human right of privacy, one that directly contradicts traditional Taiwanese notions. This positive attitude toward individual privacy is also reflected in the Taiwan Constitutional Court's decisions regarding privacy right protections (see Section III). ***Second***, the privacy culture argument oversimplifies Taiwanese society's reactions to the trade-offs between privacy and health security and overlooks the essential role of democratic values in building social trust in the digital COVID-19 measures. Studies have shown that a strong democracy is key to boosting social trust in institutions in the face of a pandemic (Yeh and Cheng, 2020). Therefore, focusing on whether Taiwanese society's high acceptance of the restrictive digital COVID-19 measures arises from its local privacy culture misses the real point, which is the question of what role the democratic process, the Taiwan government has worked to maintain during the pandemic, has played in building social trust (Yang and Tsai, 2020).

For instance, to ease concerns about human rights encroachment and the rule of law during the pandemic and to deepen social trust, the Taiwan government has avoided issuing emergency decrees with broad delegations to its administrative agencies and instead attempted to maintain its democratic legitimacy during the pandemic by expeditiously asking the legislature to pass the COVID-19 Special Act, which serves as a legal framework under which democratic processes can function to respond promptly while ensuring accountability (Lin, Wu, and Wu, 2020). The Act, regardless of its controversial open-ended delegation, reflects the government's effort to fulfill the minimum requirement of the rule of law (Huang, 2020). Additional measures have also been adopted to strengthen the democratic legitimacy of the government's decisions during the pandemic. For example, the CECC has adopted an open and responsive communication system that aims to actively provide information to the public, to improve transparency, and to ensure social trust (Lin, Wu, and Wu, 2020). The effort to balance risk assessment (carried out by scientific experts) and risk management (assigned to ensure democratic legitimacy) also plays an important role in ensuring society's trust in democratically elected and appointed bureaucrats (Pacces and Weimer, 2020). This combination of democratic and technocratic legitimacy has helped to facilitate social cohesion and compel community cooperation in the midst of the pandemic.[32] Furthermore, because COVID-19 Special Act Article 7 has been criticized for being overly broad and violating the nondelegation doctrine (see Section VI(1)), the CECC has acted with restraint relative to the power granted by the provision so as to avoid potential violations of the rule of law (Chang and Lin, 2021). These efforts have helped to build trust within the community, and the success of Taiwan's digital COVID-19 measures, whose effectiveness can still be maintained while the policy remains largely voluntary, is largely attributable to such trust.

Nevertheless, although Taiwan has endeavored to comply with the values of democracy and the rule of law while executing the digital COVID-19 measures to combat the pandemic, the democratic government's actions may still impact the privacy right and in turn diminish democratic values (Liu, Li, and Tu, 2020). For example, studies have shown that the legislature's access to the digital COVID-19 response policies has been limited while technocrats and experts tend to have an upper hand in shaping the policies due to the society's trust (Lin, Wu, and Wu, 2020, Yang and Tsai, 2020). There are also concerns that the violations of the personal data protection principles in the implementation of the digital COVID-19 measures may be overlooked by society in a context where the legal interpretation of necessity and intrusiveness may be influenced by the broader issues of social trust (Liu, Li, and Tu, 2020).

Therefore, in addition to reinforcing the aforementioned democratic mechanism and to support compliance with the rule of law, it is important to ensure that the government does not abuse its high "regulative support" from Taiwanese society by introducing overly stringent digital measures (Yang and Tsai, 2020). Furthermore, even with great social trust, there is still an urgent need to reevaluate whether the traditional democratic safeguards such as due process, proportionality, and judicial review can suffice to manage the privacy challenges imposed by the novel digital techniques. For example, although not required by law, the Taiwan government should actively, periodically assess whether the data sharing and data surveillance practices are as effective as claimed.

Conclusion

Privacy has been a prominent issue during the pandemic because digital technologies, which can be used to collect and process a great amount of personal data, have been broadly adopted for the first time in history as an effective tool to combat the novel virus. To safeguard individuals' privacy rights and to avoid authoritarian control, privacy challenges imposed by the digital COVID-19 measures need to be carefully scrutinized for their adherence to the personal data protection principles. Although the relative balance between privacy and public health may vary according to the dynamic context of the pandemic locally, Taiwan's experiences have shown that democratic governance, which promotes civic participation, fosters consensus building, and facilitates a functioning personal data protection framework, is the key to mitigating potential privacy concerns and to boosting social trust in institutions during the pandemic. It is misguided to evade privacy protection by simply arguing health security or cultural differences in privacy perceptions.

Notes

1 Yang, S.-M., *Pandemic Prevention Upgrade: Wuhan Travel History Can be Seen by Doctors After Inserting the National Health Insurance Card During Hospital Visit* (in Chinese), accessed May 2, 2022, at Central News Agency (January 27, 2020) at https://www.cna.com.tw/news/firstnews/202001270072.aspx.

2 Cheung, H., *Coronavirus: What Could the West Learn from Asia?*, accessed May 2, 2022, at BBC (March 21, 2020) at https://www.bbc.com/news/world-asia-51970379.

3 Chen, F.-L., 600,000 People's Footprints in Wanhua Were Secretly Monitored: Concerns Regarding Human Rights Violations Have Been Raised and the CECC Needs to Explain (in Chinese), accessed May 2, 2022, at Newtalk (May 27, 2021) at https://newtalk.tw/news/view/2021-05-27/579859.

4 *COVID-19 FAQs*, Taiwan Center for Disease Control, accessed November 20, 2020, at https://www.cdc.gov.tw/En/Category/QAPage/SbkmnM5v0OwdDMjJ2tI_xw.

5 See e.g., Hui, M., *How Taiwan Is Tracking 55,000 People Under Home Quarantine in Real Time*, accessed May 2, 2022, at Quartz (April 1, 2020) at https://qz.com/1825997/taiwan-phone-tracking-system-monitors-55000-under-coronavirus-quarantine/.

6 The instant photo comparison system was temporarily suspended in November 2021 due to privacy concerns. Hu, S.-N., M-Police's Instant Photo Comparison System Was Cancelled and Will Be Restored After the Law Is Improved, Stated by the National Police Agency (in Chinese), accessed August 2, 2022, at United Daily News (December 26, 2021) at https://www.chinatimes.com/realtimenews/20211226002896-260402?chdtv.

7 *Police Cloud – M-Police Mobile Computer System*, accessed May 2, 2022, at Smart City: Summit & Expo, at https://en.smartcity.org.tw/index.php/en-us/posts/news/item/47-police-cloud-m-police-mobile-computer-system.

8 Everington, K., *Taiwan Launches New QR Code for Real-Name Registration System*, accessed May 2, 2022, at Taiwan News (May 19, 2021) at https://www.taiwannews.com.tw/en/news/4206312.

9 Travel History of COVID-19 Patients (Divided by Administrative Districts), accessed September 2, 2022, at CDC at https://www.cdc.gov.tw/Category/List/_FFjBSOizDNbJZZV1Bosew.

10 CECC, New Life during the COVID-19 Pandemic: Guidance for the Real-Name Registration System, accessed May 4, 2022, at https://www.cdc.gov.tw/File/Get/Xj5T1E5D474RJnmOY--kkw.

11 See e.g., Liu, L., *Taiwan Launches Social Distancing App*, accessed May 2, 2022, at Taiwan News (May 2, 2021) at https://www.taiwannews.com.tw/en/news/4193136.

12 *Taiwan Social Distancing App*, AI Lab.tw, accessed May 2, 2022, at https://covirus.cc/social-distancing-app-intro.html.

13 *The Taiwan Social Distancing Application and Its Contact Tracing Algorithm*, accessed May 2, 2022, at GitHub at https://github.com/ailabstw/social-distancing.

14 Article 22 of the Taiwan Constitution, "[a]ll other liberties and rights that are not detrimental to social order or public welfare shall be guaranteed under the Constitution."

15 Tsai et al. v. National Health Insurance Administration, 106 NianDu Pan Zi No. 54, Supreme Administrative Court (Taiwan).

16 Constitutional Court Judgment No. 13 of 2022 (August. 12, 2022) (Taiwan).

17 Constitutional Court Judgment No. 13 of 2022 (August 12, 2022) (Taiwan).

18 Judicial Yuan Interpretation No. 702 (July 27, 2012) (Taiwan).

19 Agency Interpretation of the CECC, Fei-Zhong-Zhi-Zi Nos. 1090000237 and 1100001274 (September 9, 2020; September 14, 2021).

20 Agency Interpretation of the CDC, Wei-Shou-Ji-Zi No. 1100200731 (August 10, 2021).

21 *Supra* note 5.

22 Agency Interpretation of the CECC, Fei-Zhong-Zhi-Zi No. 1100001274 (September 14, 2021).

23 Syu, J.-Y., Yang, Y.-Y., and Ciou, Y.-J., *Announcing the "Detailed Address" of the Infected in the Zhonghe Community, the CECC: It Is Easier to Investigate the Relationship* (in Chinese), accessed May 4, 2022, at United Daily News (Mar. 29, 2022) at https://udn.com/news/story/120940/6200134.

24 *Id.*

25 Zeng, Y.-S., *Supervising Human Rights Protection Regarding Pandemic Surveillance* (in Chinese), accessed May 4, 2022, at Taiwan Ass'n for Hum. Rts. (December 29, 2021) at https://www.tahr.org.tw/news/3110.

26 *Supra* note 22.

27 Baker, J., *Pandemic Incites Concerns About Data-Sharing Overreach*, accessed May 4, 2022, at Int'l Ass'n of Privacy Prof'ls (March 26, 2020) at https://iapp.org/news/a/global-pandemic-incites-concerns-about-data-sharing-overreach/.
28 Agency Interpretation of the CECC, Fei-Zhong-Zhi-Zi No. 1104300088 (August 4, 2021).
29 TAHR, Statement: From the Digital Fence to the Sky Net - Can We Question the Digital PandemicSurveillance? (in Chinese), accessed May 4, 2022, at Taiwan Ass'n for Hum Rts. (January 7, 2021) at https://www.tahr.org.tw/news/2857.
30 Agency Interpretation of the CECC, Fei-Zhong-Zhi-Zi No. 1100001274 (September 14, 2021).
31 Yang, W., *How Has Taiwan Kept Its Coronavirus Infection Rate So Low?*, accessed May 4, 2022, at DW (April 9, 2020) at https://www.dw.com/en/taiwan-coronavirus/a-52724523.
32 Huang, C.-Y., Soft Regulation and Hard Compliance in Taiwan, accessed May 4, 2022, at Reg. Rev. (June 11, 2020) at https://www.theregreview.org/2020/06/11/huang-soft-regulation-hard-compliance-taiwan/.

References

Abiri, G., and Guidi, S., 2021, The pandemic constitution: Columbia Journal of Transnational Law, v. 60, p. 68–131.

Article 29 Data Protection Working Party (WP29), 2013. Opinion 03/2013 on purpose limitation (00569/13/EN (WP 203)).

Bastos, F. B., and de Ruijter, A., 2019, Break or bend in case of emergency?: Rule of law and state of emergency in European public health administration: European Journal of Risk Regulation, v. 10, p. 610–634.

Blauth, T. F., and Gstrein, O. J., 2021, Data-driven measures to mitigate the impact of COVID-19 in South America: how do regional programmes compare to best practice?: International Data Privacy Law, v. 11, p. 18–31.

Booth, P., Evers, L., Fosch Villaronga, E. L., Christoph , McDermott, F., Riccio, P., Rioux, V., Sears, A. M., Tamo-Larrieux, A., and Wieringa, M., 2021, Artountability: art and algorithmic accountability, *in* Hallinan, D., Leenes, R., and De Hert, P., editors, Data Protection and Privacy: Enforcing Rights in a Changing World, Hart Publishing, Oxford, UK, p. 45–66.

Bradford, L., Aboy, M., and Liddell, K., 2020, COVID-19 contact tracing apps: a stress test for privacy, the GDPR, and data protection regimes: Journal of Law and the Biosciences, v. 7, p. lsaa034.

Calvo, R. A., Deterding, S., and Ryan, R. M., 2020, Health surveillance during covid-19 pandemic: BMJ, v. 369, p. m1373.

Chang, C.-H., 2014, Eyes on the road program in Taiwan-information privacy issues under the Taiwan personal data protection act: John Marshall Journal of Information Technology and Privacy Law, v. 31, p. 145.

Chang, W. C., and Lin, C. Y., 2021, Taiwan: democracy, technology, and civil society, *in* Ramraj, V. V., editor, Covid-19 in Asia: Law and Policy Contexts, Oxford University Press, Oxford, UK, p. 43–56.

Chen, C., Frey, C. B., and Presidente, G., 2023, Disease and democracy: political regimes and countries responsiveness to Covid-19: Journal of Economic Behavior and Organization, v. 212, p. 290–299.

Chen, C.-L., 2020, Revisiting the boundaries of legal reservation regarding the ban on travel abroad during the pandemic (in Chinese): Law and Life Science, v. 9, p. 1–37.

Cimini, C. N., 2005, Principles of non-arbitrariness: lawlessness in the administration of welfare: Rutgers Law Review, v. 57, p. 451–530.

Dubov, A., and Shoptawb, S., 2020, The value and ethics of using technology to contain the COVID-19 epidemic: The American Journal of Bioethics, v. 20, p. W7–W11.

EDPB (European Data Protection Board), 2020a, Guidelines 03/2020 on the processing of data concerning health for the purpose of scientific research in the context of the Covid-19 outbreak.

EDPB, 2020b, Guidelines 04/2020 on the use of location data and content tracing tools in the context of the COVID-19 Outbreak.

EDPB, 2020c, Statement of the EDPB Chair on the processing of personal data in the context of the COVID-19 outbreak.

Ess, C., 2007, East–West perspectives on privacy, ethical pluralism and global information ethics, *in* Hrachovec, H. and Pichler, A., editors, Philosophy of the Information Society, ontos verlag, Frankfurt, Germany, p. 185–203.

Farrow, T., 2021, Contact tracing: where we were where we are, where we are going. The influence "privacy by design" has had on contact tracing apps and the lasting impression it will have will after the Pandemic is over: Rutgers JL & Pub. Pol'y, v. 19, p. 121.

Garrett, P. M., Wang, Y.-W., White, J. P., Kashima, Y., Dennis, S., and Yang, C.-T., 2022, High acceptance of COVID-19 tracing technologies in Taiwan: a nationally representative survey analysis: International Journal of Environmental Research and Public Health, v. 19, p. 3323.

Gil, E. D., 2021, Digital contact tracing has failed: can it be fixed with better legal design?: Virginia Journal of Law & Technology, v. 25, p. 1–37.

Gunawan, J., Choffnes, D., Hartzog, W., and Wilson, C., 2020, The COVID-19 pandemic and the technology trust gap: Seton Hall Law Review, v. 51, p. 1505–1534.

Hetherington, M., and Suhay, E., 2011, Authoritarianism, threat, and Americans' support for the war on terror: American Journal of Political Science, v. 55, p. 546–560.

Hsieh, C.-W., Wang, M., Wong, N. W., and Ho, L. K.-k., 2021, A whole-of-nation approach to COVID-19: Taiwan's National Epidemic Prevention Team: International Political Science Review, v. 42, p. 300–315.

Huang, Y.-H., 2020, The Special act for prevention, relief and revitalization measures for Severe Pneumonia with novel pathogens and the nondelegation doctrine: a comparative law perspective of French Law (in Chinese): The Taiwan Law Review, v. 303, p. 27–44.

Huang, Y.-L., and Lo, C.-C., 2021, Legal and ethical issues of COVID-19 "Digital Contact Tracing" measures in Taiwan: Taiwan Journal of Public Health, v. 40, p. 332–345.

Huynh, T. L. D., 2020, Does culture matter social distancing under the COVID-19 pandemic?: Safety Science, v. 130, p. 104872.

Knowles, S. G., 2014, Learning from disaster? The history of technology and the future of disaster research: Technology and Culture, v. 55, p. 773–784.

Kotschy, W., 2020, Article 6 Lawfulness of processing, *in* Kuner, C., Bygrave, L. A., and Docksey, C., editors, The EU General Data Protection Regulation (GDPR): A Commentary, Oxford University Press, Oxford, UK, p. 321–344.

Larkin, P. J., 2021, The Sturm und Drang of the CDC's home eviction moratorium: Harvard Journal of Law and Public Policy, v. 18, p. 1–28.

Lee, H. T., 2013, The fundamental principle of personal data protection: the purpose limitation principle (in Chinese): Law Monthly, v. 64, p. 37–61.

Li, R.-G., 2020a, The application of home electronic monitoring in epidemic prevention period and its legal sources (in Chinese): Angle Health Law Review, v. 42, p. 93–102.

Li, T. C., 2020b, Post-pandemic privacy law: American University Law Review, v. 70, p. 1681–1728.

Li, Z. S., Phusamruat, V., Clear, T., and Damian, D., 2021, Can technology and privacy co-exist in a pandemic?, *in* Ramraj, V. V., editor, Covid-19 in Asia: Law and Policy Contexts, Oxford University Press, Oxford, UK, p. 207–220.

Lin, C.-F., Wu, C.-H., and Wu, C.-F., 2020, Reimagining the administrative state in times of global health crisis: an anatomy of Taiwan's regulatory actions in response to the COVID-19 pandemic: European Journal of Risk Regulation, v. 11, p. 256–272.

Lin, M.-C., 2020, Desperate COVID-19 with desperate remedies: examining the legality of "Home Isolation" and "Home Quarantine": Taiwan Law Journal, v. 388, p. 1–11.

Lin, Y.-C., 2021, From SARS to COVID-19: Conflicts between Pandemic Control Measures and Fundamental Rights (in Chinese), master thesis on file with the National Cheng-Chi University Library, Taipei, Taiwan.

Liu, C.-Y., Li, W.-P., and Tu, Y.-P., 2020, Privacy perils of open data and data sharing: a case study of Taiwan's open data policy and practices: Washington International Law Journal, v. 30, p. 545–597.

Newlands, G., Lutz, C., Tamò-Larrieux, A., Villaronga, E. F., Harasgama, R., and Scheitlin, G., 2020, Innovation under pressure: implications for data privacy during the Covid-19 pandemic: Big Data & Society, v. 7, p. 1–14.

O'Mathúna, D. P., and Gordijn, B., 2018, Conceptualizing and assessing disasters: an introduction, *in* O'Mathúna, D. P., Dranseika, V., and Gordijn, B., editors, Disasters: Core Concepts and Ethical Theories, Springer, Cham, p. 1–9.

Pacces, A. M., and Weimer, M., 2020, From diversity to coordination: a European approach to COVID-19: European Journal of Risk Regulation, v. 11, p. 283–296.

Rozenshtein, A. Z., 2020, Digital disease surveillance: American University Law Review, v. 70, p. 1511–1576.

Syrett, K., 2007, Law, Legitimacy and the Rationing of Healthcare: A Contextual and Comparative Perspective, Cambridge University Press, Cambridge, UK.

Tzanou, M., 2013a, Data protection as a fundamental right next to privacy? 'Reconstructing' a not so new right: International Data Privacy Law, v. 3, p. 88–99.

Tzanou, M., 2013b, Is data protection the same as privacy? An analysis of telecommunications' metadata retention measures: Journal of Internet Law, v. 17, p. 20–33.

Unger, W., 2020, Katz and COVID-19: how a pandemic changed the reasonable expectation of privacy: Hastings Science & Technology Law Journal, v. 12:1, p. 39–82.

Van der Sloot, B., 2021, Expectations of privacy: the three tests deployed by the European court of human rights, *in* Hallinan, D., Leenes, R., and Hert, P. D., editors, Data Protection and Privacy: Enforcing Rights in a Changing World, Hart Publishing, Oxford, UK, p. 67–95.

Weng, W. Y.-H., 2021, Processing of data concerning national health insurance in the context of the COVID-19 outbreak: applications and limitations: Angle Health Law Review, v. 51, p. 7–19.

Whitman, J. Q., 2004, The two western cultures of privacy: dignity versus liberty: Yale Law Journal, v. 113, p. 1151–1221.

WHO (World Health Organization), 2020, Joint statement on data protection and privacy in the Covid-19 response.

Wu, C. W., 2020, From SARS to COVID-19: examining the communicable disease control act and restrictions of fundamental rights from the perspectives of Judicial Yuan Interpretation No. 690 (in Chinese): Law and Life Science, v. 9, p. 91–112.

Wurman, I., 2021, COVID-19 litigation and the rational basis test: Wayne Law Review, v. 67, p. 85–92.

Yang, W.-Y., and Tsai, C.-h., 2020, Democratic values, collective security, and privacy: Taiwan People's response to COVID-19: Asian Journal for Public Opinion Research, v. 8, p. 222–245.

Yeh, M.-J., and Cheng, Y., 2020, Policies tackling the COVID-19 pandemic: a sociopolitical perspective from Taiwan: Health security, v. 18, p. 427–434.

Zanfir-Fortuna, G., 2020, Article 15 Right of access by the data subject, *in* Kuner, C., Bygrave, L. A., Docksey, C., and Drechsler, L., editors, The EU General Data Protection Regulation (GDPR): A Commentary, Oxford University Press, Oxford, UK, p. 449–468.

6 Digital Pandemic Governance in Taiwan

Sung-Yueh Perng, Ying-Yu Chen, Mei-Fang Fan, Mei-Lin Pan and Hsin-Yi Sandy Tsai

Introduction

Reflecting upon the impact of COVID-19 on Taiwan and the effective containment of the pandemic, the Ministry of Health and Welfare (MoHW) suggests that a crucial strategy behind the success was the digitisation of pandemic response measures. As the government proclaims,

> [MoHW] have turned to big data and technology systems and utilized smartphones and the internet to deploy innovative technology systems against infectious diseases.
>
> (MoHW, 2020)

Many other countries also deployed digital innovations, for example, pandemic dashboards, contact tracing apps, quarantine monitoring systems or symptom tracking technologies. In Singapore, for example, the TraceTogether app used Bluetooth to track potential contacts, while the SafeEntry system employed the national identity database to record footprints (Das and Zhang, 2021). In South Korea, smart technologies supplemented the data generated by epidemiological investigators about the travel or contact history of infected individuals, including credit and debit card transaction records, mobile phone communication data and CCTV footage (Sonn and Lee, 2020). Regardless of the specific technologies each country chose to use, there was a clear turn to the digital in the efforts to contain the outbreak.

This widespread adoption of digital technologies for national pandemic response strategies has prompted ongoing critical examination regarding not only whether public health can be effectively protected but also what consequences societies will face. Kitchin (2020) warns of the dangerous and unnecessary dichotomy between public health and civil liberties that can legitimise control creep, surveillance capitalism and the erosion of human rights. Cinnamon (2020) cautions about the rhetoric of inevitability in using digital technologies, as the focus on the "public value" of such technologies belies the expanding political and economic stakes of the digital technology industry in public health and society. Milan (2020) raises questions concerning what sciences underpin the collection and analysis of

DOI: 10.4324/9781003438380-9

pandemic and epidemiological data and whether data analytics inherently excludes the social and biological experiences of non-Western bodies.

This chapter examines the governing with digital technologies in Taiwan between 2020 and 2022 to consider the ideals, practices, knowledges and experiences of implementing and living with digital responses to the COVID-19 pandemic. It will start with suggesting what ideals have been pursued in the shift to digital technologies for responding to COVID-19. It then discusses how these ideals have been implemented and how they have mutually constituted or complicated one another in the experiences of Taiwan. We then reflect upon these experiences to point out their ramifications for digital pandemic governance more broadly.

Digital Governance and COVID-19

We draw on recent work on digital governance to make sense of the use of digital technologies to curb the spread of COVID-19. Vanolo (2013) demonstrates various ways in which "efficiency" and "social inclusivity" have gained prominence in the discourses about data, digital technologies and the incorporation of their instrumental capabilities into digital infrastructure for improving human life. Also, Söderström et al. (2014) examines various dimensions of "governing through code" by demonstrating how software code, coupled with interrelated logics, knowledges and discourses, is integral in developing an apparatus of power to manage and regulate everyday life. A key aspect in this line of inquiry concerns the identification of techniques, discourses and knowledges that enable the exercise of power and the construction of preferable fields of action and the normalisation of certain behaviours. For example, Petersen and Lupton (1996) analyse the rationalities, discourses and practices that portray "responsible" citizens who adhere to a "desirable" lifestyle by government agencies and professionals as a governance mechanism to address looming public health concerns. Following their work, we understand digital pandemic governance as an emergent mode of governance consisting of a multitude of practices, institutions, subjects and knowledges that mobilise digital technologies, data and discourses to re-configure the "art of government" (Dean, 2010) targeting both the contagious and healthy population.

There are various logics or ideals that digital pandemic governance pursues. In the reflections of digital responses to COVID-19 so far, "efficiency", "realtimeness", "transparency" and "inclusivity" are amongst the most crucial ones. The case of the Digital India and Smart Cities programmes, as Datta (2020) explains, demonstrates how a suite of "smart" technologies was introduced and then quickly repurposed for setting up efficient pandemic response measures such as crowd monitoring by drones, contact tracing by mobile phones and quarantine enforcement. This led to what Datta terms "self(ie)-governance" or the accelerated and amplified digital surveillance of home as suggested by Maalsen and Dowling (2020), in which efficient monitoring and constant real-time surveillance have been idealised as critical means to control of the body and the outbreak. India and Australia are not alone in this development. As Sonn and Lee (2020) argue, the digitisation of the governance of pandemics cannot be understood independently from a social and political context where governments have been expanding smart infrastructure to demonstrate greater transparency as a strategy to rebuild legitimacy. Stevens and Haines (2020) point out the contradictions between the ideals and rhetoric invoked to legitimise data-driven governance and the practices deployed to enforce control. By examining the TraceTogether app and the language of social solidarity, openness and democratic participation, Stevens and Haines show that the government's design and deployment of TraceTogether betray these claims, fragment society and deepen the reliance on the government for the protection of health and privacy. Data generated through the app are enclosed and centralised, diverging from the initial design of peer-to-peer technologies, which TraceTogether is built upon, to gain trust and cultivate solidarity among those participating in the network. Furthermore, notwithstanding the claims about the potential to use smart technology to increase social inclusivity, a "vacuum of governance" has occurred during the pandemic (Datta and others, 2021) where the spread of the virus among marginal social groups and their consequent suffering become invisible to the governing institutions or the wider public due to their lack of access to digital infrastructure and services. Facing this challenge, various civil society groups had to step in to provide daily necessities and technical assistance, with the potential of initiating a form of "collaborative governance" (Ansell and Gash, 2008) to recruit public institutions and non-state stakeholders to respond to pandemics collectively.

In this chapter, we reflect upon digital pandemic governance as it unfolds in Taiwan during COVID-19. We extend recent discussions on digital governance during pandemics by analysing how various governance ideals as demonstrated above have been materialised in the context of Taiwan and what problems have been created or perpetuated thus far (see Chapter 4 for a related discussion of the normalisation of digital pandemic measures in a state of emergency and exception). From the discussions above, four ideals can be synthesised, including efficiency, real-timeness, transparency and inclusiveness. Our chapter focuses on examining how the four ideals are mutually constitutive of and complicating one another in practice. An outline of the operational logics of these ideals and examples of their implementation are provided in Table 6.1. These four ideals by no means form an

Table 6.1 Digital Pandemic Governance Ideals and Instances of their Implementation

	Efficiency	*Real-timeness*	*Transparency*	*Inclusiveness*
Ideal	Increasing the effectiveness of pandemic response through the use of digital technologies and data analytics	Increasing the speed of pandemic response through digital and social media platforms	Increasing the awareness and understanding of pandemic situations through open data and public announcements	Increasing the protection of diverse social groups and the appreciation of different skills and expertise
Implementation	Digital fences, quarantine database, analytics for crowd movement tracing	CECC chatbot, official social media accounts, short message services (SMS), cell broadcast	Daily press conferences, COVID-19 dashboard, open data portal	Diversifying communication channels, translation of updates and regulations

exhaustive list of what drives digital pandemic governance here in Taiwan or in other countries. However, they serve to open up a discussion on Taiwan's experiences of implementing digital pandemic governance, the specific sociotechnical and geopolitical contexts that shape Taiwan's experiences, and research and policy implications of Taiwan's digital pandemic governance in a global context.

Research Methods

Our analysis draws on various sources. A citizen forum and an expert panel discussion were organised in March 2021. The organisation of the citizen forum and the expert panel were intended to create opportunities for deliberation so as to prioritise dialogue and communication with a wide range of stakeholders on issues regarding the digitisation of pandemic response and the specific values realised through digital technologies, rather than assessing technical rights or wrongs (Pearse, 2020). The expert panel invited scholars from diverse academic disciplines and representatives of NGOs and civil society groups. Additionally, we conducted an in-depth interview with a government official from the MoHW who oversaw the IT department when COVID-19 started, as well as consulting technical documents and reports, news and commentaries.

As a data collection method, citizen forums offered us an opportunity to create spaces to encourage dialogues, conversations, reason-giving and mutual understanding among the wider public, beyond just expert opinions (Fan, 2021). The citizen forum adopted the World Café method in order to create an opportunity for members of the public to participate, learn, think, have a say and be heard by other citizens. World Café as a participatory method of data collection facilitates dialogues and mutual learning among participants. In World Cafés, participants engage in a meaningful and conversational exchange of their lived and varied perceptions and experiences in order to generate collective discussion and sense-making (Carson, 2011; Löhr and others, 2020).

To facilitate the dialogues and reflections on different aspects of digital governance of pandemics at the citizen forum, we organised four tables, each having a dedicated theme of discussion. Moderators were recruited and trained beforehand to facilitate discussion and take notes of the observations or consensus that each group arrived at collectively (as opposed to transcribing the full conversation of a session. The participants chose a theme at the beginning of the event and then moved to the next one, with fellow participants of the same table, after 15 minutes of discussion. The forum had four rounds of discussion, enabling the participants to share their views on the four themes we selected: technology adoption, citizen collaboration, inclusiveness and personal data collection. With these topics, the forum facilitated reflection on digital pandemic governance by creating a space where the participants could engage in deeper conversations and discover different experiences, unfamiliar ideas and new connections among themselves. Around 20 participants joined the forum. They were mainly from local communities in the Beitou District, the northernmost district of Taipei City, and comprised homemakers and retirees who are more likely to be excluded from accessing digital services and might have developed a diverse range of digital practices in everyday life or during the pandemic. Their participation could provide important, alternative viewpoints,

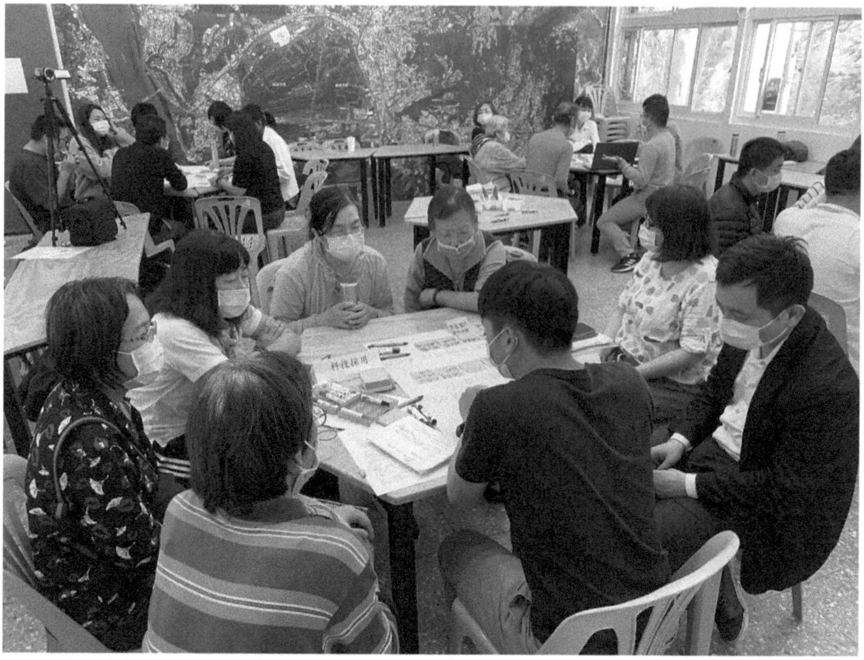

Figure 6.1 Moderators and Participants of the Citizen Forum

understandings and practices of digital pandemic response. In addition, students and other individuals in their 20s–40s also participated in the forum due to their interests in the topics (Figure 6.1).

Implementing and Living with Digital Pandemic Response

Efficiency

Efficiency has been an important motivation for government agencies to digitise their pandemic responses, aiming to reduce time and labour demands and increase the scope, speed and accuracy in the tracking and monitoring of the movement of people and viruses. As argued by the government, "a systematic and efficient big data method … may strengthen the conventional contact tracing and disease surveillance and inform the following control measures or mitigation plan" (Chen and others, 2020: 2). They further contend that the "systematic and efficient method" could be developed and implemented with equal measures of efficiency where digitally augmented contact tracing could be "quickly constructed through an innovative technology system to support timely epidemic analysis" (Chen and others, 2020: 7). But accounts and narratives such as these gloss over the material practices that are indispensable for engineering efficiency (see also Perng, 2022), which we illustrate below.

The start of COVID-19 in late 2019 and early 2020 coincided with the peak period for Taiwanese nationals living or working abroad, including China where the pandemic had already started, to return home for annual family reunions to celebrate the new year. As a result, there was a significantly increased amount of work at the border to process health declaration forms, send relevant information to various agencies involved in quarantine (public health, civil and police) and confirm the presence of passengers in their stated quarantine locations.

In the early stages of COVID-19, the data were collected using a paper-based form and had to be processed and transcribed manually onto spreadsheets, according to the interviewee. Once the data were prepared by public health workers, they then were sent to village administrators to confirm if the contact and location details were correct. During the quarantine period, village administrators (and also local public health workers, if necessary) would call those under quarantine by phone or in-person to see if they developed symptoms, had any questions or encountered any problems with which the administrators could assist them. If they appeared to be missing, the police would be informed and a search would be initiated.

The Ministry of Health and Welfare soon found that manual data processing was causing many problems. As the interviewee recounted, handwriting could be difficult to decipher, the information provided might be incomplete or wrong, or the information provided on the forms was not standardised. Consequently, processing the paper forms was time-consuming and labour-intensive. Complicating the matter further, without accurate information, village administrators could not confirm contact and location details, nor could they perform subsequent visits.

Faced with these challenges, the MoHW sought to increase the efficiency and accuracy of data collection by replacing the paper-based form with an information collection system, that is, "Quarantine System for Entry". Mobile phone numbers collected by the MoHW through the system were then incorporated into digital fences to monitor people under quarantine (including those undergoing at-home isolation, at-home quarantine and group quarantine to ensure that they stay at home during the quarantine/isolation period). To obtain the location data of these phones, digital fences used mobile geolocation data, which were generated from mobile phone towers receiving contact from phones when initiating phone calls or sending texts. Based on the information collected by the digital quarantine system, the MoWH informed relevant mobile operators of the numbers to track and the area within which the phone holders should stay. If mobile phone signals appeared to be outside of the designated area or disappear, mobile operators would notify public health agencies and village administrators to contact the persons in question.

Digital fences were expanded in early 2021 to prevent infection from spreading at the events celebrating the Lunar New Year. In what was termed "digital fences 2.0", cell towers surrounding the events were identified and mobile operators were given mobile phone numbers of those under quarantine to monitor if the phones made contact with these cell towers.

Although digital fences were designed to increase efficiency and accuracy while reducing time and human labour consumed by case monitoring, these goals could not be achieved by data feeds and digital technologies alone. Instead, a wide range of infrastructure and various social, technological, administrative and material practices (and labour) were required to negotiate and enable an increased level of efficiency and accuracy. The use of mobile geolocation data in digital fences illustrates the negotiation that was required. Mobile geolocation data are less accurate than the GPS data from mobile phones because they only show the geographic area covered by a cell tower when it is contacted by phones and cannot record the movement of phones in real-time. But they were preferred by the MoHW because of societal and regulatory considerations. Location triangulation, for example, was an alternative method to produce accurate location information. It was abandoned by the government because it was intended for criminal investigation and it was considered inappropriate for public health purposes. In comparison, mobile geolocation data were less intrusive and maintained privacy to a certain degree, which was why the MoWH chose it instead (Chen and others, 2020; Jyan and others, 2020).

Additionally, there were a number of collaborative practices that developed to ensure the efficient running of digital monitoring. The National Health Insurance (NHI) played a key part in the monitoring of symptoms in the early stages. But when the pandemic worsened and the scope of digital monitoring had to be expanded, the MoWH did not seek to link the NHI claims system with other databases, which ran the risk of control creep. Instead, according to our interview, inter-agency communication and collaboration were developed to incorporate essential and front-line workers, such as teachers, fishers, pilots, flight attendants and migrant workers, into the system for monitoring symptom developments.

Furthermore, the operation of digital fences required maintenance work by many front-line workers, including local police, public servants, and public health personnel. The use of mobile geolocation data complicated the efficiency and accuracy of digital monitoring. Due to the reduced granularity of the data, there could be a mixture of reasons for alarms to be triggered and on-the-ground personnel dispatched to verify if quarantine breaches did occur. These could be as mundane as mobile phones running out of battery and disappearing from the system. Also, if people underwent quarantine in cities, there were situations where the houses, apartments or rooms they stayed in during quarantine had poor reception due to the urban landscape (particularly concrete high rises). Conversely, rural areas might suffer from poor and unstable mobile coverage and degraded data quality, resulting in mobile phone signals appearing to be outside of designated areas or being dropped entirely even though no breach had occurred. Incidents such as these all required on-the-ground workers to either call on landlines or make in-person visits for verification and for digital fences to operate "efficiently".

Real-timeness

The desire for real-time collection and analysis of data to inform decision-making, particularly for the prediction and preemption of risks, has also driven the development of digital governance (Kitchin, 2014; Leszczynski, 2016). The requirement of swift identification and containment of the virus during COVID-19 incentivised continued attempts to devise digital measures for real-time analysis and responses to unpredictable pandemic situations. Despite the emphasis on real-timeness and much like how smart and algorithmic temporalities are multiple and intersecting (Kitchin, 2019), the lived experiences of real-timeness in receiving, perceiving and acting upon COVID-19 updates were complex. These experiences were shaped as much by digital platforms, algorithms embedded in them and the materiality of data as everyday information practices that could be dramatically different from one social group to another. In this section, we draw on our discussion in the citizen forum to demonstrate how the ideal of real-timeness was negotiated in everyday experiences of processing COVID-19 updates.

There was an emphasis on providing real-time information through digital platforms by the MoWH and other government agencies. The Taiwan Centers for Disease Control (TCDC), for example, streamed daily press conferences on video sharing platforms, broadcast announcements on social media sites, and disseminated the latest updates using a chatbot in a popular instant messaging app. The live stream of TCDC's press conferences was watched by estimated 800,000 to 1,000,000 viewers during May 2021 when daily confirmed cases sky-rocketed. The chatbot not only provided constant pandemic updates but also responded immediately to user's queries to verify information or dispel rumours.

However, there has been a complex making of "algorhythms" (Miyazaki, 2012; Coletta and Kitchin, 2017) in the everyday experiences of interacting with these platforms and technologies as illustrated in the experiences of the citizen forum participants. In the citizen forum, a recurrent theme was the dissatisfaction with the lack of updates and, related to this, the inaccuracy of the information. On the surface level, these complaints were about the government's failure to fulfil its responsibility to provide prompt and adequate information. Mask maps and crowd prediction systems were telling examples. During the early months of the pandemic when surgical masks were in short supply, mask maps showing stock availability at different shops and pharmacies were included in the government's digital repertoire for resource distribution and people were encouraged to use one of the various versions of the maps to obtain information about nearby pharmacies that had masks in stock. However, many citizen forum participants reflected upon their experiences of a lack of or inaccurate updates of mask stock levels. As they recalled, there were instances of stock information remaining the same throughout the day and, therefore, they did not feel that timely and accurate information was provided. They also shared with us experiences of seeing masks available for purchase on online maps only for them to find at pharmacies that masks had already sold out. Consequently, they often had to make multiple trips before a successful purchase. Similarly, these participants also reported a similar problem where the government's crowd prediction systems where tourist sites were marked as safe and not crowded by the system but had already been flooded by tourists.

However, it is useful to consider the lack of real-time feedback the participants experienced vis-à-vis the assemblage of digital technologies. This will produce a better understanding of the temporal slippages that are the results of "inter-related sets of digital technologies [that] work together or in conflict, perform synchronization and interact through diverse calculations and repetitions" (Coletta and Kitchin, 2017: 5). With regard to mask maps, to synchronise mask sales and stock information on maps, an assemblage of relevant technologies and data had to be appropriately aligned. Mask stock data had to be generated and released as open data, while a stock application programming interface (API) had to be set up to allow software engineers to feed the data into maps and other mobile applications. Additionally, the server that hosted the dataset had to have bandwidth sufficient to withstand the traffic accessing the dataset. However, the first iteration of such an assemblage failed to have enough bandwidth for the traffic from those eager to obtain stock-level information. When the system was revamped, other practices joined the assemblage uninvitedly. Pharmacies started to arrange their own sale procedures, for example, distributing queue tickets to customers in the early morning for them to return to buy masks later in the day. Accordingly, while mask maps could show that masks were still available for purchase at a particular pharmacy, people looking to buy them on the spot might find that masks had already sold out.

Temporal slippages could also occur when accessing technologies and services that aim to provide real-time information. In our discussion with the citizen forum participants, a sense of delay and confusion was prevalent when it came to pandemic updates on social media. There could be hours or days of delay when relevant updates and posts finally appeared on the participants' timelines. The delay could distort the participants' understanding of the sequence of events, or the participants could be misguided regarding the latest guidelines to follow. Senior citizens were among those who might be the most affected. They relied heavily on a close circle of family members and friends to receive updates, whether through social media directly or other messaging apps, and might not have other information sources they trusted.

To make sense of the temporal slippages and the lived experiences of processing pandemic information on social media as recounted by the citizen forum participants above, it is important to go beyond an individual approach and avoid attributing the slippages simply to limited digital competencies. Instead, it is necessary to take into account the logics underlying the operation of digital platforms that complicated the temporality of pandemic information processing. The TCDC and many municipalities included social media and instant messaging apps in their digital repertoire of constant and immediate information updates. Official social media accounts were not the sole sources of information for the participants since updates from families, friends or other public figures they followed all competed for visibility on social media timelines. However, as Bucher (2012) demonstrates well, algorithms contribute to a contested game of visibility on social media platforms where being seen on the platforms is temporary, unequally distributed and not guaranteed. To become visible to others and in real-time, one has to become participating, contributing and interactive on the platform so as to meet the algorithmic logic embedded in the technical architecture.

Such platform operational logics have complications for real-time pandemic information processing. Public health agencies and municipalities had to comply with these platform operational logics if their messages were to be seen earlier than other individuals or institutions competing for visibility. Consequently, "important" and "up-to-date" pandemic updates posted by government agencies were not guaranteed to appear first on one's timeline, and the real-timeness the agencies wanted to achieve was compromised by platform logics. As confirmed by the experiences of the forum participants, the updates that caught their eyes first were not necessarily the latest and were equally likely to be from their families, friends or public figures they followed, which resulted in the confusion they described and the temporal slippages amid pursuing real-time information dissemination by public health agencies.

Real-timeness mediated by digital platforms thus is complicated by the competition for visibility. The temporality of pandemic updates on social media is neither linear nor fixed, but is a result of negotiation among various parameters and algorithms that determine the popularity, relevance, interactivity and timeliness of social media posts. Algorithmically constructed visibility, in other words, significantly disrupts the ideal of real-timeness that underlies the incorporation of digital tools in pandemic updates. The lived temporal experiences of information sharing on digital platforms thus demonstrate how the government's attempt at real-time pandemic communication had to negotiate with algorithmic operations to earn a prominent spot on social media timelines, as well as gaining people's attention and trust.

Transparency

From open data to open government initiatives, the release of government data in publicly available and computationally accessible format has been considered an indispensable instrument for increasing government transparency and accountability. As Fink describes (2018: 1454), through releasing and re-using government data, open government initiatives attempt to establish new forms of governance that prioritise transparency, collaboration and participation, with the "[g]oals of open government [to] improv[e] efficiency and accountability, and increas[e] public engagement". This way of perceiving and pursuing transparent governance through open data has been heralded as the key to digital governance where opening up previously closed data would embolden a "future moral state" that "accelerat[es] towards more sophisticated, accountable and transparent structures of governance" (Datta, 2019: 398).

However, it is problematic to assume that more data equate to better knowledge and greater transparency. This transparency ideal rests upon the belief of modern sciences that data transcend individual viewpoints and reveal the "true essence of a system", which is the precondition for "a just and harmonious society", as Ananny and Crawford (2018: 974–975) draw on Daston to argue. Further, raw data are never raw. Before their public release, data are subjected to iterations of preparation, or "rawification", and should be better characterised as fragile and complex informational artefacts shaped by negotiated expectations, standards, data labour and infrastructures (Denis and Goëta, 2017).

In Taiwan's response to COVID-19, the transparency ideal also plays a significant part in the mobilisation of data for transparent governance, but the practical means to achieve it complicate its effects. Take case monitoring as an example. From reporting local and imported cases to publishing their footprints, the publication of pandemic data contributes to and compromises transparency in equal measure, and the pursuit of transparent governance of the pandemic engulfed relevant government agencies in frequent controversies. A critical aspect of being transparent for the agencies rested upon complying with existing legal and regulatory frameworks so as to ensure their mobilisation and publication of pandemic data were conducted in accountable ways. As our interviewee expressed:

> Of course, we know the [data analytics] techniques we use can serve surveillance purposes. So, you have to use them in the right way, backed by laws. We can use these techniques only if we have legal authorisations.
>
> (MoWH 2020)

However, for civil society groups, an important piece of information missing from the government's pandemic communications has been an adequate description of the data processing procedures devised to analyse and protect personal data. Different civil society groups raised this issue in the expert panel we conducted and their argument can be illustrated by the excerpt below:

> The purposes of the government's communication should not be limited to explain legal compliance. For pandemic prevention purposes, [the government] wants people to use [pandemic] technologies and this is an issue of social trust and credibility. You have to make sure that the procedure of using technologies can be explained [to the public].

The expert panel's suggestion explained the dissatisfaction expressed by the citizen forum participants about what they deemed as the "selective" release of footprints information by the government. Because the government did not fully explain the data processing procedures, some of the participants suspected that the government deliberately hid footprints information, even though it was actually published in accordance with a standard anonymisation procedure intended to protect privacy.

Several controversies occurred during the COVID-19 pandemic, and among them the one over daily PCR test results data was the most contentious. The controversy revolved around the retrospective adjustment to the number of confirmed cases after the CEEC processed a large backlog of tests during the spike in cases that led to the Level 3 alert in May 2021. On 22 May, amid heightened public anxiety and uncertainty, the CEEC announced that it "retroactively added 400 cases to the total number of COVID-19 cases calculated over the past week". The announcement shocked those who had been following the daily press conferences during the Level 3 alert and the rising numbers of confirmed cases. The CEEC explained the revisions as a result of the sudden surge in PCR tests that had to be analysed by the designated labs starting on 15 May. And it took until 22 May for the labs to complete their analysis of more than 10,000 samples accumulated over the short period. To sceptics, CEEC's explanation of the backlog was far from convincing and was considered merely a cover-up of the government's inability to control the outbreak. Hence, they reasoned, the data of confirmed cases released by the CEEC and the government itself could not be trusted.

The scepticism that continued demonstrated how the transparency ideal was complicated by the publication of pandemic data. During the controversy, many attempts were made to explain and render visible the epistemic, technological and social mechanisms involved in generating and publishing test data. Public health professionals offered their knowledge about why backlogs were difficult to avoid and what other data should also be taken into consideration. They pointed out that there could be a "reporting delay" occurring in the process from a patient starting to show symptoms to being diagnosed, as well as from being confirmed as infected to being included in the daily tally. Therefore, the data of daily confirmed cases should not be used as the sole indicator for evaluating pandemic situations. There were other data that should be taken into account. Illness onset dates, for example, could be less affected by the reporting delay and used as a standard way to understand epidemic curves. However, illness onset dates could not adequately show the latest changes due to the reporting delay. Therefore, they urged that daily counts of confirmed cases should not be overly relied upon to interpret epidemic trends and caution should be exercised when accounting for illness onset data for the most recent cases.

Additionally, medical technicians offered their knowledge of the inner working of the test reporting system by indicating several issues with regards to its infrastructure to justify why PCR results data could not fully be prepared, updated or published in time for the daily press conferences. In addition to the prolonged time to collect, prepare and analyse a sample resulting from the sudden increase in cases, logging a test result into the government's infectious disease reporting database was a laborious, time-consuming and brittle process. There were more than 20 fields to fill in manually before a test result could be uploaded. Further, the combination of the increased number of tests taken after the Level 3 alert and the simultaneous uploads of test results by different labs resulted in high network traffic volumes that the original design of the system could not withstand. The system became unresponsive; errors also occurred; case details that were only partially entered into the database were sometimes lost; consequently, the data required for completing a case report would have to be submitted again. It was also claimed that the unresponsiveness of the system was actually a long-standing problem that had been identified but never entirely fixed.

In contesting, explaining, justifying or critiquing the delay of PCR test results, the concept of transparency was invoked and expanded. The public outcry of "cover-up" turned to the transparency ideal that focuses on representation and truth to justify the demand for "more data". However, in response to the demand, the meaning and practice of transparency were also expanded. When tracing "across" sociotechnical systems striving for transparency, as Ananny and Crawford (2018) suggest, we also observe how necessary social, epistemic and infrastructural arrangements form interconnected systems that enact and complicate transparency. The various explanations offered by professionals and technicians can be seen as moving away from uncovering more data as a measure of transparency to understanding the inner workings of interconnected sociotechnical systems. In this way, transparency is not merely about data and truth; instead, drawing on Mackenzie (2019), transparency is about recognising the inevitability of indeterminacy in technological ensemble and its effects on what can be rendered knowable by test infrastructure and results. The accounts provided by the professionals and technicians were a way of redrawing professional and epistemic boundaries by rendering previously unknown systems knowable to the wider public.

The expansion of the transparency ideal led to complex consequences. The publication of PCR results data as part of transparent governance only had limited effects on developing a shared understanding of the unfolding crisis, or a sense of trust for relevant government agencies and different members of society. However, through the controversy, the public had an opportunity to become familiar with the specialist knowledge and technological systems related to PCR tests. But this was not transformed into further debates to consider whether, or to what extent, these systems should also be made accountable for the delay after knowing the inner workings of the systems. The lack of such discussions was a lost opportunity to establish procedural, regulatory and infrastructural arrangements for enacting more collaborative sense-making, trouble-shooting and recovery from breakdowns (Perng and Büscher, 2015).

Inclusiveness

Over the course of developing digital pandemic governance, inclusiveness has become a critical issue. In India, citizens are required to upload selfies at specified times on a daily basis, which ignores everyday rhythms that are different due to social, cultural and religious backgrounds (Datta, 2020). More generally, the design and use of digital technologies for containing the pandemic have been hardwired with exclusionary visions and Silicon Valley-inspired myths, as Milan (2020) contends. While scholarly and public outreach work has continuously sought to publicise these problems, it is not easy to address them effectively. In the citizen forum we organised, we sought to make the issue explicit and also to explore social and technical means to address them.

As noted by the citizen forum moderators, the participants shared their opinions about what might be the most effective or important technologies during COVID-19 and how they accessed information about the pandemic. The technologies mentioned by the participants included technologies utilised in the public space such as the "real-name registration" (實名制), "body temperature sensor" and the "alert system for crowded places" (景點人潮警示). In addition, social media platforms like LINE and Facebook were also critical to them, including the TCDC Facebook fan page, the CDC-related LINE chatbots (both the official chatbots of the TCDC [疾管家] and the MoHW) and other social groups on LINE (e.g., their family groups, communities). As for information update, both digital technologies and traditional media were used. Some participants relied on LINE notifications or the live streaming of TCDC's press conferences on TCDC's Facebook page, while others watched YouTube channels to stay informed of the status of the pandemic. Some participants depended on traditional media (such as television or newspapers) and personal networks (interpersonal communication). For elderly participants, traditional approaches were especially critical.

Traditional tools such as mass media and personal relationships then still played important roles even in Taipei as a highly connected city. To further explore what other measures might be useful for the forum participants, we encouraged them to envision how marginal social groups might be better included in digital pandemic response. Some suggestions were more technologically oriented. For example, the participants noticed that the elderly did not open apps as frequently as others and suggested adjusting the design of notification delivery. They also suggested that website designs, such as font sizes, could be more responsive to users of different age groups. Other suggestions were concerned with effective ways of embedding digital technologies into the networks of marginal groups. For example, to better include migrant workers in digital pandemic prevention measures, the participants suggested that not only should apps and updates be provided in the native languages of migrant workers, but they should also be introduced to their communities by people or institutions that were already familiar to them.

Another important issue is the access and resources that different social groups had for countering the "infodemic", the global and local influx of misinformation, disinformation or fake news regarding COVID-19. In the context of Taiwan, an important grassroots effort to combat misinformation engages in the development and maintenance of "Cofacts", a collaborative system built upon a LINE chatbot and an openly accessible database containing confirmed or disputed information. However, as the forum participants reminded us, for people who did not have regular access to the Internet, it was difficult to perform fact-checks on the information they have received. They suggested that it was also crucial for the government and other groups to co-produce pandemic technologies to protect those who were not yet included in today's digital society from the influence and potential harm of misinformation.

These suggestions might be motivated by different observations or viewpoints, and formulated with different understandings of tech design and development. Indeed, these differences might be due to particular social characteristics one possesses in terms of ages, genders, social and economic backgrounds, ethnicities, language proficiencies or access to digital technologies and services. And yet, regardless of how the differences might be considered as results of individual characteristics or competencies, these suggestions together provide useful resources to uncover what barriers still exist to exclude marginalised groups from being protected by existing pandemic response measures and the visions or imaginaries for future digital pandemic response.

Considering these suggestions further, they highlight another crucial aspect of inclusiveness, namely the inclusion of expertise, skills, experiences and practices that are not readily "digitised" into the implementation of digital governance of pandemics. Over the course of the COVID-19 pandemic, technical skills, particularly coding and design, have continuously been described in celebratory tones in reports on how the public can contribute to digital pandemic response measures, such as the mask inventory API or SMS-based contact tracing. But this way of perceiving the public and how they could contribute to pandemic response runs the risk of excluding other practices that are equally effective and important. Apart from queuing for mask purchases or the emotional labour required during quarantine that have already been discussed, other practices to care for marginal groups include printing contact tracing QR codes for shops in remote areas or setting up temporary Internet access stations for places with limited Internet connections for vaccination appointments. These all speak to the importance of prioritising considerations for the protection of civil liberties and the technical arrangements to materialise them over the technical architecture only for "efficiency" or "real-timeness". Furthermore, civil liberties groups repeatedly demanded to know the scope, process and relevant regulations related to data collection and analysis for pandemic prevention purposes, echoing the observations and concerns raised in the citizen forum and in the expert panel we organised. But these details and the relevant regulations and guidelines were rarely provided at the time when new technical arrangements for data collection were introduced. The government's lack of timely response highlights that the practices, discussions and deliberations that are not contributing directly to implementing digital pandemic responses could, like caring practices, be marginalised or silenced (c.f. Murphy, 2015).

Democratic Digital Governance of Pandemics

The experiences and criticisms detailed above are valuable, as they are "lessons learned" in a rapid, ongoing and large-scale government experiment to digitise pandemic response. Although they may seem commonplace, the scope of raising these issues is not guaranteed, which can be made explicit by contrasting Taiwan's strategies with that of authoritarian states. In such countries, surveillance measures and technologies were widespread and caused human and civil rights concerns. In Singapore, the app TraceTogether developed by the Ministry of Health, SG United and GovTech Singapore caused increased social fragmentation and distrust (Stevens and Haines, 2020). China's Health Code and the extensive collection of personal health data linked with other data held by the government to place people under quarantine and enforce epidemic surveillance. Such a system allowed the state to quickly expand its tentacles for "seeing and intervening in society" and people's everyday life based on algorithmic evaluation (Liu, 2021). But as Liu also contends, Health Code has legibility limits and potential social risks and costs. Further, Health Code uses the same system employed by the Chinese government for ethnic surveillance, which lacks mechanisms for privacy and human rights protection and has been under constant criticism by human rights groups (Wang, 2020).

Unlike authoritarian states, Taiwan sought to activate its pandemic response based on a democratic framework. Efficient and real-time pandemic responses were possible owing to the long-term development of public health infrastructure, including the National Health Insurance, fibre-optic cable networks connecting medical providers and other reporting systems (蘇湘雲, 2021). Also, transparency and inclusiveness were supported and required by law. Taiwan has learned from the 2003 SARS epidemic, and the government has strengthened not only its public health infrastructure but also relevant laws and regulations. These include the Communicable Disease Control Act which provide the legal basis for the activation of the CECC and related emergency measures. Furthermore, Taiwan did not enlist digital technologies for achieving total control of the pandemic and society. Instead, its digital pandemic governance is based on the dynamic and collaborative state-society relationship and ongoing dialogues among multiple actors in the process of increasing responsiveness, accelerating institutional adjustments and addressing disconnects between citizens and policymaking.

However, it is crucial to acknowledge that legal and procedural requirements surrounding pandemic measures and privacy concerns may become blurred as digital technologies continue to emerge. Wu (2021) points out that concerns about privacy, individual free will and freedom, and the abuse of power still led to controversies and debates even when Taiwan sought to maintain democratic governance of the pandemic. Vague, unclear boundaries of the government's power during the emergency to loosen privacy protection regulations and allow broader access to personal data, were questionable. The government failed to disclose comprehensively what personal data has been collected, how it was collected and processed, and for what purposes the data was used. As also seen in Chapter 4, the effectiveness, necessity and ultimately legitimacy of digital pandemic measures are called into question. This lack of transparency undermined public trust and the scope to scrutinise the government's emergency measures. This was most evident during the first outbreak of local transmissions in Taipei City, which occurred between May 2020 and June 2021 and resulted in over 10,000 infections and almost 300 deaths. During the period, the CECC provided the phone numbers and location data of all residents in the Wanhua District, where the outbreak started, to a laboratory without informing data subjects. The laboratory analysed residents' digital footprints and added special notations to their NHI cards. These measures were later criticised for expanding the CECC's emergency powers without sufficient justification.

Accordingly, the incorporation of digital technology for pandemic response cannot proceed without the rights protected by laws and regulations to raise concerns or voice criticisms against government measures that could erode privacy, transparency, accountability and social trust. During the course of COVID-19, different individuals, grassroots organisations and civil society groups have pointed out where Taiwan's technological, social and governance approaches should be critiqued and improved. The protection of the freedom of speech ensures that criticisms and rights claims can be made and the civil society can actively participate in enunciating dissent.

Conclusion

In this chapter, we examined in detail the ideals behind various digital "art of government" to meet pandemic challenges and suggest to pay greater attention to the diverse practices and lived experiences in the new digital regimen of pandemic governance that complicate these ideals. In the discussion above, we demonstrate how various digital governance ideals permeate pandemic response so as to render it more efficient, responsive (in real-time), transparent and inclusive. And we also show how such transformation requires more-than-digital work, engenders slippages, creates contradictions and calls for future measures to address existing gaps and barriers in the protection of the health and vulnerable population. The citizen forum we organised facilitated making these challenges explicit and contributed to co-envision potential ways to improve digital pandemic response measures. At the same time, concerns, criticisms and suggestions vehemently raised publicly further attest to the expanding scope of digital pandemic governance and the diverse perspectives and experiences that have to be taken into account to avoid future harms. We further suggest that the significance of Taiwan during COVID-19 has been its continued efforts to base digital pandemic response in democratic governance and to seek a better balance between emergency response demands and necessary protections of civil liberties. As we have shown, public deliberation on digital pandemic response measures holds great potential to enable residents to speak for the needs and concerns of elderly people and the marginalised, facilitate voicing the discursive narratives in public space to the government, contribute to epistemic inclusiveness and improve the democratic quality of pandemic governance (cf. Fan and Sung, 2022).

As pandemics become "data-intensive", everyday life and social interactions affected by the government's public health measures are and will be a core concern for democratic societies and designers of not only technologies and services but also policies and regulations. To support a better transition towards digital pandemic governance, we suggest that future research can benefit from looking into how data and digital systems used and generated by the public could be designed to highlight the concerns and opposing beliefs among different actors. Also, it is critical that governments review the responses and experiences related to COVID-19 so that various ideals and the consequences of materialising them could be thoroughly examined. Digital medical innovation to support staff, diagnoses and treatments, and patients living in remote areas is useful, but we also suggest that a focus on improving interactions with digital infrastructure, including its constituent technologies, maintenance practices and various social, regulatory and legal frameworks supporting it, will provide opportunities for effective planning and improvisation to respond to uncertainties in future pandemics. Moreover, given that ICT technologies play essential roles in digital governance during pandemics, it is important to increase digital adoption rates and to design accessible and inclusive technologies and services for marginal social groups. Finally, it is productive to provide data and digital literacy training to enhance personal capabilities, such as discerning misinformation and disinformation, and it is equally important to create opportunities for collaborative sense-making and troubleshooting to meet challenges posed by future pandemics in collective and inclusive ways.

Acknowledgements

We would like to thank the participants of the expert panel and the citizen forum, as well as Beitou Community College for facilitating the forum. The chapter is supported by the Research Center for Epidemic Prevention of National Yang Ming Chiao Tung University (MOST 111–2321-B-A49-007) and the Ministry of Science and Technology, Taiwan (MOST 109–2410-H-010–001-MY3).

References

蘇湘雲, 2021, 一張健保卡，串聯防疫戰線「疫」起善用健保卡, 衛生福利部季刊, v. 25, p. 10–15.

Ananny, M., and Crawford, K., 2018, Seeing without knowing: Limitations of the transparency ideal and its application to algorithmic accountability: New Media & Society, v. 20, i. 3, p. 973–989.

Ansell, C., and Gash, A., 2008, Collaborative governance in theory and practice: Journal of Public Administration Research and Theory, v. 18, i. 4, p. 543–571.

Bucher, T., 2012, Want to be on the top? Algorithmic power and the threat of invisibility on Facebook: New Media & Society, v. 14, i. 7, p. 1164–1180.

Carson, L., 2011, Designing a public conversation using the World Café method: Social Alternatives, v. 30, i. 1, p. 10–14.

Chen, C.-M., Jyan, H.-W., Chien, S.-C., et al., 2020, Containing COVID-19 among 627,386 persons in contact with the Diamond Princess cruise ship passengers who disembarked in Taiwan: Big data analytics: Journal of Medical Internet Research, v. 22, i. 5, p. e19540.

Cinnamon, J., 2020, Platform philanthropy, 'public value', and the COVID-19 pandemic moment: Dialogues in Human Geography, v. 10, i. 2, p. 242–245.

Coletta, C., and Kitchin, R., 2017, Algorhythmic governance: Regulating the 'heartbeat' of a city using the Internet of Things: Big Data & Society, v. 4, i. 2, p. 1–16.

Das, D., and Zhang, J. J., 2021, Pandemic in a smart city: Singapore's COVID-19 management through technology & society: Urban Geography, v. 42, i. 3, p. 408–416.

Datta, A., 2019, Postcolonial urban futures: Imagining and governing India's smart urban age: Environment and Planning D: Society and Space, v. 37, i. 3, p. 393–410.

Datta, A., 2020, Self(ie)-governance: Technologies of intimate surveillance in India under COVID-19: Dialogues in Human Geography, v. 10, i. 2, p. 234–237.

Datta, A., Aditi, A., Ghoshal, A., et al., 2021, Apps, maps and war rooms: On the modes of existence of "COVtech" in India: Urban Geography, v. 42, i. 3, p. 382–390.

Dean, M., 2010, Governmentality: Power and Rule in Modern Society: Sage, London.

Denis, J., and Goëta, S., 2017, Rawification and the careful generation of open government data: Social Studies of Science, v. 47, i. 5, p. 604–629.

Fan, M.-F., 2021, Deliberative Democracy in Taiwan: A Deliberative Systems Perspective: Routledge, London.

Fan, M.-F., and Sung, S.-C., 2022, Indigenous political participation in deliberative systems: The long-term care service controversy in Taiwan: Policy Studies, v. 43, i. 2, p. 164–182.

Fink, K., 2018, Opening the government's black boxes: Freedom of information and algorithmic accountability: Information Communication & Society, v. 21, i. 10, p. 1453–1471.

Kitchin, R., 2014, The real-time city? Big data and smart urbanism: GeoJournal, v. 79, i. 1, p. 1–14.
Kitchin, R., 2019, The timescape of smart cities: Annals of the American Association of Geographers, v. 109, i. 3, p. 775–790.
Kitchin, R., 2020, Civil liberties or public health, or civil liberties and public health? Using surveillance technologies to tackle the spread of COVID-19: Space and Polity, v. 24, i. 3, p. 362–381.
Leszczynski, A., 2016, Speculative futures: Cities, data, and governance beyond smart urbanism: Environment and Planning A: Economy and Space, v. 48, i. 9, p. 1691–1708.
Liu, C.-C., 2021, Seeing like a state, enacting like an algorithm: (Re)assembling contact tracing and risk assessment during the COVID-19 pandemic: Science, Technology and Human Values, v. 47, i. 4, p. 698–725.
Löhr, K., Weinhardt, M., and Sieber, S., 2020, The "World Café" as a participatory method for collecting qualitative data: International Journal of Qualitative Methods, v. 19, p. 1–15.
Maalsen, S., and Dowling, R., 2020, Covid-19 and the accelerating smart home: Big Data & Society, v. 7, i., p. 1–5.
Mackenzie, A., 2019, From API to AI: Platforms and their opacities: Information, Communication & Society, v. 22, i. 13, p. 1989–2006.
Milan, S., 2020, Techno-solutionism and the standard human in the making of the COVID-19 pandemic: Big Data & Society, v. 7, i. 2, p. 1–7.
Ministry of Health and Welfare (MoHW), 2020, The Taiwan Model for Combating COVID-19: The Ministry of Health and Welfare, Taipei, Taiwan.
Miyazaki, S., 2012, Algorhythmics: Understanding micro-temporality in computational cultures: Computational Culture, v.2, http://computationalculture.net/algorhythmics-understanding-micro-temporality-in-computational-cultures/.
Murphy, M., 2015, Unsettling care: Troubling transnational itineraries of care in feminist health practices: Social Studies of Science, v. 45, i. 5, p. 717–737.
Pearse, H., 2020, Deliberation, citizen science and COVID-19: The Political Quarterly, v. 91, i. 3, p. 571–577.
Perng, S.-Y., 2022, Materialities of digital disease control during Covid-19 in Taiwan: Big Data & Society, v. 9, i. 1, p. 1–12.
Perng, S.-Y., and Büscher, M., 2015, Uncertainty and transparency: Augmenting modelling and prediction for crisis response: Proceedings of the ISCRAM 2015, Kristiansand, Norway.
Petersen, A., and Lupton, D., 1996, The new public health: Health and self in the age of risk: Sage: London.
Sandvik, K. B., 2020, 'Smittestopp': If you want your freedom back, download now: Big Data & Society, v. 7, i. 2, p. 1–11.
Söderström, O., Paasche, T., and Klauser, F., 2014, Smart cities as corporate storytelling: City, v. 18, i. 3, p. 307–320.
Sonn, J. W., and Lee, J. K., 2020, The smart city as time-space cartographer in COVID-19 control: The South Korean strategy and democratic control of surveillance technology: Eurasian Geography and Economics, v. 61, i. 4–5, p. 482–492.
Stevens, H., and Haines, M. B., 2020, TraceTogether: Pandemic response, democracy, and technology: East Asian Science, Technology and Society: An International Journal, v. 14, i. 3, p. 523–532.
Vanolo, A., 2013, Smartmentality: The smart city as disciplinary strategy: Urban Studies, v. 51, i. 5, p. 883–898.
Wang, M., 2020, China: Fighting COVID-19 with automated tyranny: The Diplomat, April 1.
Wu, C.-F., 2021, Covid-19 and data privacy challenges in Taiwan, accessed 10 May, 2023 at Lex-Atlas: Covid-19. https://lexatlas-c19.org/covid-19-and-data-privacy-challenges-in-taiwan/.

Part 3

Self-Governance and Individual Citizens

7 To Stay or to Leave? A Study of Noncompliance of COVID-19 Quarantine Regulations in Taiwan

Hsuan-Wei Lee, Chih-Han Leng and Chi-Shiun Tsai

The authorship of this chapter shall be jointly and equally vested among the three contributors. The data collected from this study is not representative. People were recruited from various social media to join the online survey of this research. Therefore, there might be sampling bias in data collection in terms of gender, age, and homogeneity. When resorting to the conclusions of this research, one must be aware of this potential risk and research limitations.

Introduction

Governance is the determinant of the development of a nation, which includes health development (Kirigia and Kirigia, 2011). According to Fidler (2004), "governance" is how societies react to the challenges they encounter, and "germ governance" refers to how societies organize their responses to pathogenic threats both within and outside of national borders. The uncertainties of abrupt changes bring challenges to emergency governance and crisis management. Governance capacity and legitimacy are the building blocks of a well-functioning crisis management system. Governance capacity is the preparedness to provide effective crisis management, and governance legitimacy is the trust of people in the government (Christensen and Lægreid, 2020). As for governance legitimacy, the first priority is building the trust of people in the government. During the coronavirus crisis, the governance capacity and legitimacy of each nation were put to the test. Besides, it also posed challenges to global health governance due to the contagion spreading across countries. While governance is crucial during the pandemic, people's compliance plays an important role as well. Without people's compliance with policy, containment measures would not work. Scholars have studied the factors that drive compliance with COVID-19 containment measures, including trust in government and risk communication (Clark *et al.*, 2020; Devine *et al.*, 2021; Nivette *et al.*, 2021; Six *et al.*, 2021). Studies have also shown that additional sanction for violations does not reduce the noncompliance rate (Ryu *et al.*, 2022). There are different types of noncompliance, such as direct, indirect, active, passive, aware, and unaware (Gofen, 2015). These types of noncompliance are all conspicuous. What if the government could understand how to prevent people from violating the measures before noncompliance behaviors take place? We would like to explore

DOI: 10.4324/9781003438380-11

reasons behind possible noncompliance behavior so that the government could get prepared in advance. Moreover, the government could tailor the quarantine regulations for future public health crises.

COVID-19 (coronavirus) has been sweeping the world since early 2020. To limit its spread, multiple preventive measures and regulations were adopted by governments. For the most part, the regulations were correlated with restricting residents' freedom. When government policy is implemented with the aim of keeping people healthy, conflicts between public health and individual rights inevitably arise. During the coronavirus pandemic, this issue has become more important and it has been widely discussed by scholars. When the public feels that individual rights are sacrificed, they might not be willing to follow the regulations. Therefore, striking a balance between public health and individual rights is crucial when coming up with policies relevant to the containment of the pandemic. There are several common measures and regulations for the government to put into practice during the pandemic, many of which could compromise individual freedom. One of the common governmental measures is to recommend or require people to wear masks in public. Despite this recommendation, there are people who do not want to wear masks because they feel that it violates their freedom of choice. Studies have shown that hyper-individualists refuse to wear masks (Blum *et al.*, 2020). Other studies have also mentioned that preventive behaviors, such as mask-wearing, could be influenced by political identities (Pereira and Stornelli, 2022).

Many countries have been enforcing compulsory lockdowns in cities and other populated areas. Studies have shown that lockdown has been successful in containing the pandemic and mitigating the pressure on healthcare units (Cauchemez *et al.*, 2020). However, the impact on mental health has also been discussed in other studies. High rates of negative emotions were found when the lockdowns were implemented (Hiremath *et al.*, 2020). Considering that personal freedom would be deprived, how did governments convince their citizens to be quarantined or constrained at home? Besides, what do people experience when facing mandatory quarantine? Based on this experience, what would induce the intention of violating the quarantine regulations?

Countries around the world have also implemented travel restrictions and quarantine measures for inbound travelers. The measures are correlated with the severity of COVID-19 pandemic. Most countries share similar restrictions, with a difference in the length of quarantine. In short, the length of quarantine in Western countries is shorter than in Asian countries. Among these countries, China and Taiwan are the ones with the longest quarantine periods. However, as of June 15, 2022, Taiwan has shortened the quarantine period to seven days. The Central Epidemic Command Center (CECC) has decided to terminate the prior seven-day self-health management.

Compared to the WHO statistics, Taiwan only had 742 confirmed cases and seven deaths on December 15, 2020 (Taiwan CDC, 2020), the seven-day rolling average of daily new confirmed COVID-19 cases were less than 0.1 per million people, which suggested that Taiwan succeeded in combating the COVID-19 pandemic. Still, until December 15, 2020, there were 1,201 cases of violation of quarantine regulations: such as leaving the designated quarantine facility during home quarantine or home isolation. However, in May 2021, the number of daily new confirmed cases in Taiwan suddenly rose to the triple digits, forcing the Central Epidemic Command Center (CECC) to raise the warning level for Taipei City and New Taipei City to level 3. The public were requested to follow and comply with level 3 epidemic prevention and control measures. The CECC also increased the number of testing sites, quarantine hotels, and facilities across the whole country to ensure that the medical supply was adequate. Although the CECC told the public not to panic, the worsening conditions did worry the people. It influenced people's feelings toward coronavirus containment policies, particularly the quarantine.

Comparing the number of people violating the quarantine regulation with the number of people getting infected with coronavirus during different periods of the pandemic in Taiwan could help us understand noncompliance behavior in different scenarios. From January 2020 to April 2021, the number of people who had experienced home quarantine or home isolation was 650,797. Among those people, 602 were infected with coronavirus, and there were 1,801 people who have reportedly been fined for violating the quarantine measures. During this period of time, there were more people infected with coronavirus than those who violated the measures. As for May 2021 to September 2021, the number of people who had been through home quarantine or home isolation was 240,666. Among these, there were 7,254 people infected with coronavirus, while 510 people have been fined for violation of the obligation to stay in quarantine. In comparison with the previous period when the pandemic was less severe, the rate of people violating quarantine regulations was relatively small when the percentage of people getting infected with coronavirus was higher.

A number of studies have examined the impact of quarantine. One of the main impacts of quarantine is the influence on mental health. As mentioned by Benke et al. (2020), higher restrictions were associated with more severe mental health consequences. Being in self-quarantine was associated with a level of anxiety, and contacting loved ones who were at risk of getting infected was related with health anxiety. Moreover, young people, those with a higher level of education, and people with lower income were more likely to have mental health problems, including depression, anxiety, and insomnia (Wang *et al.*, 2021). School closures and quarantine during the COVID-19 pandemic increased the level of anxiety among young people as studied by Kılınçel et al. (2021). In addition to the impact on the youth, Yildirim et al. (2021) found that the anxiety levels of the elderly who were in quarantine during the epidemic exacerbated the severity of depression. Another impact related to mental health during the pandemic is job loss. People who lost their jobs had a higher risk of feeling stress compared to those who kept their jobs (Ruengorn *et al.*, 2021). Therefore, scholars have stated that the government should provide job security and income replacement programs to fulfill the basic requirements of those in quarantine. With job security or stable financial aid from the government, people in quarantine would be more willing to comply with regulations (Rothstein and Talbott, 2007).

Moreover, based on the quarantine experience during the 2003 SARS epidemic in Toronto, Canada, "do not go out of one's house to socialize" was the most challenging quarantine regulation to comply with (Reynolds *et al.*, 2008). Though a quarantine period of two weeks may seem small, few studies have explored the factors causing the violation of this regulation. Is it simply a case of rebellious behavior or are there significant factors causing burnout? Consequently, we conducted this study to mainly investigate the following research question.

> RQ: Why do quarantined people have the desire to leave or escape from their quarantined places?

This mixed-method study aims to explore the triggers of people's noncompliance during the quarantined days. In contrast to Dr. Tseng's study in Chapter 8, which used in-depth interviews, we use daily questionnaires and statistical and contextual analysis to figure out what the overall effect of quarantines is on people. We aim to examine people's inclination so that the government could prevent violations of regulations in advance. The study focuses on 2020 and 2021, which marked the onset of the COVID-19 pandemic and the sudden rise of COVID-19 cases in Taiwan. During these most tense phases of the pandemic, the COVID-19 outbreaks drastically disrupted life and caused widespread concern among the populace of Taiwan. To measure the noncompliance, we use a self-evaluation of the thoughts of leaving the quarantined place as the reference. The triggers are hypothesized to contain demographic characteristics, living environment, negative emotion, social support, social responsibility, and the attitude toward the government's related information. Thus, we regress people's noncompliance on the triggers using an ordinal logistic regression model. Since past studies indicated most factors affecting the inclination of noncompliance were about individuals' mental health as mentioned above, among all the mental health issues, we focus on finding what people were anxious about as the anxiety resulted from various aspects (Ehlers and Clark, 2000). We also collect and analyze the responses from people who had just experienced quarantine. Lastly, we compare different groups of people who had quarantine experiences during the first and second waves of pandemics in Taiwan, trying to portray and distinguish their attitudes toward the quarantine policies and other government measures. Therefore, we could understand individual differences in attitudes regarding quarantine regulations. We hope to provide insights into the framing of government capacity and legitimacy during the pandemic and come up with policy implications based on the results of our study.

Methods

Participants

In late March 2020, as COVID-19 began spreading in the United States of America and Europe, a significant number of people who studied or worked abroad returned to Taiwan resulting in the most severe and nervous time of the pandemic. During this period, 152 currently quarantined people (113 females), all over 20 years old and with Taiwan as their nationality, were recruited from social media (e.g., Facebook and Line) and unspecified email mailing lists, by the Institute of Sociology, Academia Sinica, Taiwan (Fu and Lee, 2020) for a one month long longitudinal study. Participants were rewarded with a fixed payment ($2,500 TWD, roughly $85 USD) if they completed at least 23 days of the questionnaire in a month, and they also had a chance to win a lottery (not fixed payment) based on the level of detail of their response. The survey period was from March 30 to May 8, 2020, when Taiwan had experienced its first wave of local COVID-19 outbreak.

Before attending our study, participants needed to provide their copy of the official home quarantine or home isolation notice for identity verification. After approval, participants were required to use a web-based platform, named "Click Diary", for recording their contacts and answering a daily life survey during their quarantine days. After the quarantine, participants needed to complete the post-quarantine survey. In the post-quarantine survey, people were required to make a holistic report of their quarantine experience. At the end of the survey, they were asked to write down how they felt about the quarantine or any incidents relevant to the pandemic that they had encountered. We discuss the details of the variables measured by each survey in the following paragraphs. Notably, since participants entered our study on different days during their quarantine, we did not have complete data of their two-week-long daily life survey. Therefore, we only had 908 records in total.

Besides, it is important to have a comprehensive understanding of the issue to identify potential barriers and opportunities for compliance. We would like to recognize how people feel toward coronavirus containment policies and measures. By considering different experiences and perspectives across various groups, we can gain valuable insights into why some people or groups might be more likely to violate the regulations. This knowledge can inform the development of more effective policies and measures that take into account the diverse needs and perspectives of the population. To examine public opinion and attitudes toward policies relevant to coronavirus containment when the number of confirmed COVID-19 cases in Taiwan rose in 2021, we set up a survey website named "Social Distancing Survey". People who were over 20 years old and living in Taiwan, regardless of their nationalities, could be the participants. The survey was conducted during the first two weeks (May 15–28, 2021) of Taiwan's mid-2021 outbreak, when the level 3 alert was issued and the number of confirmed cases reached its peak. Participants were recruited through multiple social media platforms such as Facebook, LINE, WhatsApp, Twitter and different unspecified email mailing lists. In this survey, participants were not rewarded with a fixed payment, but they had a chance to win gift cards with different values if they finished the survey. The survey questions included attitudes toward policies, such as satisfaction with the response of the government to the pandemic, opinion on restricting individual freedom to contain the epidemic, tracking the movement of people, releasing the personal information of those infected with COVID-19, and how trustworthy the information provided by the government was. In the survey period, 1,151 participants (70 with quarantine experience) filled out the survey.

Measures

(a) Demographic characteristics: The demographic characteristics contain gender (male/female), age, marital status (single/ married), and income.
(b) Inclination to leave: Participants were asked whether they felt like leaving the designated quarantine area. People with a high score of this item would have a strong desire to leave the quarantine place. The question was stated as following: Do you have thoughts about leaving the designated quarantine place today?
(c) Cumulative number of quarantine days: This variable was the cumulative number of participants' quarantine days.
(d) Sunlight exposure: This was a dummy variable asking whether the participants had exposure to sunlight in the quarantined place.
(e) Loneliness: People with a high score of this item would feel lonely during the quarantine.
(f) Worry about job loss: People with a high score of this item might be worried about their job during the quarantine.
(g) Anxiety of losing interpersonal connections: This item measured participants' anxiety about losing touch with others. The higher the score, the higher the anxiety.
(h) Anxiety of being known by others: This item measured participants' anxiety about others knowing that they were quarantined. The higher the score, the higher the anxiety.
(i) Anxiety of worsening personality: This item measured participants' anxiety about their personalities worsening during the quarantine. The higher the score, the higher the anxiety.
(j) Anxiety of being fragile: This item measured participants' anxiety about emotional being fragility during the quarantine. The higher the score, the higher the anxiety.
(k) Daily contacts: This variable was the estimate of the total number of participants' daily contacts. These contact records included physical and online contact.
(l) Friend support: This item measured participants' confidence about receiving help from friends if they were at risk. The higher the score, the higher the assurance of receiving friends' support.
(m) Social responsibility: This item measured participants' attitudes toward the helpfulness of the quarantine policy. Participants with a high score of this item would think the quarantine was helpful for stopping the spread of the COVID-19 virus.
(n) Government support: This item measured participants' confidence about receiving help from the government if they were at risk. The higher the score, the higher the assurance of receiving the government's support.
(o) Information transparency: This item measured participants' attitudes toward the transparency of the government's information. The higher the score, the higher the trustworthiness of the government's policy.

Variables (b)–(e) were measured in the daily life survey, and variables (f)–(o) were measured in the post-quarantine survey. Variable (d) measured the living environment, variables (e) and (f)–(j) measured the negative emotion, variables (k)–(l) measured the social support, variable (m) measured the social responsibility, and variables (n)–(o) measured the attitude toward the government's related information.

As for "Social Distancing Survey", which examined people's attitudes toward government policies, there were five questions to measure how people felt about their government and their attitudes toward certain policies relevant to COVID-19 containment:

1 Satisfaction with the government: In general, how satisfied are you with your government's response to the coronavirus outbreak?
2 Restricting individual freedom: Do you agree that the government should restrict individual freedom in order to control the coronavirus outbreak? (e.g., quarantine, mobility, and gathering restrictions).
3 Tracking people's movement: Do you agree that the government should track people's movements in order to control the coronavirus outbreak? (e.g., using location data from cell phones).
4 Releasing personal information: Do you agree that the government should release personal information of coronavirus patients for the sake of enhancing people's understanding of the coronavirus outbreak? (e.g., gender, age, location, and occupation).
5 Information provided by the government: During the coronavirus outbreak, how trustworthy is the information provided by your government about the development of the epidemic?

Analyses

Statistical Analysis

We conducted all analyses using R software in version 4.1.1 and used ordinal logistic regression to build the model. We built two models to explain quarantined people's inclination to leave the quarantine place under a significance level of 0.05. In the two models, females were the reference group of "gender", single status was designated as the reference group of "marital status", and no sunlight exposure was set as the reference of "sunlight exposure". Specifically, in the first model, variables (g)–(j) were added up into one variable–anxiety in the model, as they were moderately interrelated with correlation coefficients greater than 0.4. We hypothesized that participants' inclination to leave the quarantine place would rise with a poor living environment, intense negative emotion, low social support, low social responsibility, and low attitude toward the government-related information. In the second model, variables (g)–(j) were divided and incorporated into the model to explore their contribution to the inclination, respectively.

Content Analysis

A summative content analysis was carried out to examine how participants in our study felt about the quarantine experience and the government in terms of quarantine policy (Hsieh and Shannon, 2005). We first counted the occurrence of each word in their responses by using the programming language R, and focused primarily on the words relevant to quarantine, government and policy, such as "quarantine", "isolation", "Taiwan", "government", and "policy". Then we categorized their responses into topics based on word usage and the content.

Results

Demographic Characteristics

As shown in Table 7.1, most of our participants were female (74.34%), aged 29 years old on average, and single (85.53%). About two-fifths of them had income within the range of 1,700–3,399 US dollars a month (42.11%).

Associated Factors of the Inclination to Leave

Table 7.2 recorded people's inclination to leave the quarantine place. According to the table, 11.67% of people had a neutral inclination to leave the quarantine place. Furthermore, 11.12% of people strongly desired to leave the quarantine place.

Moreover, in terms of the living environment, 57.27% of participants had exposure to sunlight during the quarantine. In regards to the negative emotions, 42.73% of participants recorded low feelings of loneliness. Most participants were strongly worried about job loss (30.92%), lowly anxious about losing links

Table 7.1 Demographic Characteristics of 152 Participants

Characteristic	*Total No. (%)*
Overall	152 (100)
Gender	
Male	39 (25.66)
Female	113 (74.34)
Age Mean±SD	29.42± 5.94
Marital status	
Single	130 (85.53)
Married	22 (14.47)
Income	
≤329 USD/month	4 (2.63)
330–989 USD/month	9 (5.92)
990–1,699 USD/month	27 (17.66)
1,700–3,399 USD/month	64 (42.11)
3,400–6,799 USD/month	40 (26.32)
≥6,800 USD/month	8 (5.26)

Table 7.2 The Inclination to Leave the Quarantine Place of 152 Participants on a Total of 908 Days

Characteristic	*Total No. (%)*
The inclination to leave	
Very low	321 (35.35)
Low	355 (39.10)
Neutral	106 (11.67)
Strong	101 (11.12)
Very strong	25 (2.75)

(48.03%), lowly anxious about being known by others (32.89%), about worsening personality (40.13%), and about being fragile (31.58%). Still, more than 10% of people were (very) strongly anxious about losing interpersonal connections (14.47%), being known by others (19.74%), worsening personality (15.79%), being fragile (29.61%). Regarding social support, 42.76% of participants contacted 1–4 people and 45.39% contacted 5–9 people per day on average during quarantine. Most participants thought their friends would support them when they were in trouble (79.61%). Regarding social responsibility, about half of the participants agreed that the quarantine measure helped prevent the spread of the COVID-19 virus (55.26%) and that the government's information was transparent (46.71%).

Statistical Analysis

Tables 7.3–7.5 summarized the two ordinal logistic models of the inclination to leave the quarantine place. As shown in Table 7.3, that is, Model I, among demographic characteristics, the inclination of males to leave the quarantine place was 0.56 times that of females. Older people had a strong desire for noncompliance, with an increasing rate of 1.04 per age. People's unwillingness to comply with the rules increased following their income with an increasing rate of 1.14 per unit. The inclination to leave the quarantine place increased following the cumulative number of quarantine days with a rate of 1.04. Among negative emotions, people who felt lonely tended to leave the quarantine place with an increasing rate of 2.05 per unit. Moreover, anxious individuals had a higher impulse of violating the rules with an increasing rate of 1.13 per unit. In regards to social support, individuals who contacted many people were more willing to stay at the quarantine place, with an increasing rate of 0.79. In regards to social responsibility, people who agreed with the quarantine rule were willing to follow the practice with an increasing rate of 0.78. In regards to the attitude toward the government's related information, people who were confident of the government's support were willing to comply with the regulations with a rate of 0.71 per unit. In contrast, people who thought the government's policies were transparent did not want to stay at the quarantine place with a rate of 1.27 per unit. However, when we checked the correlation coefficients among the variables, as shown in Figure 7.1, the relationship between the inclination to leave and the information transparency was negative; thus, it might show

Table 7.3 Model I: Ordinal Logistic Regression Model of the Inclination to Leave

Variable	*Estimate*	*O.R.*	*95% C.I.*	*Signif.*
Demographic characteristics				
Gender, male	−0.59	0.56	(0.40, 0.78)	
Age	0.04	1.04	(1.01, 1.07)	**
Marital status, married	−0.21	0.81	(0.51, 1.28)	–
Income	0.10	1.11	(0.98, 1.26)	–
Cum. number of quarantine days	0.03	1.04	(1.00, 1.08)	–
Living environment				
Sunlight exposure	−0.22	0.80	(0.62, 1.05)	–
Negative emotions				
Loneliness	0.72	2.05	(1.72, 2.45)	
Worry about job loss	0.09	1.09	(0.97, 1.23)	–
Anxiety	0.12	1.13	(1.08, 1.18)	
Social support				
Daily contacts	−0.23	0.79	(0.66, 0.94)	**
Friend support	0.04	1.04	(0.79, 1.38)	–
Social responsibility				
Social responsibility	−0.25	0.78	(0.63, 0.96)	*
Attitude toward the government's related information				
Government support	−0.34	0.71	(0.55, 0.92)	**
Information transparency	0.24	1.27	(1.03, 1.57)	*

Significance levels are indicated as follows: $p < 0.001$; **: $p < 0.01$; *: $p < 0.05$.
The abbreviations are indicated as follows: O.R.: odds ratio; C.I.: confidence interval; Signif.: significance.

that the information transparency was a suppressor in Model I. We, therefore, built a new model, namely Model I-2, without the information transparency as shown in Table 7.4 and compared the new model with Model I using the likelihood ratio test (LRT). The result demonstrated that the performance of Model I was better than Model I-2 [$\chi^2_{(1)} = 5.05$, $p < .05$]. We, therefore, used the result of Model I in the following study.

Additionally, the model in Table 7.5 considered anxiety in separate aspects, called Model II. The results demonstrated that an anxious individual with a worsening personality had a higher tendency to leave the quarantine place with a rate of 1.49 per unit, which determined that anxiety was the most significant contributor. Yet, as we re-operated the model, in demographic characteristics, people with higher income had a higher motivation to leave the quarantine place with a rate of 1.14 per unit. Also, the inclination to leave increased with the cumulative number of quarantine days.

However, when further looking at the correlations between "the inclination to leave the quarantine place" and independent variables, as plotted in Figure 7.1,

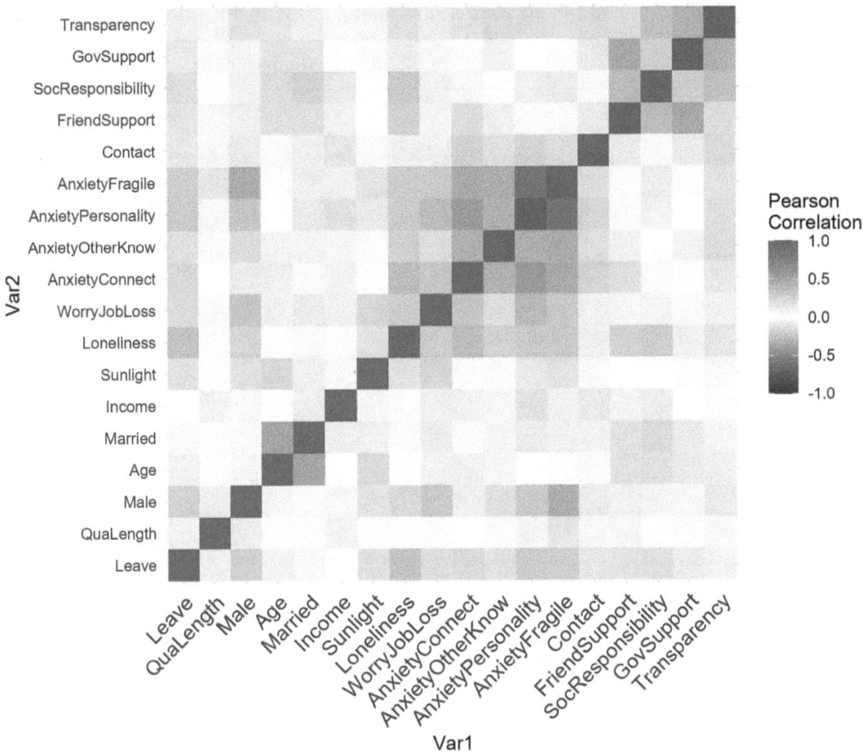

Figure 7.1 Heat Map of the Variables' Correlation Matrix

information transparency was negatively correlated to the inclination. This negative correlation was opposed to the above models, which may indicate that the transparency was a suppressor in the model. The slightly low correlation between the transparency and the inclination shrunk when the contribution of the transparency was shared by other independent variables.

Content Analysis

Among the 152 participants that took part in our study, there were 108 people who shared with us their quarantine experience and incidents that they came across at the end of the survey (71.05%), while the other participants chose not to answer the question (28.95%). Based on content analysis, their responses were categorized into two main topics: personal feelings and government performance.

Personal Feelings

Twenty people stated that the quarantine experience did not make much difference to their life (18.51%). Among these, five people mentioned that they did not feel

Table 7.4 Model I-2: Ordinal Logistic Regression Model of the Inclination to Leave

Variable	*Estimate*	*O.R.*	*95% C.I.*	*Signif.*
Demographic characteristics				
Gender, male	−0.66	0.52	(0.37, 0.72)	
Age	0.04	1.04	(1.01, 1.06)	**
Marital status, married	−0.18	0.84	(0.53, 1.33)	–
Income	0.09	1.09	(0.96, 1.24)	–
Cum. number of quarantine days	0.03	1.03	(0.99, 1.08)	–
Living environment				
Sunlight exposure	−0.24	0.79	(0.60, 1.02)	–
Negative emotions				
Loneliness	0.71	2.04	(1.71, 2.43)	
Worry about job loss	0.08	1.08	(0.96, 1.21)	–
Anxiety	0.12	1.12	(1.07, 1.17)	
Social support				
Daily contacts	−0.20	0.82	(0.69, 0.97)	*
Friend support	−0.02	0.98	(0.75, 1.29)	–
Social responsibility				
Social responsibility	−0.18	0.83	(0.68, 1.02)	–
Attitude toward the government's related information				
Government support	−0.23	0.80	(0.63, 1.01)	–

Significance levels are indicated as follows: $p < 0.001$; **: $p < 0.01$; *: $p < 0.05$.
The abbreviations are indicated as follows: O.R.: odds ratio; C.I.: confidence interval; Signif.: significance.

discriminated against and their family and friends supported them during the quarantine (4.62%). One of them said:

> Nothing special. My family and friends are very supportive.

However, another five participants said that their emotions were influenced by the quarantine experience (4.62%). Two people stated that they felt depressed (1.85%). One of them mentioned:

> During the quarantine period, I indeed felt depressed, I became more concerned about the news about the pandemic, and at the same time I became more sensitive to how the public felt.

Another participant mentioned:

> I felt bored during the last three days of the quarantine. I would have felt better if balcony and gardens had been provided.

Table 7.5 Model II: Ordinal Logistic Regression Model of the Inclination to Leave

Variable	*Estimate*	*O.R.*	*95% C.I.*	*Signif.*
Demographic characteristics				
Gender, male	−0.68	0.51	(0.36, 0.72)	
Age	0.05	1.05	(1.02, 1.08)	
Marital status, married	−0.32	0.72	(0.45, 1.16)	–
Income	0.14	1.14	(1.01, 1.30)	*
Cum. number of quarantine days	0.04	1.04	(1.00, 1.09)	*
Living environment				
Sunlight exposure	−0.23	0.8	(0.61, 1.04)	–
Negative emotion				
Loneliness	0.72	2.05	(1.71, 2.46)	
Worry about job loss	0.04	1.04	(0.92, 1.18)	–
Anxiety of losing interpersonal connections	0.17	1.19	(1.00, 1.42)	–
Anxiety of being known by others	0.06	1.07	(0.93, 1.23)	–
Anxiety of worsening personality	0.40	1.49	(1.18, 1.88)	
Anxiety of being fragile	−0.10	0.91	(0.74, 1.12)	–
Social support				
Daily contacts	−0.24	0.79	(0.66, 0.94)	
Friend support	0.07	1.07	(0.80, 1.44)	–
Social responsibility				
Social responsibility	−0.26	0.77	(0.61, 0.96)	*
Attitude toward the government's related information				
Government support	−0.34	0.71	(0.55, 0.92)	*
Information transparency	0.25	1.28	(1.04, 1.58)	*

Significance levels are indicated as follows: *: p<.05; -: insignificant.
The abbreviations are indicated as follows: O.R.: odds ratio; C.I.: confidence interval; Signif.: significance.

In addition, there were ten people who expressed their worries about getting affected by the coronavirus or affecting their family and friends, indicating that they did feel the risk of getting infected (9.26%).

Government Performance

Thirteen people claimed that the government did well in containing the pandemic and they were grateful to the government for keeping Taiwan safe (12.03%). Two of them mentioned that their friends from other countries were amazed at how well Taiwan had done (12.03%). One of the participants stated:

> I think the government of Taiwan has done an excellent job, and all my foreign friends are envious.

However, three people stated that the quarantine policy made them feel worse (2.78%). One of them suggested that the government treated those who had been quarantined as "criminals", while another said it made them "feel like being monitored by the government".

To sum up, there were mixed feelings about the quarantine experience. Most people felt that quarantine did not cause any impact on their daily life, while some did experience depression, were afraid of being affected by COVID-19, and stigmatization. Our findings are consistent with those of Dr. Tseng in Chapter 8, which demonstrate that the experience of quarantine is essentially heterogeneous for various people and that different people experience stigmatization from others to varying degrees. Moreover, those who had negative emotions were the ones that described their quarantine experience in detail. As for the responses relevant to the performance of the government, most people appreciated the actions of the government, feeling blessed as citizens of Taiwan. However, there were still a few people expressing their worries about the impact of quarantine measures on their social relationships and the fear of being tracked by the government.

Attitudes toward Policies

As shown in Table 7.6, there was not much difference between those who had and had not been quarantined in terms of attitudes toward government policies. Both found the performance of the government satisfying. Restricting individual freedom to contain the pandemic was also acceptable for people who had and had not been quarantined, indicating that those with quarantine experience felt the need for quarantine regulations. As for contact tracing, both acknowledged that it was necessary, with small differences in the share of people agreeing. However, when it comes to releasing information about the people affected with COVID-19, the two groups did not feel the need necessary enough to contain the pandemic. Most participants found the information provided by the government to be trustworthy. This could be compared with the participants who took part in "Click Diary" as most of them found the information provided by the government to be transparent.

Discussion

This study examines the noncompliance behavior in response to the quarantine regulation of "do not leave the quarantine place" the living environment, negative emotion, social support, social responsibility, and attitude toward the government's related information. Notably, this study was conducted from late March to early May, which was the most challenging public health governance situation in 2020. Considering the significance of this period, we explored compliance behavior in relation to the quarantine experience so as to improve the government's response to the pandemic while maintaining quarantined people's well-being. In addition, to gain a more comprehensive understanding of people's attitude toward policies, we also incorporated the attitudes toward policies of people who have

Table 7.6 Attitudes Toward Policies (Between May 15 and May 28, 2021)

	No. (%)	*No. (%)*
Quarantine experience	Never quarantined 1081 (93.92)	Quarantined 70 (6.08)
Satisfaction with the government		
Very dissatisfied	31 (2.87)	4 (5.71)
Dissatisfied	94 (8.70)	5 (7.14)
Neither dissatisfied nor satisfied	235 (21.74)	15 (21.43)
Satisfied	573 (53.01)	38 (54.29)
Very satisfied	148 (13.69)	8 (11.43)
Restricting individual freedom		
Strongly disagree	1 (0.09)	0 (0.00)
Disagree	12 (1.11)	3 (4.29)
Neither agree nor disagree	73 (6.75)	14 (20.00)
Agree	631 (58.37)	32 (45.71)
Strongly agree	364 (33.67)	21 (30.00)
Tracking people's movement		
Strongly disagree	16 (1.48)	3 (4.29)
Disagree	141 (13.04)	11 (15.71)
Neither agree nor disagree	252 (23.31)	20 (28.57)
Agree	507 (46.90)	25 (35.71)
Strongly agree	165 (15.26)	11 (15.71)
Releasing personal information		
Strongly disagree	142 (13.14)	15 (21.43)
Disagree	330 (30.53)	21 (30.00)
Neither agree nor disagree	281 (25.99)	14 (20.00)
Agree	266 (24.61)	13 (18.57)
Strongly agree	62 (5.74)	7 (10.00)
Information provided by the government		
Very untrustworthy	16 (1.48)	2 (2.86)
Moderately untrustworthy	44 (4.07)	1 (1.43)
Neither trustworthy nor untrustworthy	185 (17.11)	10 (14.29)
Moderately trustworthy	591 (54.67)	42 (60.00)
Very trustworthy	245 (22.66)	15 (21.43)

been quarantined and those who have never been quarantined when the number of confirmed cases increased in 2021. By examining attitudes toward policies during a time when the number of confirmed cases increased, we can also gain insights into how attitudes may shift in response to changes in the situation.

First, demographic characteristics are associated with noncompliance. According to our results, females relatively tended to violate the regulation. However, as reported by Clark et al. (2020), women were more willing to follow the government's rules than men during this pandemic, which contradicted our findings. Therefore, our study may have a confounding variable moderating or mediating the relationship between gender and noncompliance. Take anxiety, for instance. Our results indicated that women were more anxious than men, which was consistent with the findings of Parlapani et al. (2020). Furthermore, since the anxiety triggered the inclination of noncompliance (Parlapani *et al.*, 2020), the noncompliance of women may be promoted by their anxiety, which needed a further study for validation. Additionally, we found that older individuals had a higher impulse to leave the quarantine place than younger individuals. Since the relationship was unknown, older individuals may have a different belief about the rule of "do not leave the quarantine place" from the younger individuals, which required researchers to do a follow-up study on them. Furthermore, people who earned more were less likely to follow the rules, which was consistent with a past study on a tax program which indicated that the noncompliance increased as income increased (Young, 1994). Whereas, according to Wright et al. (2020), poor people were also less likely to follow the government's regulations. Therefore, the relationship between noncompliance and the economy might not be linear, which could be investigated in further studies. Besides, noncompliance became more frequent during the last quarantine days. This relationship might relate to increasing anxiety or the increasing expectancy for relief.

Second, noncompliance is connected with negative emotions. According to our results, people who felt lonely had a higher tendency to violate the quarantine rules. Although quarantine and social distancing could prevent the spread of the virus, they might also lead people to be socially isolated and thus have adverse effects on their mental health (Hwang *et al.*, 2020). Therefore, people's compliance would undoubtedly be lower. Besides, our data being consistent with past studies, suggested the quarantine experience would impact people's health and lead to mental issues (Hawryluck *et al.*, 2004). Therefore, we observed that over 10% of people were anxious about losing connections with others (14.47%), being known by others that they were quarantined (19.74%), worsening personality (15.74%), and being fragile (29.61%). Especially, anxiety about worsening personality raised people's inclination to escape from the quarantine, as negative emotions would lower people's compliance (Clark *et al.*, 2020).

Additionally, noncompliance is correlated to social support. According to our results, people with a large number of daily contacts had a lower impulse to leave the quarantine place. As people contacted more people, they were less likely to feel socially isolated (Office *et al.*, 2020) and had fewer mental issues (Mind, 2004). Therefore, similar to "loneliness", it would lower noncompliance.

Lastly, social responsibility and attitude toward government-relevant information are connected with noncompliance. According to Blendon et al. (2006), majority of people in Taiwan supported quarantining people during a public health emergency. However, it is still unknown whether people would follow the regulations when they are quarantined. The results of our study can fill this gap. People who found the quarantine policy helpful were more likely to comply with regulations. Based on this, it should be a top priority for the government to persuade people into understanding the need for quarantine regulations. When people feel that the quarantine policy is beneficial to society, people will be more willing to comply with the regulations. Therefore, it will be much easier for the government to control the public health crisis as the government would not have to monitor people as long as most of them stay in the quarantine place. Attitude toward the government is associated with noncompliance as well. People who believed that the government would provide assistance were more willing to follow the regulations. During quarantine, people feeling lonely and anxious need support, whether it is from family, friends, or the government. With confidence in the support provided by the government, people will be more likely to comply with the regulations. The government should ensure that people in quarantine have access to government support. However, Models I and II demonstrated that people who found the government's information transparency tended to leave the quarantine place. Although our models demonstrated that "transparency" promoted noncompliance, when checking the correlation between transparency and noncompliance, the relationship was slightly negative, consistent with past studies that transparency is discussed as an indispensable factor of successful COVID-19 containment (Yeh and Cheng, 2020; Yen, 2020). For this, this problem of the opposite sign may relate to the issue of the suppressor, where the high correlations among the independent variables led the suppressor "information transparency" with a low relationship with the dependent variable to change the direction of the relationship in the model. Nevertheless, due to the suppressor, the contribution of the other variables that highly correlated with the suppressor increased, such as social responsibility and government support, as demonstrated in Model I-2. Also, the performance of Model I was better than Model I-2 when tested using the LRT. Therefore, we chose to retain the variable "information transparency" in the model.

This study was limited in several ways. First, our participants from both surveys were recruited from social networks, so our study was restricted to social media users. In addition, since most of Taiwan's quarantined people were overseas-returned students or workers, most of our participants were young and relatively homogeneous in demographic attributes. Moreover, consistent with the past report (Eysenbach and Wyatt, 2002), since women were more patient with our data collection process, most of our participants who finished the survey were females. Therefore, there could be a sampling bias in data collection in terms of gender, age, and homogeneity. Besides, we failed to consider the quarantined people's opinions on the quarantine regulations. Their intention of leaving the quarantine site might also result from "control aversion" (Schmelz, 2021) to the government policies. Future studies need to measure the quarantined people's perspectives on the government's quarantine regulations. Besides, the participants were asked about whether they had "thoughts about leaving the designated place". We did not specify any particular settings in the questionnaire, such as legal issues or ethical concerns. Participants would answer based on their pure feelings on the day they took the survey, and we could not identify different degrees of desire to leave. Lastly, the negative emotions survey did not indicate that there was a psychological impact on people's mental health but indicated that people did have negative emotions in quarantine. Therefore, as most people would have had their quarantine in Taiwan, future studies could consider assessing their mental health post-quarantine since this could prove to a traumatic experience.

Policy Implications

Providing governmental and societal support for people in quarantine is vital during the pandemic, both physically and psychologically (Goethals *et al.*, 2020). Based on the results of this study, governance capacity of Taiwan has sound foundations and governance legitimacy could be seen as successfully connected to the public because most participants were satisfied with the government and they trusted the information provided by the government. Besides discussing the general principle of providing those in quarantine with adequate support, we will suggest future directions and details for policymakers to consider when coming up with quarantine regulations in the future as the COVID-19 pandemic evolves. Moreover, this study could ensure the government to tailor quarantine regulations so that people's inclination to leave the quarantine place could decline.

First, support should be provided to those with a higher tendency to leave the quarantine places. Due to limitations in government resources, coordination for effective usage is crucial, especially in times of public health crisis. According to the results of our study, the elderly tended to leave the places more than the youth. Besides, they are more likely to be infected with COVID-19, and they are also more vulnerable to mental health issues (Petretto and Pili, 2020). Therefore, the government should prioritize the needs of the elderly by providing social support networks (Cugmas *et al.*, 2021).

Second, extra care should be provided to people with mental health issues and providing them with social support. The government should pay more attention to people with mental health issues since they are more prone to violating the quarantine regulations more easily, especially those who are lonely or with anxieties about worsening personalities. According to the results of our study, people who have been quarantined could provide their feelings and details of how others treated them during the quarantine. The responses from family and friends are influential on the mood of quarantined people. Therefore, the government should come up with ways to strengthen the social support of those in quarantine so that they could better cope with negative emotions (Hou *et al.*, 2021).

Lastly, the government should ensure that the information received by quarantined people is accurate. Based on the findings of this study, people who believed that the quarantine policy was helpful to society followed the regulations. Therefore, it is critical for the government to inform the public of the necessity and helpfulness of the quarantine policy. Our results suggest that most people support the policy of restricting individual freedom when the pandemic was getting worse. However, the results also show that people in quarantine were concerned about being monitored by the government and that they were being treated unequally. As a result, it is the government's responsibility to make people feel secure when being quarantined to avoid communication crisis (Gollust *et al.*, 2020).

Conclusion

The COVID-19 pandemic and its subsequent considerable impact have imposed new challenges on governments around the world in terms of public health governance, such as resource allocation and communication with the public. Facing this severe public health crisis, quarantine is one of the most extreme prevention mechanisms, which can limit one's personal freedom in the pursuit of collective safety. Understanding people's attitudes toward quarantine is crucial for policymakers.

Many people returned to Taiwan at the beginning of the COVID-19 pandemic in late March 2020, resulting in one of the most challenging situations the country had ever faced. Using a cross-sectional survey, we studied the impacts and possible reasons for noncompliance of people who were in quarantine during the first wave of the COVID-19 outbreak from March to May 2020. To prevent the spread of the virus, these people with a potentially higher risk of infection were required to be quarantined. Their primary requirement was "not to leave the quarantine place". Yet, according to our results, their inclination toward noncompliance was relatively higher if they were women and elderly. Furthermore, high income and increasing number of quarantined days increased the motivation to leave. Among negative emotions, the higher the loneliness and anxiety, the higher the inclination toward noncompliance. Among the factors influencing anxiety, the anxiety about worsening personality contributed the most. With regards to social support, similar to loneliness, people with higher contacts were less likely to have the inclination to noncompliance. In the attitude toward government-related information, people who thought they were supported by the government and thought the government-related information was transparent had a lower inclination toward noncompliance.

We furthermore summarized their text responses and found that there were mixed feelings of gratitude, loneliness, and fear of stigmatization when they expressed feelings about their quarantine experience. Most of them did not feel much about the impact of quarantine on their life, while some were concerned about the risk of being affected by coronavirus and how others treated them. Additionally, many of them were satisfied with the government, showing appreciation in their words. While some expressed their concerns about their privacy and stigmatization. Lastly, we compared the level of government support when the mid-2021 outbreak happened in Taiwan. The severity of the pandemic could affect people's attitude toward the government greatly. However, the effect of previous quarantine experience didn't have much influence on people's attitude toward government information. The majority felt that government information was transparent when the number of confirmed COVID-19 cases was low. When the pandemic hit Taiwan in 2021, most people still found the information provided by the government trustworthy. By combining the findings of the first and second studies, we can obtain further insight into attitudes toward epidemic prevention, the quarantine mentality, and how these attitudes may vary across groups and over time. This can aid in the identification of potential barriers to compliance with epidemic prevention measures and inform the development of more effective strategies to promote compliance with these measures.

Through the findings of this study, we suggest that it is important for governments to focus on providing support to those with a higher tendency to leave quarantine places, providing extra care to people with mental health problems and providing them with social support, and ensuring that the information received by people is accurate, especially those in quarantine. To tackle challenges and crises, it is critical for governments to establish strong governance structure. Building capacity and legitimacy is an essential step toward accomplishing this goal. Capacity involves preparing necessary skills and resources to effectively govern and manage crises, and legitimacy involves establishing trust and support from the people. In addition to enhancing governance systems to face unforeseen changes, governments should also focus on the impact of governance on individuals. The implications of this study also echo Dr. Chen's study in Chapter 9, where he emphasizes the significance of having heterogeneous and distributed strategies and policies in order to achieve effective and sustainable change in society. Therefore, instead of relying on a single approach to governance, the efforts of various actors and institutions should be coordinated to create a more comprehensive and diverse strategy. For example, current dimensions that describe types of governance could be expanded to take into account the needs and weaknesses of individuals. These elements should be changed to suit the needs and priorities of the people, thus fostering a broader sense of social inclusion. We hope that the present study could shed light on the attitudes and difficulties of individuals in quarantine and may provide governments with an empirical and dynamic base to design tailored strategies to respond to epidemics.

References

Benke, C., Autenrieth, L. K., Asselmann, E. and Pané-Farré, C. A. (2020). Lockdown, quarantine measures, and social distancing: Associations with depression, anxiety and distress at the beginning of the COVID-19 pandemic among adults from Germany. *Psychiatry Research*, vol 293, pp. 113462.

Blendon, R. J., DesRoches, C. M., Cetron, M. S., Benson, J. M., Meinhardt, T. and Pollard, W. (2006). Attitudes toward the use of quarantine in a public health emergency in four countries: The experiences of Hong Kong, Singapore, Taiwan, and the United States are instructive in assessing national responses to disease threats. *Health Affairs*, vol 25, no supp 11, pp. W15–W25.

Blum, D., Smith, S. L. and Sanford, A. G. (2020). Toxic Wild West syndrome: Individual rights vs. community needs. In *COVID-19*, pp. 122–133. London: Routledge.

Cauchemez, S., Kiem, C. T., Paireau, J., Rolland, P. and Fontanet, A. (2020). Lockdown impact on COVID-19 epidemics in regions across metropolitan France. *The Lancet*, vol 396, no 10257, pp. 1068–1069.

Christensen, T. and Lægreid, P. (2020). Balancing governance capacity and legitimacy: How the Norwegian government handled the COVID-19 crisis as a high performer. *Public Administration Review*, vol 80, no 5, pp. 774–779.

Clark, C., Davila, A., Regis, M. and Kraus, S. (2020). Predictors of COVID-19 voluntary compliance behaviors: An international investigation. *Global Transitions*, vol 2, pp. 76–82.

Cugmas, M., Ferligoj, A., Kogovšek, T. and Batagelj, Z. (2021). The social support networks of elderly people in Slovenia during the Covid-19 pandemic. *PloS One*, vol 16, no 3, pp. e0247993.

Devine, D., Gaskell, J., Jennings, W. and Stoker, G. (2021). Trust and the coronavirus pandemic: What are the consequences of and for trust? An early review of the literature. *Political Studies Review*, vol 19, no 2, pp. 274–285.

Ehlers, A. and Clark, D. M. (2000). A cognitive model of posttraumatic stress disorder. *Behaviour Research and Therapy*, vol 38, no 4, pp. 319–345.

Eysenbach, G. and Wyatt, J. (2002). Using the internet for surveys and health research. *Journal of Medical Internet Research*, vol 4, no 2, pp. e13.

Fidler, D. P. (2004). Germs, governance, and global public health in the wake of SARS. *The Journal of Clinical Investigation*, vol 113, no 6, pp. 799–804.

Fu, Y. C. and Lee, H. W. (2020). Daily contacts under quarantine amid limited spread of COVID-19 in Taiwan. *International Journal of Sociology*, vol 50, no 5, pp. 434–444.

Goethals, L., Barth, N., Guyot, J., Hupin, D., Celarier, T. and Bongue, B. (2020). Impact of home quarantine on physical activity among older adults living at home during the COVID-19 pandemic: Qualitative interview study. *JMIR Aging*, vol 3, no 1, pp. e19007.

Gofen, A. (2015). Reconciling policy dissonance: Patterns of governmental response to policy noncompliance. *Policy Sciences*, vol 48, no 1, pp. 3–24.

Gollust, S. E., Nagler, R. H. and Fowler, E. F. (2020). The emergence of COVID-19 in the us: A public health and political communication crisis. *Journal of Health Politics, Policy and Law*, vol 45, no 6, pp. 967–981.

Hawryluck, L., Gold, W. L., Robinson, S., Pogorski, S., Galea, S. and Styra, R. (2004). SARS control and psychological effects of quarantine, Toronto, Canada. *Emerging Infectious Diseases*, vol 10, no 7, pp. 1206–1212.

Hiremath, P., Kowshik, C. S., Manjunath, M. and Shettar, M. (2020). COVID-19: Impact of lock-down on mental health and tips to overcome. *Asian Journal of Psychiatry*, vol 51, pp. 102088.

Hou, J., Yu, Q. and Lan, X. (2021). COVID-19 infection risk and depressive symptoms among young adults during quarantine: The moderating role of grit and social support. *Frontiers in Psychology*, vol 11, pp. 577942.

Hsieh, H. F. and Shannon, S. E. (2005). Three approaches to qualitative content analysis. *Qualitative Health Research*, vol 15, no 9, pp. 1277–1288.

Hwang, T. J., Rabheru, K., Peisah, C., Reichman, W. and Ikeda, M. (2020). Loneliness and social isolation during the COVID-19 pandemic. *International Psychogeriatrics*, vol 32, no 10, pp. 1217–1220.

Kılınçel, Ş., Kılınçel, O., Muratdağı, G., Aydın, A. and Usta, M. B. (2021). Factors affecting the anxiety levels of adolescents in home-quarantine during COVID-19 pandemic in Turkey. *Asia-Pacific Psychiatry*, vol 13, no 2, pp. e12406.

Kirigia, J. M. and Kirigia, D. G. (2011). The essence of governance in health development. *International Archives of Medicine*, vol 4, no 1, pp. 1–13.

Mind. (2004). *Not alone?: Isolation and mental distress*. London, UK: Mind.

Nivette, A., Ribeaud, D., Murray, A., Steinhoff, A., Bechtiger, L., Hepp, U., Shanahan, L. and Eisner, M. (2021). Non-compliance with COVID-19-related public health measures among young adults in Switzerland: Insights from a longitudinal cohort study. *Social Science & Medicine*, vol 268, pp. 113370.

Office, E. E., Rodenstein, M. S., Merchant, T. S., Pendergrast, T. R. and Lindquist, L. A. (2020). Reducing social isolation of seniors during COVID-19 through medical student telephone contact. *Journal of the American Medical Directors Association*, vol 21, no 7, pp. 948–950.

Parlapani, E., Holeva, V., Voitsidis, P., Blekas, A., Gliatas, I., Porfyri, G.N., Golemis, A., Papadopoulou, K., Dimitriadou, A., Chatzigeorgiou, A.F. and Bairachtari, V. (2020). Psychological and behavioral responses to the COVID-19 pandemic in Greece. *Frontiers in Psychiatry*, vol 11, pp. 821.

Pereira, B. and Stornelli, J. (2022). Collective health versus individual freedom: Goal centrality and political identity shape COVID-19 prevention behaviors. *Journal of the Association for Consumer Research*, vol 7, no 1, pp. 17–26.

Petretto, D. R. and Pili, R. (2020). Ageing and COVID-19: What is the role for elderly people? *Geriatrics*, vol 5, no 2, pp. 25.

Reynolds, D. L., Garay, J., Deamond, S., Moran, M. K., Gold, W. and Styra, R. (2008). Understanding, compliance and psychological impact of the SARS quarantine experience. *Epidemiology & Infection*, vol 136, no 7, pp. 997–1007.

Rothstein, M. A. and Talbott, M. K. (2007). Encouraging compliance with quarantine: A proposal to provide job security and income replacement. *American Journal of Public Health*, vol 97, no Supplement_1, pp. S49–S56.

Ruengorn, C., Awiphan, R., Wongpakaran, N., Wongpakaran, T., Nochaiwong, S. and Health Outcomes and Mental Health Care Evaluation Survey Research Group (HOME-Survey). (2021). Association of job loss, income loss, and financial burden with adverse mental health outcomes during coronavirus disease 2019 pandemic in Thailand: A nationwide cross-sectional study. *Depression and Anxiety*, vol 38, no 6, pp. 648–660.

Ryu, S., Hwang, Y., Yoon, H. and Chun, B. C. (2022). Self-quarantine noncompliance during the COVID-19 pandemic in South Korea. *Disaster Medicine and Public Health Preparedness*, vol 16, no 2, pp. 464–467.

Schmelz, K. (2021). Enforcement may crowd out voluntary support for COVID-19 policies, especially where trust in government is weak and in a liberal society. *Proceedings of the National Academy of Sciences*, vol 118, no 1, pp. e2016385118.

Six, F., De Vadder, S., Glavina, M., Verhoest, K. and Pepermans, K. (2021). What drives compliance with COVID-19 measures over time? Explaining changing impacts with goal framing theory. *Regulation & Governance*, vol 17, no 1, pp. 3–21.

Taiwan CDC. (2020). *Press Release*. Retrieved October, 11, 2020, from https://sites.google.com/cdc.gov.tw/2019-ncov/Taiwan

Wang, C., Song, W., Hu, X., Yan, S., Zhang, X., Wang, X. and Chen, W. (2021). Depressive, anxiety, and insomnia symptoms between population in quarantine and general population during the COVID-19 pandemic: A case controlled study. *BMC Psychiatry*, vol 21, no 1, pp. 1–9.

Wright, A. L., Sonin, K., Driscoll, J. and Wilson, J. (2020). Poverty and economic dislocation reduce compliance with COVID-19 shelter-in-place protocols. *Journal of Economic Behavior & Organization*, vol 180, pp. 544–554.

Yeh, M. J. and Cheng, Y. (2020). Policies tackling the COVID-19 pandemic: A sociopolitical perspective from Taiwan. *Health Security*, vol 18, no 6, pp. 427–434.

Yen, W. T. (2020). Taiwan's COVID-19 management: Developmental state, digital governance, and state-society synergy. *Asian Politics & Policy*, vol 12, no 3, pp. 455–468.

Yildirim, H., Işik, K. and Aylaz, R. (2021). The effect of anxiety levels of elderly people in quarantine on depression during COVID-19 pandemic. *Social Work in Public Health*, vol 36, no 2, pp. 194–204.

Young, J. C. (1994). Factors associated with noncompliance: Evidence from the Michigan tax amnesty program. *The Journal of the American Taxation Association*, vol 16, no 2, pp. 82.

8 Negotiating the Risk-Stigma Assemblage

Quarantine Experiences of Returnees to Taiwan during the COVID-19 Pandemic

Fan-Tzu Tseng

Introduction

Since 2020, coronavirus disease (COVID-19) has swept the globe, causing more than 765 million confirmed cases and 6.9 million deaths worldwide as of April 30, 2023. This unanticipated pandemic has compelled countries to employ various public health measures to combat the disease, while attempting to strike a balance between mitigating virus transmission and maintaining everyday social activities. Taiwan was among the few countries to maintain stringent border controls and quarantines throughout much of the pandemic. When the outbreak originated in Wuhan, China, the Taiwanese government immediately launched quarantine protocols to minimize the possibility of virus introduction, given the frequency of cross-strait travel and the lessons learned from the mismanagement of the 2003 severe acute respiratory syndrome (SARS) outbreak. As COVID-19 spread globally, the quarantine target population broadened from solely inbound travelers from Wuhan to encompass all arrivals. These individuals, classified as "people at risk of infection," were mandated to undergo a 14-day quarantine (later augmented with seven days of self-health management). This prolonged requirement persisted until early March 2022, when the government began phasing out its zero-COVID policy. Subsequently, the quarantine duration was gradually shortened, culminating in its complete elimination in October 2022. These border controls and quarantine measures were often acknowledged as a key factor in Taiwan's ability to avoid large-scale, uncontrolled community transmission (Soon 2021; Steinbrook 2021) in 2020 and 2021. Public health scholar and former Taiwanese Vice President Chen Chien-jen lauded the quarantined individuals as "unsung heroes" in Taiwan's battle against the pandemic who relinquished their personal freedom for the sake of enabling the majority to lead a conventional life (Wen, Gu, and Ye 2020).

Contrary to the positive official narrative, individuals returning from abroad were subjected to intense stigmatization. At the start of the outbreak in early 2020, Taiwanese returnees from mainland China quickly encountered cyberattacks and faced a social backlash that put them under enormous pressure. Instances of returnees not complying with social distancing measures was publicly exposed, and the identification of a businesswoman returning from Wuhan as the first case of COVID-19 in Taiwan triggered strident protests on the Facebook page of the

DOI: 10.4324/9781003438380-12

Central Epidemic Command Center (CECC). The returnees were labeled as "selfish" and even referred to as "suicide bombers" threatening Taiwan. As the pandemic spread globally, citizens returning from different countries faced similar condemnations, and opposition to the return of overseas Taiwanese came to the fore. Although there were media reports of discrimination against returnees and community opposition to the presence of home quarantinees (e.g., Taipei Times 2020), critical reflection on this stigmatization rarely appeared in the public sphere.

Disease and morality are intrinsically intertwined, affecting not only the experience of those infected but also shaping society's response to associated risks. Bayer (2008) candidly acknowledges that as modern states take increasingly systematic action to prevent and control infectious diseases, stigmatization of specific subjects is almost inevitable. In order to effectively minimize the risk of disease transmission, the management of potential virus carriers becomes necessary. However, it is well known that the stigmatization accompanying such policies can cause them to backfire by pushing the potentially infected to hide their risk status to avoid unfair treatment. Therefore, conducting an in-depth examination of how such stigmatization influences the perspectives and experiences of individuals in quarantine, along with its potential implications for national pandemic governance, has become a crucial concern in the COVID-19 era.

This study draws on the case of Taiwan's quarantine of citizen-returnees during COVID-19 to contribute to the literature on stigma and public health governance. Beyond the analysis of policy discourse, I delve into the quarantine experiences of these individuals to see how they dealt with the government-imposed risk status and the related social stigma. Considering that infectious disease control always requires a combination of individual costs and social collaboration, this study argues that the commitment of returnees to strict quarantine is not merely a product of obedience to authority or individual conscience, but is enacted within a heterogeneous assemblage that has emerged to combat the pandemic. This heterogeneous assemblage brings together various elements of government risk regulation and social sanctions, and is conceptualized in this chapter as a "risk-stigma assemblage." I will use this concept to illuminate how the risk management and stigmatization experiences of the quarantined are mutually constituted within this assemblage. This intertwined configuration, in turn, prompted returnees to strengthen their self-governance both to minimize the probability of infection and transmission and also to legitimize their return during the pandemic and allow them to reclaim their moral membership in the Taiwanese community.

Taiwan's Quarantine Policy and Its Evolution

Quarantine is not a novel epidemic management technique but can be traced back to the restrictive measures used against people from infected areas when the Byzantine Empire was threatened with plague in the sixth century AD (Little 2007). In contemporary liberal countries, however, depriving people who are merely potentially infected of their rights can easily lead to ethical and legal disputes (Gostin, Bayer, and Fairchild 2003); therefore, quarantine has seldom been a favored prevention measure. The 2003 SARS outbreak prompted several East Asian countries, including Taiwan, to introduce mandatory quarantine as a means of controlling the epidemic, sparking debates about its effectiveness in infectious diseases management (Day et al. 2006; Barbisch, Koenig, and Shih 2015). In the case of Taiwan, over 150,000 individuals were quarantined, of whom only 46 were subsequently identified as probable SARS patients (Chen et al. 2005). Such discrepancies led sociologists to criticize the scientific basis for the policy's loose definition of risk.

As an island nation, Taiwan's natural geographical separation from the rest of the world enables the implementation of rigorous border controls and mandatory quarantine measures, forming the core strategy of its pandemic governance. In response to the COVID-19 outbreak, the CECC issued in April 2020 a "Tracking and Management Mechanism for People at Risk of Infection" (see Figure 8.1), which outlined specific requirements for individuals undergo "home isolation" as close contacts and "home quarantine" for inbound travelers.[1] These requirements included: (1) mandatory 14-day confinement at home or a designated location without leaving the premises, (2) regular health monitoring by authorities, and (3) seeking medical care only through health agencies if symptoms are suspected. The government allocated quarantine subsidies (around $35 per day) and assigned district/village-level officials to closely monitor the health and movements of those under quarantine, providing support and resources as needed (Yen and Liu 2021). Furthermore, an "electronic security monitoring system" was launched as early as February 2020, utilizing mobile phone positioning technology to track the whereabouts of quarantinees; violators would be subject to forced placement and fines under the Communicable Disease Control Act. These regulations reflected the government's approach of treating all overseas arrivals as potentially high risk, necessitating quarantine and daily health monitoring during the COVID-19 incubation period. At the same time, compliance concerns for these individuals required enhanced management through mobile phone signal tracking.

Throughout 2020 and 2021, as COVID-19 spread worldwide and the virus continued to mutate, Taiwan's quarantine policy adhered to the principle "better too tight than too loose" that had characterized SARS governance (Wu and Tseng 2006),

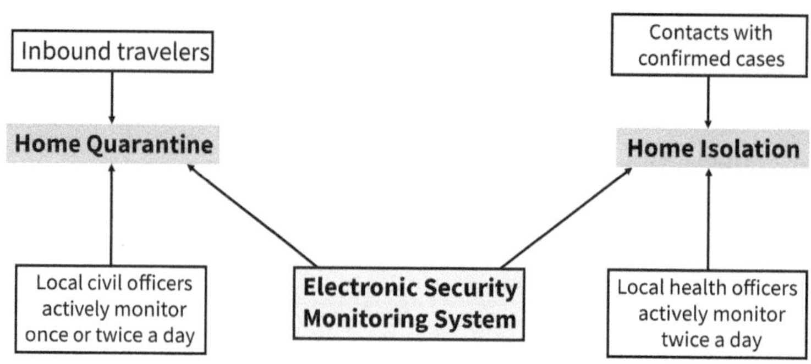

Figure 8.1 Tracking and management mechanism for people at risk of infection

without the flexibility to adjust requirements based on country-specific epidemic situations or the vaccination records of individual arrivals. Moreover, the quarantine regulations became increasingly stringent. In spring 2021, returnees were no longer allowed to quarantine in households where non-quarantinees were present, even if they were able to maintain sufficient social distance; home quarantine was then completely banned at the end of June 2021 as it was blamed for causing Taiwan's first Delta outbreak. Subsequently, arrivals from countries deemed high risk were directed to government facilities for quarantine, whereas others were mandated to stay in designated hotels at their own expense. In addition, all quarantinees were obligated to present a negative test result before being released, or they would be transferred to a hospital for isolation as confirmed cases. Over the next few months, the frequency and type of required testing increased. At the end of 2021, CECC had to reopen the option of home quarantine in anticipation of the upcoming influx of returnees for Lunar New Year celebrations during the global Omicron surge. However, cohabitants were required to engage in enhanced self-health management and self-funded rapid screening, essentially placing them in a state of "quasi-quarantine" solely because they lived under the same roof with actual quarantinees. Arguably, the escalating price of freedom for those quarantined under the zero-COVID policy framework presented greater challenges for them to shed their risk status and the associated stigma of being perceived as potential carriers of the virus.

Despite the implementation of stringent measures, the government faced the infiltration of the highly transmissible Omicron variant in spring 2022 and had to shift from the "zero-COVID" strategy to a new paradigm of "living with the virus." This transition led to a significant loosening of regulations, which in tandem with a rapid surge in daily Omicron cases, led to a greater number of new cases within a fortnight than the total number of cases recorded over the preceding two years. Considering that over 99% of confirmed patients were asymptomatic or mildly symptomatic, CECC insisted on the path of opening up and progressively loosened the mandatory quarantine requirements until their complete elimination in October 2022. Nevertheless, the relaxation of quarantine measures for new arrivals had been significantly slower compared to the reduction in home isolation periods for locally infected residents. For example, while the home isolation period for confirmed patients was reduced to three days in late April 2022, the home quarantine duration for new arrivals was not similarly shortened until mid-June, although they were still required to present negative test results before boarding a plane. Therefore, although the policy shift meant that Taiwan was no longer a largely COVID-free haven, overseas returnees were still considered an alien threat requiring differentiation, labelling, and discriminatory treatment.

Stigma and Infectious Disease Governance

Throughout the history of infectious diseases, quarantine measures for epidemic control have been intertwined with the stigmatization of individuals who might transmit diseases. Stigmatization, in this context, refers to the social process of excluding those perceived as potential disease sources, posing a threat to society's normal functioning (Bhanot et al. 2021). It has even been argued that quarantine-related stigmatization may be considered an "appropriate" form of stigma (Lee et al. 2005), as it produces "a marking off, the creation of a boundary to ward off a feared biological contaminant lest it penetrate a healthy population" (Musto 1986, p. 98). It is worth noting that not all diseases controlled through quarantine evoke the same level of stigma (compared to chickenpox, for example). In addition to the biological nature of the disease itself (e.g., its perceived lethality or contagiousness), equally important is the perceived moral responsibility of those infected (e.g., the infection's controllability, personal responsibility, and culpability for contracting the disease) (Williams, Gonzalez-Medina, and Le 2011). In Taiwan's public perception of COVID-19, widespread media coverage of the catastrophic global pandemic reinforced its gruesome image as a deadly disease, while personal hygiene and social distancing to curb transmission emphasized individual responsibility for infection and transmission. However, the higher stigmatization experienced by even non-diagnosed quarantinees in Taiwan compared to other advanced countries (Hale 2022) remains unexplained by these accounts.

Mary Douglas's early work on purity and danger set the stage for further inquiry into the function and meaning of stigma for the social collective (Douglas 1966; Douglas and Wildavsky 1982). She argued that the social perception of impurity stemmed from the confusion of established categorical boundaries, which in turn was perceived as dangerous, triggering anxiety and attempts to avoid or even suppress it in order to reestablish and stabilize the pre-existing symbolic order. Douglas emphasized that this cognitive framework was by no means unique to primitive societies: Even though contemporary societies replaced the identification of danger with the ostensibly scientific and neutral language of "risk," it was still essentially about blame allocation and moral concern, and both served to protect a set of values relevant to a particular way of life. Many empirical studies continue this line of thought by arguing that the condemnation of particular subjects that results from epidemics is not only motivated by people's fear of contagion, but also reflects a quest for order and certainty to reduce the sense of vulnerability. After all, condemning others "defines the normal, establishes the boundaries of healthy behavior and appropriate social relationships, and distinguishes the observer from the causes of fear" (Nelkin and Gilman 1988, p. 363). Stigma can thus be viewed as a social engineering tool to eliminate aliens, clarify and reaffirm important community values, consolidate self-identity, and strengthen coherence among members.

Lupton (2013) highlights the critical status of emotion in Douglas's analysis of individual and group reactions to the Other, and their desire to maintain social groups and demarcate symbolic and physical boundaries; she further develops the concept of the "emotion-risk assemblage" to show that how people respond to risk is motivated by emotion, and therefore public health discourses and practices often purposefully use emotional appeals to identify and contain risk. Notably, although Lupton uses the neutral, umbrella term "emotion" to construct a more general conceptualization of the relationship between risk and emotion, she also points out that the emotions mobilized in public health campaigns are often negative, such as shame, guilt, disgust, and fear, and are often deployed through strategies that "incite or reproduce" the stigmatization of the target group (Lupton 2013, p. 634).

These studies inspire us to look beyond the disease itself to other material and non-material factors that foster the stigmatization of potential transmitters. For example, exclusionary public health practices used to combat disease may themselves reinforce fears of these "others" (Brooks et al. 2020). Quarantine, in particular, consists of a set of institutional practices that mark difference, link stereotypes, differentiate others, and create status gaps and discrimination, all of which are essential elements of stigmatization (Link and Phelan 2014). Moreover, Taiwan's response to COVID-19 witnessed strong moralistic criticism that went beyond the socially disadvantaged groups typically described in the literature as excluded during community crisis to target Taiwanese citizens returning from overseas.[2] These returnees, once seen as relatively privileged people capable of living or traveling abroad, were now regarded as a potential threat of virus transmission to this otherwise safe and secure island. This stigmatization of citizen-returnees reflects not so much a fear of the virus that transcends class boundaries as an attempt by those living on the island to redefine who belongs to "us" as an imagined community united against the pandemic. Such identity work is most active and intense when the social gap between the stigmatizers and the stigmatized is less pronounced (Crawford 1994), and leads to the mobilization of specific moral boundaries to exclude the perceived Other. Given the Taiwanese authorities' reliance on border control and quarantine, it is worth exploring what moral tensions shape returnees' engagement with quarantine regulations and how they may influence the outcome of pandemic governance.

In addition, while critical social science approaches have recognized that risk is not simply a matter of probabilistic knowledge, but is linked to specific categories, values, and timeframes (such as emergencies or long-term threats) (Heyman 2010; Brown 2020), further theorization is needed to understand the interrelation of these factors. Building upon the insights of Douglas and Lupton's analysis of the intersection of categories, values, and emotions in individuals' responses to risk, this study goes further to explore how the timeframe of quarantine, which sets a defined and relatively short-term duration for the presence of risk, affects individuals' perception and reactions to risk and stigma. This temporal aspect distinguishes quarantine-related stigmatization from other forms of social exclusion based on more permanent attributes such as race, class, or chronic illness. By highlighting this temporary nature, I believed that quarantine will be a more productive case for elucidating the configuration of these risk-related elements and unraveling their interactions.

This chapter proposes the concept of "risk-stigma assemblage" to describe the unique arrangements and complex dynamics experienced by quarantinees in Taiwan. The concept formally draws on the work of Lupton (2013), but uses the more direct term "stigma" rather than "emotion" to name the primary elements that shape each other with risk. The term "assemblage" indicates that the relationship between risk and stigma is not fixed, but fluid and variable in the interplay of its ideological, material, human, and non-human heterogeneous elements (Marcus and Saka 2006). This concept thus serves to distinguish between different types of stigmas concerning risk (although they may evoke similar emotions) and to clarify which stigmas relate to the disease itself, which result from particular ways of governing, and which represent the struggle of "separating, placing boundaries, making visible statements about the home that we are intending to create" (Douglas 1966, p. 85) in the midst of community crisis. I also describe the engagement of these returnees in quarantine practices and the negotiation of moral boundaries and membership in their quest to be re-accepted as part of the Taiwanese community. Finally, the concluding section suggests the potential contributions of this concept and highlights the implications of the timeframe of quarantine.

Methods and Data

The main analysis is based on in-depth interviews with 50 individuals who returned to Taiwan from abroad in 2020–2021. Although some residents who did not travel also required quarantine due to potential contact with local COVID patients, these experiences are not included in this study because community transmission in Taiwan was quite low during most of the study period, and their perspectives on infection risk, expectations and preparedness for quarantine, and social stigma encountered may differ from those of returnees.

Of the participants in this study, 18 were recruited through an online survey on daily contacts during quarantine, conducted from March to May 2020 (Fu and Lee 2020). An additional 14 participants were referred by these initial interviewees, and the rest were sourced from the author's personal network. Participants experienced a total of 56 instances of quarantine. Notably, 26 of these instances took place in March 2020, coinciding with the escalation of the pandemic in Europe and the United States. This period witnessed a significant influx of overseas students and workers into Taiwan, leading to the first wave of imported COVID-19 cases and presenting challenges to the government's quarantine management system and community acceptance. Furthermore, 21 instances were scattered between April and December 2020, with an additional nine instances occurring in 2021. The last recorded instance took place in December 2021. Additionally, 17 of these instances occurred in institutions such as the quarantine hotels or government-run group quarantine facilities, while the remaining instances were conducted in homes or other private residences.

The participants included 31 females and 18 males, aged 22–57 years. The largest age group was 30–39 years (26 participants), followed by 20–29 years (17 participants). Nearly all participants (48 out of 49) had a university degree or higher, with 27 holding a bachelor's degree and 21 having a master's degree or higher. In terms of occupation, there were 12 students, 7 unemployed individuals, 7 working part time, and 23 full-time workers.

Interviews for this study covered topics including the reasons behind individuals' departures and returns, their journey home and quarantine process, interactions with government regulatory systems, assessment of and response to infection risks, and encounters with stigma. The interviews, lasting approximately one to two hours, were recorded with participants' consent and transcribed verbatim. This chapter is organized based on core categories derived from coding and the richness of the collected data, focusing on the quarantinees' navigation of the risk-stigma assemblage and their negotiation strategies to mitigate its effects. Participants are referred to using pseudonyms with dates and sites of quarantine to facilitate the contextualization of their experiences in the evolving landscape of the pandemic and the corresponding quarantine measures. To this end, I additionally collected relevant policies, regulations, and documents published by the CECC and local governments, media reports, popular comments, and official statements, and I also attended related academic workshops and conferences to gain a comprehensive understanding of the evolution of institutional requirements and quarantine measures during the pandemic.

Being a "Walking Virus" in the Eyes of Society

During the first two years of the pandemic, COVID-19 was widely perceived in Taiwan as a deadly and highly destructive disease to society. This image of the disease instilled a sense of fear in the population and legitimized the government's adherence to a strict strategy to "keep the virus out" through strict border controls and mandatory quarantine measures in order to achieve the policy goal of "zero COVID." As part of these measures, people returning from overseas were classified as "at risk of infection" and subjected to mandatory movement restrictions and health monitoring for more than two weeks. These measures appeared to reinforce the perception that these individuals posed a potential threat to Taiwanese society. Although many of the participants in this study mentioned being almost moved to tears when hearing "welcome home" from customs officers upon entry, they were still concerned about hostility toward their return. As Renee (2020-10/Institution) said, "[People] won't be happy to see someone like you come back." For this reason, Renee chose to quarantine at a hotel instead of at home to avoid the neighbors' complaints.

> I think Taiwanese folks simply want zero imported cases, so they can feel at ease. They just can't wrap their heads around the idea of having infected individuals detected and treated here. So, instead of getting frustrated with why they are like this, just adjust yourself.

"Adjusting yourself," as Renee suggested, essentially means minimizing the potential harm to others. For returnees, utilizing the risk management techniques provided by the government was one of the few available strategies. For example, prior to December 2020, Taiwan did not require all arrivals to present a negative COVID test; only those displaying symptoms were tested at the airport. Some returnees, in order to reduce the risk of "bringing back the virus," pretended to be unwell upon entry to undergo state-funded testing. Shelly (2020-03/home) mentioned her sister's concerns about her returning home for quarantine, fearing it could endanger their parents. As a result, Shelly opted to request a test upon arrival to demonstrate her "cleanliness":

> My sister … she thought I WAS a walking virus…. so I went for the test, that is, I told the border agent that my throat was itchy. (Q: Did you really have an itchy throat?) No, I really didn't. She kept going on about how asymptomatic infections are terrible… and it made me so mad. I said to myself, "Fine, I'll get tested right at the border… (Q: Were you afraid of testing positive?) Not really, but I did have a slight allergy, yeah, so maybe there was like a 5% chance? … But as soon as I got the test results, I told my sister, "See! I'm negative."

The characteristics of COVID-19, such as its incubation period, resemblance to other respiratory illnesses, and the potential for asymptomatic infection, make it challenging to rely solely on apparent health status as an indicator of infection. Medical technology is necessary to detect the presence of the virus in the body. However, before comprehensive arrival testing was implemented, border controls depended on the cooperation of individuals who were potentially infected to aid in virus detection and management. The same applied to symptom monitoring during quarantine, where quarantinees were required to report their health status through daily phone calls or the CECC's digital system, but ultimately had to self-monitor their physical condition and decide what information to disclose to the authorities. Joyce (2020-03/home), for example, had a runny nose during quarantine and chose to request testing:

> I thought it was an allergy, but I wasn't sure. That's why I had to take such an action, otherwise I could go out and endanger others later, in case I really had it.

Most returnees in this study acknowledged their risk status and willingly engaged in national pandemic prevention measures to manage it. Beyond their genuine concern for others' well-being, they also sought to avoid the stigma of being perceived as a "walking virus" by their neighbors and even their own family members. Unfortunately, Joyce's responsible decision to report her symptoms led to the revelation of her quarantine status when an ambulance arrived at her doorstep to take her for a hospital test, exposing her family to community ostracism and gossip. Despite testing negative, Joyce continued to stay home for nearly another month after her quarantine period ended, opting to "play it safe." She had heard of cases with incubation periods of "up to 21 days" and worried about being blamed for an infection if someone contracted the virus after she had been outside. These experiences highlight how returnees' perceptions and responses to their risk status were strongly influenced by the stigma they perceived and encountered. This led them to employ elements of the risk-stigma assemblage, such as configuring space (e.g., staying in a quarantine hotel), time (e.g., prolonged self-quarantine), or adopting virus detection techniques to enhance self-governance.

Despite these efforts, many returnees noted that the stigma could persist for a period of time even after they fulfilled their mandated quarantine obligations. Tony (2021-08/hotel) was denied entry to a clinic after 21 days of quarantine and self-health management because his NHI card still indicated his quarantine record. Additionally, a notice was posted at his regular barber shop refusing service to customers who had been in Taiwan for less than a month. Similarly, Hela (2021-12, hotel) was forced by her employer to take additional weeks of unpaid leave simply because a client discovered that the quarantine hotel Hela was staying at happened to have a cluster infection, even though she was not involved and had multiple negative test results. "For me, the pressure from Taiwanese people is greater than the virus itself," Hella remarked. Notably, while other participants who quarantined in 2020 had similar experiences of stigmatization, the local outbreak in May 2021 heightened domestic anxieties regarding infection risks and further exacerbated the rejection of returnees. Although experts continue to debate the origins of this outbreak, public opinion attributed it to insufficient quarantine enforcement (Zennie and Tsai 2021). This suggests that returnees were collectively scapegoated for causing the outbreak of domestic transmission that resulted in over 800 deaths.

Suffering from the Unintended Stigmatization of National Prevention Measures

As Joyce and Tony's experience illustrated, returnees could be inadvertently exposed to social stigma due to imperfect government procedures or technical errors, despite fulfilling their quarantine obligations. One example was the government's detailed epidemiological investigations for COVID-19 cases, along with the accompanying press releases with basic profiles of newly detected patients and their whereabouts during their infectious period. While such measures were intended to enable the public to identify potential social contacts, in the context of society's pursuit of achieving "zero COVID," any information disclosure could amplify public scrutiny of these patients' movements as people searched for any sign of "immorality," which sometimes even sparked online manhunts to uncover their true identities. Kevin (2020-3/home) admitted feeling "scared" during his return journey and subsequent quarantine, which I initially attributed to fear of being infected. However, he later explained that his anxiety stemmed from the possibility of becoming the target of an online manhunt if he tested positive:

> It's scary… At that time, the returnees were witches and everyone was hunting for them. So, we all felt very anxious. No one wanted to be the target of a multitude of arrows.

While most of the quarantinees did not believe they were actually infected, the uncertainty surrounding the incubation period of COVID-19 made it challenging for them to ease their concerns. Even with negative PCR tests before departure or during quarantine, the possibility of sudden diagnosis remained a source of anxiety, especially considering that recovered individuals could still test positive weeks later. Julia (2020-3/home) expressed her reluctance to leave her room even during the self-health management period following the two-week quarantine, which she hoped would lead to a more sympathetic media portrayal if she were diagnosed: "They would just say she stayed home all the time." Another participant, Hella (2021-12/hotel), shared a similar sentiment. These self-imposed restrictions aimed to completely eliminate the risk of endangering others and the subsequent social condemnation. During a COVID-19 workshop, I encountered an attendee who expressed a preference for being infected abroad, as he believed he would go unnoticed among the countless confirmed cases. The sole participant in this study who was diagnosed during quarantine faced accusations from his own family. Despite the limited personal details provided in the CECC's announcements of confirmed cases, relatives who knew his return schedule were able to identify him in the news. They blamed his parents for allowing him to return and accused him of acting recklessly and neglecting his duty to "take care of himself":

> [They] said things like "Oh, how could you be so careless?" "How could this happen? Weren't you wearing protective gear properly?" "You must have been wandering around" or "[I] told you not to eat [on the plane], but you didn't listen!"

In addition, technical errors often occurred in the electronic fences set up by the government that caused quarantinees to be misidentified as having gone out without permission, leading to police visits and thus exposing their identities to the neighbors. For example, during quarantine Ingrid (2020-3/home) was eating dinner in her room when she received a text message claiming that she had been detected leaving her home and should return immediately. Before she could contact the system to explain the situation, the police had appeared at her door and asked Ingrid to prove that she was home:

> I opened the window from upstairs to talk to them and let them see me … and then I felt upset because my home is in kind of a small rural area and whenever a police car drives by the whole street will know about it.… At the moment, I saw many people running out to see why the police were there, and we had to shout from afar, … I was like, "well, now the whole street knows I am here in quarantine."

Although Ingrid did not experience direct stigmatization from her community following the incident, she experienced a sense of "felt stigma" (Scambler 2004) and discomfort regarding the disclosure of her quarantine status. This feeling was exacerbated by her mother being asked to take leave from work during Ingrid's home quarantine as a precautionary measure against potential virus transmission. Ingrid became acutely aware of the stigma associated with individuals returning from abroad and their families, which intensified her fears of societal condemnation if she were to contract the disease. Her heightened perception of risk was further influenced by encountering online criticism directed towards returnees during her quarantine period. Consequently, Ingrid became more vigilant towards any potential symptoms and constantly worried about her own infection, despite her anxiety not being based on actual evidence:

> I think that was psychological … [because] every day I read some news and some discussions and then a lot of people posted about how horrible these things were and about how annoying it was for people back in this country, and it worried me.

While returnees achieved self-governance through investing in government risk techniques, these techniques sometimes brought about unintended stigma. This demonstrates the fluid and contingent nature of the various elements and relationships within the risk-stigma assemblage. As the pandemic progressed, some infection control measures improved the protection of privacy; for example, quarantinees were later allowed to take their own vehicles to seek medical treatment without alerting neighbors, as long as they had prior permission from the authorities. The gradual opening of Taiwan in 2022, coupled with the fact that the number of locally infected patients far exceeded imported ones due to the domestic Omicron outbreak, meant that the CECC was no longer able to conduct detailed case investigations and provide briefings on individual cases at daily press conferences. Against the backdrop of these changes, it could be inferred that the stigmatization of returnees would be significantly diminished, even though they still carried the risk of infection. After all, in comparison to the thousands of new cases diagnosed daily on the island, even if someone "brought the virus back to Taiwan," as mentioned earlier, they were just "one of the countless confirmed cases and no one would even notice."

Negotiating the Othering of the Taiwanese "National Health Insurance Community"

As social science research on epidemics has shown, classification and stigmatization arise not only from the biological risks of disease, but also from efforts to preserve social groups and reinforce established values. New Zealand, which instituted similar border controls to Taiwan for most of the pandemic, also witnessed stigmatization of individuals returning from overseas. This phenomenon prompted anthropologist Susanna Trnka (2021) to observe the redefined boundaries of community in the context of the pandemic: The identities of those who were once "us" were "erased," repositioned as "strangers" or "potential COVID-19 carriers," and symbolized "an irresponsible state that failed to get things right."

Such pervasive xenophobic sentiment was arguably an inevitable by-product of the stringent border controls the state implemented to combat the epidemic. While the government prioritized its own citizens, allowing individuals with citizenship to enter and benefit from the state's care and protection, legal membership alone was not enough to neutralize societal hostility. Returnees were systematically categorized as potential infectious risks, and their exclusion was often driven by factors beyond the mere biological threat of the disease. The online attacks targeting returning Taiwanese individuals exemplified how they were branded as opportunistic individuals seeking to exploit Taiwan's healthcare resources and benefit from the collective efforts of other Taiwanese in containing the epidemic. Tiffany (2020-03/home), who temporarily returned to Taiwan due to visa problems while in the process of emigrating abroad, vividly expressed the overwhelming stigma she experienced.

> At that time, we felt as if we were sinners, that is, when we came back, it was as if we wore a sign that we were abusing Taiwan's health care, or [we] were the kind of people who, for example, revere everything foreign and pander to overseas powers, and only now think of the goodness of our own country, this and that. So this is the kind of pressure that we inexplicably carry and can only bear in silence.

Vivian (2020-03/home), who worked abroad and returned to Taiwan due to concerns about the severity of the outbreak and her own chronic cough symptoms, also described feeling "guilty" when she decided to return:

> When I came back, if I had such … a little guilt, I think we should all have, that is, I wondered if it would cause a waste of resources in Taiwan. Or, like I [later] did three [negative] tests, in fact, I think these costs were additional expenses for this country's epidemic prevention costs, … it was not something I deserved or took for granted.

Just as COVID-19 is often likened to a social mirror reflecting pre-existing tensions, this type of stigma suggests the long-standing debate over whether overseas Taiwanese are abusing Taiwan's NHI system and the deeper anxiety over who is one of "us" in the context of Taiwan's ambiguous national status (Lee 2020). The condemnation of "abuse" is reminiscent of frequent media reports of Taiwanese expatriates suspending their payment of Taiwanese NHI premiums, only to return to Taiwan and resume coverage when they need expensive medical services. A 2017 proposal on the government-run Public Policy Network Engagement Platform that "people who have lived overseas for many years should be ineligible for the NHI system" quickly garnered more than 5,000 supporters in two days, indicating that the issue has long been contentious. The proposal stated that "health insurance should provide coverage for those who live and work in Taiwan, and not for those who only have ROC nationality" (Yang 2017). Such a distinction clearly delineated who should be a member of the community connected by health insurance, that is, who can be considered "one of us," sharing our health risks and helping each other live, and who is a "[citizenship] speculator," "an American (or a Chinese) when things go well, and a Taiwanese when things go wrong" (Lee 2020).

Therefore, most of the participants in this study had to employ specific discursive re-moralization techniques to negotiate their status as the Other in the eyes of Taiwanese society. Interestingly, these individuals capable of living or working abroad (especially in Western countries) were originally seen in Taiwan as "symbols of success, indicators of upward mobility, and dreams of the underclass" (Huang 2007, p. 19), enjoying what Ong (1997) calls a "flexible citizenship" in an era of globalization. However, when it comes to the allocation of limited national healthcare resources in the pandemic, the image of these transnational migrants as adept at utilizing "strategic making-do that seeks access to as many rights as possible whilst falling prey to as few responsibilities" (Miller 2002, p. 231) can expose them to the challenge of attribution of membership in a community whose borders coincide with a nation-state.

To reconnect with the people of Taiwan, returnees often employed a discursive strategy of distancing themselves from the privileged global elite. They emphasized their lack of comprehensive health insurance coverage in their host country, highlighting the potential financial burden of contracting a disease and the uncertainty of accessing healthcare during the pandemic. The high risks associated with hospitals further deterred them from seeking medical attention when experiencing symptoms. In addition to accusing Taiwan's critics of "not understanding the dangers overseas," they positioned themselves as "vulnerable Taiwanese overseas" in a bid for greater public acceptance and sympathy. Yvonne (2020-05/home), who had accompanied her husband to study in the United States, expressed indignation over her Taiwanese friend's refusal to allow his overseas-working brother to return home in order to prevent a potential "epidemic prevention breach" in Taiwan. She said:

> We were really scared to get sick because even if you have insurance, these costs were really too high for you to get treatment. If I got diagnosed there, there could be millions of dollars in medical bills … And we wouldn't be able to come back, so how the hell would I raise the money there? I couldn't afford it even if I sold my house. Right … When you counted that possibility, you thought you wouldn't even qualify to be sick there. It's very painful, and you just had to be very careful about living like that. That kind of pressure was huge and everyone felt that way … how could you complain about us when we lived that kind of life abroad?

In contrast to previously mentioned types of risk-stigma, the focal concern here pertained to the linkage between returnees' biological vulnerability and their deservingness for inclusion in Taiwan's NHI system. Functioning as a compulsory redistributive social insurance framework, the NHI system was ethically rooted in the perception of shared responsibility among participants to assume risks and provide mutual care. However, the genesis of collective solidarity, whether grounded in civic nationalism forged by shared ordeals of oppression or in the pragmatic realities and values of public communal life facilitated by NHI implementation (Yeh and Chen 2020), did not readily extend to Taiwanese expatriates. The health burden imposed by the pandemic and the ensuing threat to the sustainability of the already strained NHI system further accentuated Taiwanese' desire to demarcate boundaries, thus positioning returnees as marginalized others.

Striving to Rejoin the "Epidemic Prevention Community"

In this study, individuals who quarantined after "non-essential" vacations abroad experienced heightened moral stigma and were considered the least qualified members of the "epidemic prevention community" during the global crisis. This inferior status was evident in explicit government regulations that excluded them from state quarantine subsidies, unlike other returnees. Furthermore, they were denied government-funded medical treatment if they contracted COVID-19, indicating that community membership relied on fulfilling the moral obligation to protect and care for others in the crisis. Participants quarantined after such vacations were acutely aware of the challenges in gaining full legitimacy. Consequently, they expressed acceptance of their stigmatized status in interviews, emphasizing their willingness to take responsibility for quarantine to mitigate the risk of endangering others. Through these actions, they sought to reaffirm their moral eligibility to reintegrate into the epidemic prevention community. For instance, Emily (2020-03/Home) self-mockingly referred to her overseas vacation at the onset of the epidemic as "inviting trouble" and publicly announced on her social media platforms her commitment to adhere to the 14-day quarantine period. Similarly, Howard (2020-03/Home) candidly accepted the ridicule from friends who labeled him an "epidemic prevention breach":

> I did come back from abroad; [so] I did run the risk of carrying the pathogen. [But] as long as I stayed home and eliminated that risk after that period of time, then there's no problem. So it should be about letting [returning] people know that they need to do their own process well.

Howard's passage concisely elucidates a pivotal attribute of risk-stigma encountered by all returning individuals—its temporary nature. Essentially, although there is indeed a risk of spreading the virus, this can be eliminated by avoiding social contact during the incubation period of the disease, implying that stigma is not enduring. Consequently, the quarantine period can be regarded as a symbolic "rite of passage." By successfully undertaking this process, individuals can substantiate their transformation from being perceived as a risky and morally inferior outsider to being deserving of reintegration into the community.

Further, obedience to quarantine transcends mere apprehension of stigma. This study aligns with previous research, highlighting that sometimes people's willingness to sacrifice their own interests to protect the public good is not simply a matter of normative obedience, but stems from a moral experience grounded in a deep concern for the relational nature of what constitutes "us" (Zigon and Troop 2014). This sense of interconnectedness may extend to one's family, neighborhood, society, or even the state, and influence their inclination towards altruistic choices.

Eason (2020-09/Institution) explained his willingness to adhere to quarantine measures despite acknowledging that the government's regulatory system was far from thorough:

> I think it's "reciprocal", that is, the government thinks that our people are on average at this level, so there's no need to control it in an overly oppressive way. [Like] I think I do it because I'm aware of the risks of the disease, not because I'm just afraid of walking out and getting fined hundreds of thousands of dollars.

In contrast to Eason's positive statement, another participant, Albert, was the only person in this study who expressed regret about his "good behavior" during his quarantine. Because the dental clinic refused to provide him with services after his quarantine expired, he felt that his efforts to restrain himself to protect the society were not rewarded. "Had I known that, I would have slipped away during the 14-day quarantine period," he said. "After all, if I was already infected, then … it was a risk to everyone else but not to me."

Although the two participants presented varying perspectives on their own compliance with the quarantine, both underscored the significance of the governed's commitment to controlling their personal risks in order to "protect others." Albert's experience further underscored how this commitment, manifested through adhering to movement restrictions and enduring social stigma, stemmed from the belief that their efforts would eventually lead to acceptance back into the community. Thus, in addition to functioning as an assemblage that places risk status and moral stigma on returnees, the quarantine also serves as an institutional ritual that enable returnees to reintegrate into Taiwan's "epidemic prevention community." By diligently following the quarantine measures to minimize potential risks, returnees had the opportunity to demonstrate their dedication to the duty of caring for others, thus establishing themselves as deserving members of the collective civic solidarity shared by all residents on the island.

Conclusion

This chapter examines civic engagement in national pandemic governance, specifically focusing on a distinct population category: Taiwanese who returned from abroad and were thus considered to be "at risk of infection." Unlike Lee et al.'s (Chapter 7 of this book) analysis of quarantine compliance through a quantitative approach, this study contributes to the literature on risk and morality by delving into experiences of quarantine and stigma, while echoing Chen's discussion of Taiwan's "thick governmentality" in the context of a vaccine-free strategy (Chapter 9 of this book). For much of the pandemic, Taiwan was seen as a success story in the fight against COVID-19, and most Taiwanese were proud of their "normal" life, with little attention paid to how overseas returnees were constructed as an external risk by the nation's infectious disease prevention system and consequently subjected to intense restrictions and high levels of stigmatization in the name of protecting the domestic population. Understanding their quarantine process and the associated social interactions allows us to see the nature of risk governance in Taiwan under the zero-COVID policy and reveals who primarily bore what consequences.

These new population categories, regulatory practices, and the redefined social relations during the pandemic constitute what I call a "risk-stigma assemblage" that contains multiple actors: Not only government agents and the risk technologies they operate, but also civilians and internet users who exercise neighborhood monitoring and moral sanctions. Returnees are certainly involved in this heterogeneous collection of governance, configuring various temporal, spatial, discursive, and material elements to manage risk and resist stigmatization, whether it is about the threat of bringing the virus back to endanger others, or being challenged as citizenship opportunists interested only in exploiting Taiwan's already distressed medical resources, or being perceived as not fulfilling their obligations as community members to protect and care for each other. Such efforts, this study argues, often lead returnees to strengthen their self-policing of risk, which is simultaneously considered as a means of de-stigmatization.

The empirical findings of this study suggest that returnees' engagement with national risk governance was driven by their concern for the well-being of others and their desire for de-stigmatization. I would like to further emphasize the impact of the timeframe of quarantine on these risk perceptions and feelings of stigma. The quarantine system, as an epidemic prevention measure to control virus transmission during the incubation period, specifies a defined timeframe. This means that once the quarantine period is completed, returnees can be relieved of their risk status and the associated stigma and thus be reintegrated into society. The temporary nature of these risks and stigmas, coupled with the expectation of social inclusion after the required period (despite potential delays), endows the strict quarantine measures with positive meaning and value for those under its governance. Additionally, Taiwan's comparatively rigorous quarantine protocols established a "bubble of normality" throughout much of 2020 and 2021, in contrast with the chaos experienced in other pandemic-affected regions. This comparison strengthened returnees' willingness to comply with quarantine in exchange for the prospect of a future free from the fear of the coronavirus, a life believed to hinge precisely on the adherence of all individuals undergoing quarantine.

This chapter also demonstrates that the risk-stigma assemblage is a useful concept for analyzing quarantine practices and experiences. It is the heterogeneity, fluidity, and contingency of the assemblage itself that enables quarantine systems to impose risk status and stigma on the governed, while providing them with the means to eliminate threats and demonstrate morality. Furthermore, it can enforce classification and hierarchical values while simultaneously promising a desired civic solidarity. Nonetheless, this study draws attention to the adverse consequences that particular configurations of risk-stigma may have on the governed. Despite the temporary nature of the suffering, the stigma still placed a significant physical and psychological burden on returnees that exceeded the quarantine obligation itself, compelling them to bear excessive costs to safeguard society from the menace of COVID-19.

Notes

1 Although the government has classified "home isolation" and "home quarantine" as separate categories for administrative purposes, both pertain to individuals without a confirmed diagnosis. This chapter follows academic convention by using the term "quarantine" for state management measures for undiagnosed individuals and "isolation" for measures concerning diagnosed individuals.

2 The focus on citizen-returnees is due to the discriminatory border control policies in Taiwan, which granted them priority while imposing restrictions on the majority of foreigners, including migrant workers and even unmarried foreign partners of native residents/citizens, by barring them from entering the country for nearly two years (Tuohy 2022).

References

Barbisch, D., Koenig, K. L., and Shih, F.-Y., 2015, Is There a Case for Quarantine? Perspectives from SARS to Ebola: Disaster Medicine and Public Health Preparedness, v. 9, p. 547–553.

Bayer, R., 2008, Stigma and the Ethics of Public Health: Not Can We but Should We: Social Science & Medicine, v. 67, p. 463–472.

Bhanot, D., Singh, T., Verma, S. K., and Sharad, S., 2021, Stigma and Discrimination during COVID-19 Pandemic: Frontiers in Public Health, v. 8, p. 577018.

Brooks, S. K., Webster, R. K., Smith, L. E., Woodland, L., Wessely, S., Greenberg, N., and Rubin, G. J., 2020, The Psychological Impact of Quarantine and How to Reduce it: Rapid Review of the Evidence: Lancet (London, England), v. 395, p. 912–920.

Brown, P., 2020, Studying COVID-19 in Light of Critical Approaches to Risk and Uncertainty: Research Pathways, Conceptual Tools, and Some Magic from Mary Douglas: Health, Risk & Society, v. 22, p. 1–14.

Chen, K.-T., Twu, S.-J., Chang, H.-L., Wu, Y.-C., Chen, C.-T., Lin, T.-H., Olsen, S. J., Dowell, S. F., and Su, I.-J., 2005, SARS in Taiwan: An Overview and Lessons Learned: International Journal of Infectious Diseases, v. 9, p. 77–85.

Crawford, R., 1994, The Boundaries of the Self and the Unhealthy Other: Reflections on Health, Culture and AIDS: Social Science & Medicine, v. 38, p. 1347–1365.

Day, T., Park, A., Madras, N., Gumel, A., and Wu, J., 2006, When is Quarantine a Useful Control Strategy for Emerging Infectious Diseases?: American Journal of Epidemiology, v. 163, p. 479–485.

Douglas, M., 1966, Purity and Danger: An Analysis of the Concepts of Pollution and Taboo: Penguin, London.

Douglas, M., and Wildavsky, A., 1982. Risk and Culture: An Essay on the Selection of Technical and Environmental Dangers: University of California Press, Berkeley.

Fu, Y.-C., and Lee, H.-W., 2020, Daily Contacts under Quarantine Amid Limited Spread of COVID-19 in Taiwan: International Journal of Sociology, v. 50, p. 434–444.

Gostin, L. O., Bayer, R., and Fairchild, A. L., 2003, Ethical and Legal Challenges Posed by Severe Acute Respiratory Syndrome Implications for the Control of Severe Infectious Disease Threats: JAMA, v. 290, p. 3229–3237.

Hale, E., 2022, How Taiwan Used Simple Tech to Help Contain COVID-19: BBC News, accessed May 29, 2023, at https://www.bbc.com/news/business-60461732.
Heyman, B., 2010, The Concept of Risk, in Heyman, B., Alaszewski, A., Shaw, M., and Titterton, M. editors, Risk, Safety and Clinical Practice: Healthcare through the lens of risk: Oxford University Press, Oxford, p. 15–36.
Huang, T.-Y. M., 2007, The Cosmopolitan Imaginary of Global City-Regions: Articulating New Cultural Identities, in Taipei and Shanghai: Router: A Journal of Cultural Studies, v. 4, p. 9–40. (In Chinese).
Lee, S., Chan, L. Y. Y., Chau, A. M. Y., Kwok, K. P. S., and Kleinman, A., 2005, The Experience of SARS-related Stigma at Amoy Gardens: Social Science & Medicine, v. 61, p. 2038–2046.
Lee, Y., 2020, Is Taiwan 'Using the Pandemic for Independence'? The Thriving Nation Health Insurance Community in the Midst of the Pandemic: Initium Media, accessed May 29, 2023, at https://theinitium.com/article/20200408-taiwan-epidemic-nationalism/. (In Chinese).
Link, B. G., and Phelan, J., 2014, Stigma Power: Social Science & Medicine, v. 103, p. 24–32.
Little, L. K., editor, 2007, Plague and the End of Antiquity: The Pandemic of 541–750: Cambridge University Press, Cambridge.
Lupton, D., 2013, Risk and Emotion: Towards an Alternative Theoretical Perspective: Health, Risk & Society, v. 15, p. 634–647.
Marcus, G. E., and Saka, E., 2006, Assemblage: Theory, Culture and Society, v. 23, p. 101–106.
Miller, T., 2002, Cultural Citizenship, in Isin, E. F., and Turner, B. S., editors, Handbook of Citizenship Studies: Sage, London, p. 231–245.
Musto, D. F., 1986, Quarantine and the Problem of AIDS: The Milbank Quarterly, v. 64, p. 97–117.
Nelkin, D., and Gilman, S. L., 1988, Placing Blame for Devastating Disease: Social Research, v. 55, p. 361–378.
Ong, A., 1997, Flexible Citizenship: The Cultural Logics of Transnationality: Duke University Press, Durham and London.
Scambler, G., 2004, Re-framing Stigma: Felt and Enacted Stigma and Challenges to the Sociology of Chronic and Disabling Conditions: Social Theory & Health, v. 2, p. 29–46.
Soon, W., 2021, Why Taiwan is Beating COVID-19 – Again: The Diplomat, accessed May 29, 2023, at https://thediplomat.com/2021/07/why-taiwan-is-beating-covid-19-again/.
Steinbrook, R., 2021, Lessons from the Success of COVID-19 Control in Taiwan: JAMA Internal Medicine, v. 181, p. 922–922.
Taipei Times, 2020, EDITORIAL: Virus Discrimination Continues: Taipei Times, April 1, p. 8.
Trnka, S., 2021, BE KIND: Negotiating Ethical Proximities in Aotearoa/New Zealand During COVID-19: Cultural Anthropology, v. 36, p. 368–380.
Tuohy, N., 2022, Personal Communication.
Wen, G.-X., Gu, Q., and Ye, S.-P., 2020, Chen Chien-jen: Tens of Thousands in Home Quarantine are Unsung Heroes in the Fight against the Pandemic: Focus Taiwan, accessed May 29, 2023, at https://www.cna.com.tw/news/firstnews/202003240402.aspx. (In Chinese).
Williams, J. L., Gonzalez-Medina, D., and Le, V. Q., 2011, Infectious Diseases and Social Stigma: Medical and Health Science Journal, v. 7, p. 58–70.
Wu, C.-L., and Tseng, Y.-F., 2006, The Risk Governance of SARS: Beyond the Technical Model: Taiwanese Sociology, v. 11, p. 57–109. (In Chinese).
Yang, C.-Y., 2017, Netizens' Proposal Passed: "Long-term Residents Abroad are Not Allowed to be Enrolled in the National Health Insurance": The News Lens, accessed May 29, 2023, at https://www.thenewslens.com/article/83676. (In Chinese).

Yeh, M.-J., and Chen, C.-M., 2020, Solidarity with Whom? The Boundary Problem and the Ethical Origins of Solidarity of the Health System in Taiwan: Health Care Analysis, v. 28, p. 176–192.

Yen, W.-T., and Liu, L.-Y., 2021, Crafting Compliance Regime under COVID-19: Using Taiwan's Quarantine Policy as a Case Study: Global policy, v. 12 , p. 562–567.

Zennie, M., and Tsai, G., 2021, How a False Sense of Security, and a Little Secret Tea, Broke Down Taiwan's COVID-19 Defenses: TIMES, accessed May 29, 2023, at https://time.com/6050316/taiwan-covid-19-outbreak-tea/.

Zigon, J., and Troop, C. J., 2014, Moral Experience: Introduction: Ethos, v. 42, p. 1–15.

9 Comparing the Governance of the Pandemic between Vaccine-Free and Free Vaccine Strategies

Thick Governmentality in Taiwan

Tzung-Wen Chen

Introduction

COVID-19 posed a significant challenge for Taiwan as vaccines were not available in the first year of the pandemic and because Taiwan is not a part of the World Health Organization (WHO). On the one hand, since Taiwan has an excellent record of public health governance concerning immunization policy (Chen 2013), if there were enough effective vaccines, the positive attitude toward vaccination may have helped protect Taiwan in the beginning of the pandemic. On the other hand, since Taiwan is not included in the global allocation of resources for pandemic governance, political considerations were sometimes more significance than other factors that determine outcomes of governance. In particular, the political factor is strongly associated with China—the location of the first outbreak of COVID-19. Accordingly, the situation in Taiwan from the end of 2019 to early 2022 was unique even compared to countries with similar geopolitical conditions, such as South Korea.

Despite its unique situation, Taiwan was once the safest place in the world—the virus did not invade Taiwan and cause sustained local transmission for almost a year and a half after the beginning of the pandemic. When a "real" outbreak hit Taiwan in May 2021, at least four kinds of COVID-19 vaccines were available on the global market. However, at that time, there was a global vaccine shortage, and the Taiwanese government also struggled to acquire sufficient vaccines for the population. Taiwan suffered from problems with both production and consumption of vaccines. For a long time, most vaccines have been imported into Taiwan because the domestic vaccine industry is not mature enough. In addition, the "Chinese factor" prevented the Taiwanese government from entering into official negotiations with most vaccine makers outside Taiwan, thus making vaccine purchases even more difficult. Even so, by 2023, Taiwan's vaccination rate slightly surpassed South Korea's, with both among the most vaccinated countries in the world.

Both Taiwan and South Korea recovered quickly from initial difficulties in obtaining vaccines and managed to weather the pandemic relatively successfully. It is tempting to turn to the Foucauldian concept of governmentality in modern societies to explain how both countries achieved a new normal in pandemic control (cf.

DOI: 10.4324/9781003438380-13

Horton 2020). However, we cannot ignore the complicated "normalization" process, which combines ambiguities and conflicts in and between truth regimes, or even conflicting rationalities in an individual (Dean 1999). It is especially dangerous and difficult to explain the cases of Taiwan and South Korea with the original concept of governmentality because, in both cases, the path of economic and social transformations has been very different from those of Western countries, such as France. The concept of governmentality was, after all, first developed to describe a dimension of the long modernization history of Western societies.

In this chapter, the concept of governmentality is utilized as an ideal type, according to Max Weber's methodology of comparative study (Weber 1991). From his Western point of view, Weber applied his ideal types of authority—traditional, rational, and charismatic—to examine Confucianism and Taoism in China. Since these ideal types do not perfectly map onto religious life in China, Weber's analysis highlights the uniqueness of Confucianism, as compared with other "world religions" such as Christianity. In other words, ideal types are tools for Weber to seek differences over similarities, thus making the Chinese economy and society more comprehensible. This method is more likely to lead one to understand (*verstehen*) rather than to find social rules or laws. Based on this logic of comparative study, the case of Taiwan in the thick of the pandemic will be reexamined to uncover characteristics of governmentality, especially regarding vaccines and vaccination on the island in its specific geopolitical milieu. The question posed in this chapter is why could Taiwan recover quickly from the COVID-19 outbreak using both the strategies of no vaccines—such as border control, social distancing, and, especially, the mask-wearing policy—and mass vaccination.

In the following sections, first, the concept of governmentality and its metaphor of the social body will be discussed. Then, vaccine-free strategies in Taiwan will be examined in terms of governmentality. The transition from vaccine-free to free vaccine strategies will be discussed to highlight the problems of traditional academic approaches of vaccination. Finally, the free vaccine strategy is studied to show the complicated rationale behind the governmentality, thus introducing the specific form of thick governmentality.

Governmentality: Ideal and Realistic

Governmentality and the Social Body

To give the concept of governmentality a historical context, Michel Foucault defines two types of biopower: biopolitics and disciplinary power. He said, "Biopower is required in developing capitalism, which cannot be secured without including bodies into production machines, and harmonizing the population with economic processes" (Foucault 1994: 185). This statement indicates that both biopolitics and disciplinary power are required for a capitalist society.

He further emphasizes that disciplinary power is exerted on human bodies from the norm (*norme*), and biopolitics forms the norm from the normal (*normale*) identified through the population (Foucault 2004: 65). Therefore, biopower,

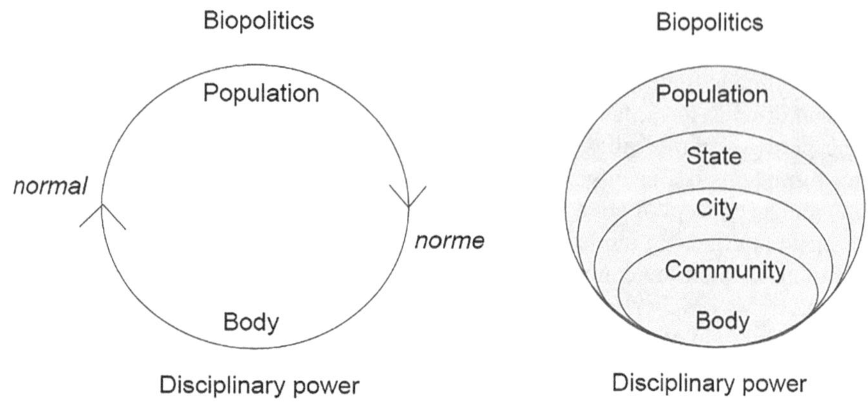

Figure 9.1 Iterative cycle of Governmentality (Left, Modified from Chen 2013) and Thick Governmentality (Right)

according to Foucault's later works, can be redrawn as an iterative cycle, as shown in Figure 9.1, in which the upper pole is biopolitics and the lower pole is disciplinary power (Chen 2013).

This figure was never explicitly proposed by Foucault but originates from the statement: "*We can even say that in most cases, the disciplinary mechanism of power and the regulatory mechanism of power, that is, the disciplinary mechanism to the body and the regulatory mechanism to the population are articulated*" (Foucault 1997: 223). Therefore, biopower oscillates between the two poles to maintain productivity in a neoliberal society. The system is acceptable to members of the group as it provides them with "rationality of governance," that is, governmentality.

Disciplinary power is exerted on individual bodies. The government is authorized to use this power by the population. For example, vaccination is the act of injecting a vaccine into an individual body, and it can be made compulsory for members of the population. Biopolitics is a regulatory mechanism used to protect a population from damage to productivity. Individual members of the population must forfeit a portion of their rights to defend society from threats. The governance over the population's safety is, therefore, based on rationality acknowledged by most individuals among the population, for example, the scientific evidence of the benefits of mass vaccination. It is the process of interpretating collective results from individuals that constitutes the rationality of government and is thus called governmentality. A dominant interpretation, mostly from scientific statements, becomes the truth regime, which is as important as the governmentality.

Foucault and his followers emphasize that governmentality is necessary for an advanced capitalist or neoliberal society to defend itself by protecting the population from damage to productivity (Foucault 1975; 1988; 1994; Rose 2007; Lemke 2011). Governmentality based on the biopower scheme of Figure 9.1 defines a social body inside the biopolitics-disciplinary power circle. According to Foucault, "*il faut défendre la société*" (society must be defended), the metaphor of the social body can precisely describe what governmentality is designed for: to protect the society against viruses to improve the productivity contributed by its members, that is, individuals and social groups in the society. Therefore, the path from *norme* to *normale* and vice versa in Figure 9.1 is the source of rationality for governing the social body. In other words, the social body must be defended to maintain "normal" by regulating each individual body with the "norm" derived from normal values of the social body. The norm of a social body is recognized by the population and serves as a "truth regime" for governmentality.

Societies Must Be Defended in the "Thick" of the Pandemic

To understand the case of Taiwan, a new form of governmentality called "thick governmentality" is proposed. Thick governmentality consists of governance behaviors at different levels, which intersect to contribute to a "solid" governmentality, as shown in the right of Figure 9.1, in contrast to the skin-deep circle shown on the left. The metaphor of "thick" in governance of a social body can be imagined as what traditional Chinese medicine calls "body constitution" (*tǐjhi̊h*)—essential conditions that characterize each person's body. Since each body is constituted differently, in case of illness the body must be treated specifically according to its particular body constitution. Similarly, when a social body is in the thick of fighting a disease, actions taken to conquer the disease must fit the body constitution. These actions must be thick enough as they consist of all parts of the body, and thus require taking the body as a whole, rather than just a part, a sector, or an organization of the social body.

Arguing that thick governmentality implies that biopower is a multi-level phenomenon, affecting different levels crossing from the individual body to the whole population, it is imaginable that governmentality is a complicated assemblage of social techniques practiced at different levels among more than one group of people in society. Besides, there may be conflicts among these social techniques. Thick governmentality is used to produce a more flexible outcome, rather than to align the techniques.

Accordingly, thick governmentality is a combination of different rationalities distributed among different layers. Habermas (1981) argued that in addition to Weberian rationalities (e.g., *instrumentelle Vernunft*), there is also communicative rationality which constitutes social lives. Some behaviors related to pandemic governance may exceed rationality or even be irrational. As shown in Figure 9.1, these rationalities and irrationalities are distributed across different layers, from the population, state, city, and community to the body. Each layer consists of its proper truth regime. Therefore, thick governmentality may not be homogeneous; there may be conflicts between layers.

Thick governmentality means that any action taken to prevent diseases may have different reasons at different levels (layers). For example, individuals wear masks to protect themselves. At the community level, this action is taken to protect others rather than for self-protection. At the city level, it becomes an issue of accessibility of public spaces. One may wear a mask for the following reasons:

self-protection, altruism, or obligation. No matter the reasons, or even if reasons conflict, they result in mask-wearing.

Contextual and Acquired Social Body Constitution

Taiwan and South Korea have long been compared due to their various similarities, such as being Japanese colonies before the Second World War, their fast economic growth from the 1980s to the 1990s, and their progress toward democracy from authoritarian governments. A more critical common factor is their geopolitical milieu: situated between China, Japan, and the United States. This factor also contributes to diverse rationalities for making choices among different layers of the social body.

Along with these similar economic, social, and political factors, emerging infectious diseases (EID), such as SARS and MERS, also shaped their public health systems in the early 21st century. These systems were critical governance structures with which both Taiwan and South Korea successfully conquered the pandemic before vaccines were available. This is especially true when discussing how healthcare systems can maintain their functions at the onset of an outbreak, for example, at the end of February 2020 in Daegu or after mid-May 2021 in Taipei.

Beyond these apparent similarities in governance experience, the actions of citizens' may have been even more consequential in preventing the further spread of the virus after the outbreaks in both Daegu and Taipei. Moreover, without much resistance to immunization programs, both societies reached very high vaccination rates once vaccines were widely available. The simple example of mask-wearing also implies that Taiwan and South Korea may have found their proper "governmentality" in the face of the COVID-19 pandemic, despite their very different governance strategies. Taiwan maintained a limited number of infections during the first year and a half of the COVID-19 pandemic, and South Korea recovered rapidly from the Daegu outbreak in February 2020.

In the cases of Taiwan and South Korea, a significant deviation from the ideal type of governmentality is that most actions taken by the citizens during the pandemic were voluntary and collective. Sometimes certain actions can have restrictions on the citizens themselves, sometimes on others: foreigners, travelers, or a group of people suspected to be infected. Besides, the actions may surpass the scope of disease control set by the central government. With the evolution of the pandemic, some actions would gradually be integrated into public policy, while others might be abandoned. That is, interactions between governmental and civil actions constantly change to co-produce a unique style of governance structure in the society.

As mentioned above, the geopolitical factor may contribute to different actions taken by Taiwan and South Korea. In short, the social bodies of Taiwan and South Korea were defended against the virus, but not necessarily according to Foucauldian governmentality. In the following sections, examples are given to explain how thick governmentality worked in Taiwan at the height of the COVID-19 pandemic.

Vaccine-free Strategies

EIDs are rarely vaccine-preventable. At least for the governance of COVID-19, no vaccine was available for nearly all of 2020. Under this condition, traditional approaches such as quarantine are more plausible to prevent the spread of viruses. However, very different approaches were utilized to tackle the COVID-19 pandemic in the first year, from "total control" to "laissez-faire" and from strict isolation to a milder form called "social distancing," depending on the situation of each society. These actions depended on the initial conditions of the virus spreading in each society.

Vaccine-free Strategies in Taiwan

Body Constitution in the Face of Potential Viruses

Taiwan suffered greatly from the SARS outbreak in 2003. This event is considered a critical factor in laying the groundwork for the successful actions taken to prevent the spread of COVID-19. But we cannot consider the SARS experience as a proper initial condition for COVID-19 control. It is undeniable that the experiences of SARS management contributed to the creation of a disease-monitoring system which pays close attention to relevant information from China. But the system could not prevent the first wave of the virus from spreading from Wuhan to Taiwan. Without immediate action taken to block the travel route from China to Taiwan, the monitoring system would have been futile. The blockage resulted from the suspicious attitude of the Taiwanese government toward China. If it had been a pro-China government, the initial reaction would have been quite different.

Border Control: Keeping Viruses Outside the Body

At the outbreak of COVID-19 in China at the end of 2019, Taiwan took immediate action, blocking cross-border traffic. This action, strongly supported by most people, worked very well, as the virus was kept outside the island for quite a long time. The rationality behind the border control is not technical only. Political considerations might have an even more important effect on decision-making. Even though thousands of Taiwanese people lived in Wuhan when the outbreak occurred, their evacuation was deemed impossible until several parties interfered in negotiations across the Taiwan Strait to reach a solution in March 2020.

The Taiwanese people in China were members of Taiwanese society but were considered outsiders of the state. Their return to Taiwan was initially blocked by the government to protect Taiwan. A large portion of them remained in China and hence their citizen's rights in Taiwan were partly deprived. However, this kind of treatment applied only to people in China. People from other regions of the world were relatively welcomed, even though situations in their places of residence were worse than in China.

Collective Quarantine: Protection Extending Deep into the Body

Another important government action was the installation of collective quarantine residences: quarantine hotels and government quarantine centers. These residences were provided for people, citizens or not, entering Taiwan through the national border or having had contact with infected cases. Collective quarantine creates a rather centralized, isolated space for those who are not yet identified as infected. The length of quarantine changed periodically according to the principles of pandemic control defined by the government. Quarantine is to maintain social distancing through an assemblage of artifacts. This governmental action was widely supported in the society during the pandemic.

Production and Distribution of Masks: Enforcement of Body Components

Initially, the preventative effects of masks on the spread of the virus were not scientifically proven. It was especially ambiguous as no evidence could be gathered in Taiwan because there were very few COVID-19 cases. Nonetheless, the governance of masks became an important issue in Taiwan because it was considered strong evidence of the society's rapid response to the global pandemic.

Mask governance is more than just wearing masks. Issues such as supply, quality control, and distribution are equally important. These issues are related to governmental, industrial, and social actors, who work together as a "national mask team" to provide a sufficient number of masks to the public and export masks to foreign countries. Taiwan launched an app to show the available stock of face masks. Also, the distribution of face masks was coordinated through the national health insurance system. As shown in Figure 9.2, people queuing outside a community drugstore to buy masks was common sight in the early stage of the pandemic in Taiwan. At that time, each person could only buy five masks per week. Given the long lines, standing outside of the drugstore itself required the consumption of one mask.

The national mask distribution system could not work without the full support of the community drugstores as well as members of the community who followed the national guideline for mask distribution. Almost all policies were made at the state level, governed by the national pandemic administration center. From all these facts, it is obvious that the collective action of mask governance tends to be centralized at the state level, supported and distributed at the community level, even though individuals tend to wear masks simply for self-protection. Considering these facts, Taiwanese society could remain "negative" because of, on the one hand, the strict control taken by the government and, on the other hand, the bottom-up self-protective actions.

Self-Protection by Vaccination

People also queued to acquire vaccinations even before the availability of COVID-19 vaccines, as shown in Figure 9.3. The two lines in Figure 9.3 are for

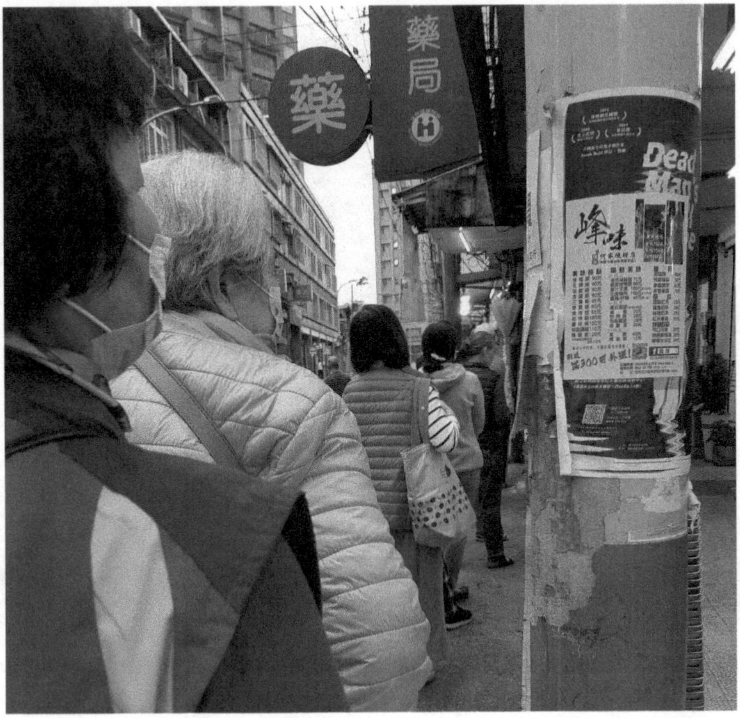

Figure 9.2 People Queuing to Buy Masks in Front of a Community Drugstore (Photo by the Author, March 18, 2020)

different vaccines. The upper line is for seasonal influenza vaccines, whereas the lower line is for scheduled children's vaccines. They were eager to get vaccinated because they hoped vaccines for flu or pneumonia would help prevent complications from COVID-19.

Taiwan has long been an excellent example of immunization programs, such as those for hepatitis B and polio prevention. The affinity to vaccines and vaccination has been studied as a combination of various metaphors across various social groups: industries, medical experts, public policymakers, and the potential vaccinees (Chen 2018). The lines pictured in Figure 9.3 are again the outcomes of multi-rationalities. Accordingly, compared with many Western countries, vaccines were much more welcomed in Taiwan (despite being mostly of foreign origin). There were very few anti-vaccine activities.

In early 2020, soon after the outbreak in Wuhan, China, some domestic pediatric clinics announced that "*even though there is no infected case so far in Taiwan, we recommend people of high-risk groups to receive pneumococcal vaccines for self-protection*" (January 17, 2020, source: http://www.gkc.com.tw/news/detail.php?id=788). This suggestion was not irrational and was also supported by certain physicians, as one said: "*Just like pneumococcal vaccines, though useless in*

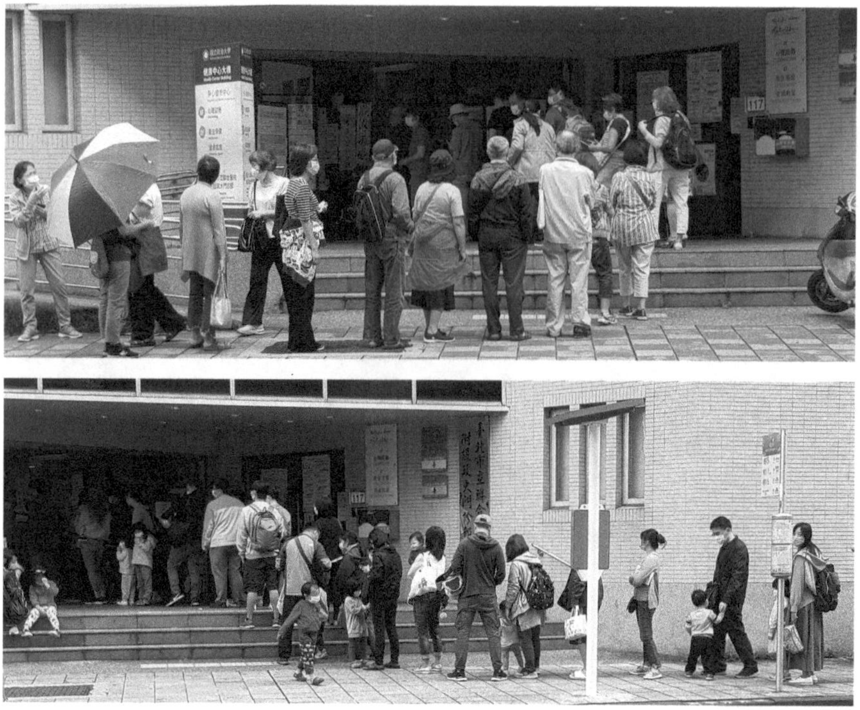

Figure 9.3 People Lined Up for Their Flu Vaccine (Top, October 8, 2020) and Children's Vaccines (Bottom, October 24, 2020) (Photo by the Author)

prevention of flu infections, can reduce the risks of severe complications caused by flu." And it is supposed that "*pneumococcal vaccines still work for COVID-19 because complications can be reduced*" (January 21, 2020, source: https://heho.com.tw/archives/64607).

Pediatricians also encouraged parents in Taiwan to protect their young children from potential complications of COVID-19 by vaccinating their young children with pneumococcal vaccines, which have been part of the childhood vaccine schedule for years (seen in the lower photo of Figure 9.3).

Personal social networks serve as another important information source. In the case of the seasonal flu, people were urged to get vaccinated by their peers, especially via social media during the pandemic. Among them, the following opinion spread: "*obviously, it is impossible to acquire Covid-19 vaccines by the end of this year (2020), so it is suggested that Taiwanese people should at best take some vaccines against respiratory infectious diseases.*" Consequently, as seen in the report below, people in the 50–64 age group were more likely to queue outside the clinic to get vaccinated:

> Fear of an outbreak of both COVID-19 and flu in the coming autumn and winter, immunization rate of government-funded influenza vaccines is

> so high that, even though [free] vaccination for the 50–64 age group was canceled, people seek to get vaccinated at their own expense. It is said that influenza vaccines will be out of stock soon by the end of October. Some experts suggested that, for prevention of COVID-19, effects of pneumococcal vaccines are better than that of flu vaccines.
>
> (October 18, 2020, Formosa News)

Combining Non-vaccine and Non-COVID Vaccine Strategies

Obligation at the city and state level, altruism at the community level, and self-protection at the individual level constitute a basic governance structure of multi-rationality. It is especially strong at the state level, as Taiwan was isolated from the world by strict border controls. The obligation upon citizens commanded by the Central Epidemic Command Center (CECC) marked a top-down governance structure, but the outcome could not be achieved without the segmented governmentality—a superposition of different governance layers. Each layer or segment has its own governmentality, oscillating between collective and individual levels, with its specific rationality.

Moreover, at the same time, people sought to protect themselves with "imported vaccines." That is, despite non-vaccine strategies, there were immunization strategies utilizing non-COVID vaccines mostly manufactured outside Taiwan. As seen in Figures 9.3 and 9.4, people queued to obtain preventive things, however, they are quite different: one is related to tools completely domestic for protecting the body from exposure to COVID-19; another is to inoculate someone with something *étranger* (foreign, strange), which is not necessarily related to COVID-19. These vaccines are for strengthening the (social) body's constitution, rather than preventing coronaviruses. In sum, the Taiwanese government's zero-COVID principle is a result of "preemptive preparation" with all strategies, which combined actions from central and local governments, communities, and individuals that had diversified rationalities.

Transition from Vaccine-Free to Free Vaccine Strategies

Again, using the metaphor of the social body, a negative social body means that the society contains very few or zero viruses. The ultimate goal of vaccine-free strategies is to prevent an invasion of viruses to maintain the negative state of the social body, or zero-COVID in the case of the COVID-19 pandemic. However, regarding the wide transmission of viruses globally, it is difficult to keep a virus outside national borders. As a result, Taiwan dropped the zero-COVID strategies in April 2022. Without border controls, the best way to prevent the social body from becoming infected is mass vaccination, if vaccines are available and effective.

However, viruses cannot be eliminated from the population, especially when mutations frequently occur. For example, the seasonal flu vaccination is not intended to eliminate the virus. Instead, it is to prevent the wider spread of the virus and reduce the severity of disease among those who become infected after vaccination, thus reducing the disease burden. This is also the case with COVID-19.

The transition from vaccine-free to mass vaccination in a society depends on vaccine availability. A lengthy process is usually required before implementing a compulsory vaccination policy. It took at least five to ten years for vaccines such as the pneumococcal vaccines to be made compulsory (Chen 2014). This period was part of a phase IV trial conducted to prove the safety and effectiveness of the new vaccines. Some vaccines failed to pass the trial and were withdrawn from the market.

In the case of COVID-19, the transition from vaccine-free to free vaccination in Taiwan could have been a difficult process, partly because of the "successful" boundary strategies that resulted in a quasi-negative society. However, as we can see below, the boundary of the social body was clear enough to prevent not only the virus but also COVID-19 vaccines. Also, there was significant hesitation from both the public and policymakers regarding the chaotic situation of global vaccine supplies and varied immunization programs in different countries. Additionally, political reasons prevented the Taiwanese government from taking a more active approach to secure vaccine purchases in advance.

However, the percentage of Taiwanese vaccinated against COVID-19 rapidly from 4% in May 2021 to nearly 80% at the beginning of January 2022. Comparing Taiwan with South Korea, even though the types of vaccines utilized and actions taken to promote mass vaccination were different, the evolution patterns of vaccination rates for both countries are very similar. The most significant difference is use of AstraZeneca vaccines. Korea stopped using AstraZeneca vaccines in June 2021, whereas Taiwan continued utilizing AstraZeneca vaccines throughout the pandemic. Therefore, we cannot evaluate the performance of the vaccination policy by the rate only. More detailed information about vaccines and vaccination is required.

COVID-19 did not invade Taiwan in 2020. Accordingly, vaccines were met with doubt among the people. However, an outbreak in Taiwan on May 19, 2021, triggered a rapid governmentality cycle, stimulating public debates over vaccines. The most significant evidence comes from key terms that appeared in public media. From a well-controlled situation in late 2020 to the outbreak in May 2021, and thereafter, the volume of vaccine-related news increases abruptly between May and September 2021. We wondered what people cared about and what the effects were among the issues.

Therefore, we further analyzed the news with word clouds. This analysis is carried out through four major phases: pre-vaccine, pre-vaccination, outbreak, and mass vaccination. Our analysis of texts relevant to vaccines in four major newspapers (*Apple Daily*, *China Times*, *Liberty Times*, and *United Daily*) in Taiwan is shown in Table 9.1.

As shown in Table 9.1, in the pre-vaccine phase, COVID-19 vaccines were still "imaginary," but public opinions tended to be objective and more scientific, as demonstrated by the popularity of terms such as clinical trials and R&D. Besides, the impact of external factors was also considered, as reflected by terms such as "China," "global," and "Trump." This indicates that before the availability of COVID-19 vaccines, reasonable discussions based on scientific rationales were more possible.

Table 9.1 Word Cloud Analysis

Phases	*Word Clouds*	*Key Terms*
Pre-vaccine phase (no vaccine available) January 2020–August 2020	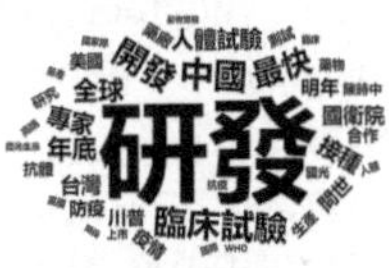	Research and Development, Clinical trials, China, development, fastest, experts, global, end of the year …
Pre-vaccination phase (very limited amounts of vaccines imported) March–May 19, 2021	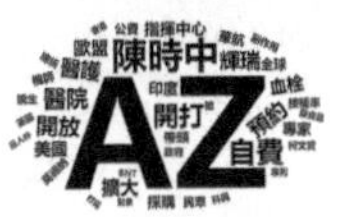	AZ, Chen Shi-chung, vaccination campaign, one's own expense, hospital, reservation, healthcare providers, Pfizer, …
Outbreak phase (strong demand for vaccines) May 20–June 15, 2021	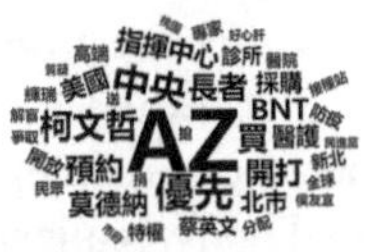	AZ, priority, Central government, Ko Wen-je (Mayor of Taipei city), elders, reservation, campaign, Moderna, purchase, CECC, USA, healthcare providers, BNT, …
Mass vaccination phase (vaccination rate climbing) June–July 10, 2021	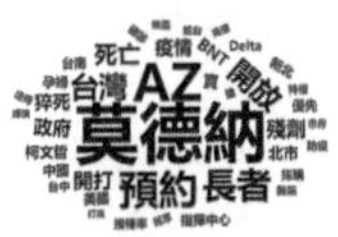	Moderna, AZ, reservation, elders, Taiwan, open, death, campaign, pandemic, leftover vaccines, government, sudden death, …
July 25–August 22, 2021	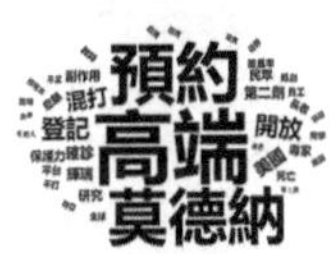	Medigen, Moderna, reservation, open, register, mixing vaccine, USA, second dose, confirmed case, Pfizer, …
August 23–September 21, 2021	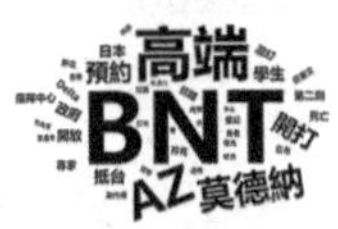	BNT, Medigen, AZ, Moderna, vaccination campaign, reservation, student, arrived in Taiwan, Japan, …
September 22–November 5, 2021	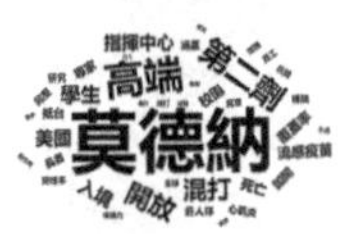	Moderna, Medigen, second dose, mixing vaccine, open, arrival, student, USA, coverage rate, influenza vaccine, …

In the pre-vaccination phase, since the society was not ready to accept mass vaccination, issues were centered around utilization and potential problems associated with AstraZeneca vaccines. Moreover, how to effectively launch the COVID-19 vaccination program was another hotly debated topic. The role of the central government is always important in public debates. Still, at this stage, the vaccine issues remained far from daily life.

Dramatic changes in public opinion occurred in the outbreak phase. Although some vaccines were still very popular, the roles and actions taken by local governments became top issues. This meant that the implementation of vaccination rather than vaccine types was more important. Also, people were concerned about vaccination priority as there were not enough vaccines. Accordingly, the categories of people prioritized for vaccination were a hotly debated topic. Another important issue was the technical terms for vaccination.

As the vaccination campaigns continued, in the mass vaccination phase, there were more discussions about the different types of vaccines. Still, the categories of people were important because each campaign targeted different groups. While the number of vaccinations increased, more and more reports about the undesirable effects of vaccinations appeared. On the other hand, since more types of vaccines were utilized, people tended to compare the vaccines: vaccine types, side effects, potential problems, and so on.

Table 9.1 shows how the "truth regime" about vaccines and vaccination shifted over the course of the four phases. This process produced a concretized state of existence for the COVID-19 vaccines in Taiwanese society. That is, COVID-19 vaccines are no longer imaginary. Rather, they are integrated into the bodies of Taiwanese people, thus forming a new social body, realized by free vaccine strategies.

Free Vaccine Strategies

Body Constitution for Vaccination

Taiwan and South Korea can be compared to see their body constitutions in association with vaccines. Taiwan and South Korea have very different vaccine industries (Chen 2015). In both societies, modern vaccine enterprises emerged in the 1980s to produce vaccines against hepatitis B, which seemed to be a good starting point. However, due to a lack of international connections, especially with the WHO, Taiwanese vaccine makers could not reach foreign markets. By contrast, Korean firms were able to provide their vaccines to third-world countries with the strong support of WHO experts. This external factor of the vaccine industry resulted in failure in Taiwan and success in South Korea.

Producing vaccines for foreign markets was most beneficial for Korean firms to join in the global supply chain of COVID-19 vaccines. At least four kinds of COVID-19 vaccines, including AstraZeneca, Moderna, Novavax, and Sputnik, were made in South Korea, by manufacturers who have their own vaccine products and have been in the industry for a long time. As these Korean companies are experienced vaccine manufacturers, they had the opportunity to make COVID-19 vaccines for large foreign firms. Having an industrial base is the first factor that set South Korea and Taiwan apart at the beginning of the COVID-19 vaccine acquisition, in both technological and commercial aspects.

Even though the Taiwanese government has had to purchase vaccines on the global market due to the inability of the domestic vaccine industry to provide a sufficient number of vaccines to meet domestic demand, immunization programs have been very successful in Taiwan for several decades. An expert group that provides professional opinions to policymakers plays an important role. A large portion of the group is clinicians specializing in infectious diseases. Moreover, the head of the Taiwanese Ministry of Health is a former medical professor, unlike in South Korea, where the position is assigned to a civil servant. The major actors in immunization policymaking in Taiwan are, therefore, very closely related to the medical community.

In South Korea, the government, industry, and medical community have more complicated interactions. Immunization policy involves compromise among various stakeholders in South Korea, as we can see from the hepatitis B vaccination experience (Chen 2013). Taiwan and South Korea launched their first campaigns for hepatitis B vaccination nearly concurrently. The immunization program in Taiwan soon resulted in herd immunity and, surprisingly, proved effective in preventing liver cancer. By contrast, due to unstable policy implementation, the prevention of hepatitis B in South Korea did not improve until the mid-1990s. Accordingly, the social context for immunization policy implementation is the second factor that makes a difference.

The aforementioned conditions were not directly related to COVID-19 vaccines as limited vaccines were available for Taiwan and even South Korea in the first half of 2021. Since Taiwan did not suffer from widespread transmission of the virus before May 2021, the global vaccine shortage seemed to be a marginal issue for pandemic governance. Consequently, the government took rather passive steps toward vaccine acquisition.

However, the situation changed dramatically in May 2021. An outbreak of COVID-19 made vaccines a hot issue in Taiwan. The volume of public discussion of vaccines rose suddenly after the outbreak, and then gradually lowered as vaccination rates rose. The decrease in public opinion volumes and increase in vaccination rates reflect more than just a change of truth regimes about vaccines and vaccination. As seen in Table 9.1, there were in fact multiple complex reasons for vaccine acceptance at different levels, as was also the case for the acceptance of vaccine-free strategies.

Emergence of Free Vaccine Strategies

The phases in Table 9.1 can be separated into two zones, as shown in Figure 9.4. In Zone 1, the Taiwanese government utilized essentially vaccine-free strategies. A small number of imported COVID-19 vaccines were only provided to "high-risk" groups for free. Everyone else had to pay. During this phase, the Taiwanese government still expected to have domestically produced vaccines. By the end of 2020, at least three Taiwanese firms had each obtained subsidies of more than 400 million NT$ for vaccine development, including Adimmune, Medigene, and UBI. The almost zero-infection situation in early 2021 allowed the government to postpone large-scale acquisition of foreign vaccines and wait for the availability of domestically made vaccines. Besides, media kept reporting safety incidents associated with the AstraZeneca vaccine in countries such as South Africa, France, Germany,

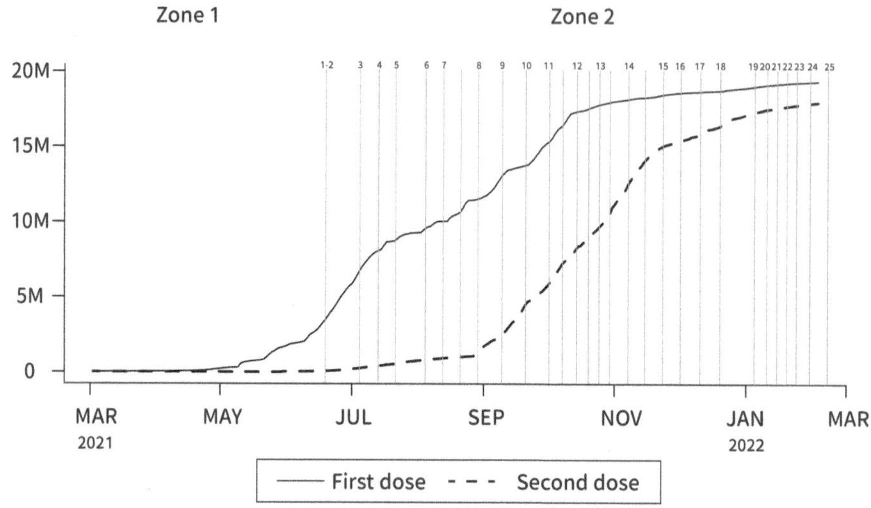

Figure 9.4 Accumulated Numbers of Vaccinated Individuals (First and Second Shots in Taiwan) and Phases of Vaccination Campaigns

Source: TCDC.

Italy, the Netherlands, Denmark, and even Thailand. These reports caused further vaccination hesitation. These factors explain why the curve in Zone 1 is flat in Figure 9.4.

The outbreak in May 2021 changed the suspicious attitudes toward COVID-19 vaccines. As shown in the word cloud analysis above, key terms in major media tended to support mass vaccination. The pre-vaccination and outbreak phases constitute the transition stage from Zone 1 to Zone 2. This means that the government modified its governance tools to include vaccination while maintaining vaccine-free strategies, which remained essential due to the shortage of vaccines.

In order to meet public demand, the government widely searched for vaccines in the global market. As Premier Su announced on June 8, 2021, at the Legislative Yuan:

> For foreign vaccines, contracts of purchase up to totally 20 million doses of vaccines have been signed with suppliers such as the COVAX platform, AstraZeneca, and Moderna. As for domestic producers, both the suppliers will provide 5 million doses according to the contract of purchase signed at the end of May.

Even though the total number of vaccines announced by Premier Su was far below the total needed to provide two doses to Taiwan's entire population, the strong demand for vaccination drove the government to launch a series of vaccination campaigns, from the first campaign in early July 2021 to the 25th campaign in early March 2022, with other campaigns following.

Since there were initially insufficient vaccines for mass vaccination, the campaigns in Zone 2 of Figure 9.4 were thus organized according to the rhythms of arrivals of foreign vaccines of diverse brands and sources. Additionally, each campaign targeted specific groups of people based on their professions, ages, and health conditions. Each segment in the incremental curve had specific reasons for vaccination, with their priority defined by the government. The curves are the outcomes of very skillful vaccination strategies based on different rationales from campaign to campaign.

Assemblage of Different Vaccines into a Social Body

The prevention of diseases with vaccines is logically different from prevention using vaccine-free methods. Vaccine-free methods create barriers against virus transmission, primarily based on social distancing by utilizing spatial arrangement and artifacts. Social distancing blocks the paths of infection and prevents face-to-face social interactions. As an artifact, the vaccine is integrated into humans and stimulates immunity within. Vaccines are designed to prevent specific viruses and one dose is only for one person. Therefore, vaccine-free methods are general purpose, as the social body is reorganized to protect individuals, whereas vaccination has a unique purpose, modifying individual bodies to change the social body.

Moreover, each individual may have been inoculated with several different vaccines from childhood to adulthood. These individual bodies make up the social body. Each kind of vaccine spans an immunity network connecting all individual bodies in the social body. This is the social base of herd immunity—immunity at the collective level.

COVID-19 vaccines are characterized by their short routes from the laboratory to the market, multiple brands with different technological platforms, and especially vaccine mixing options; one might be vaccinated with more than one type of vaccine. Taiwanese people were primarily vaccinated with four types of vaccines: AstraZeneca, Moderna, BNT, and Medigen. Except for domestically made Medigen, these vaccines were imported from different countries at different periods and distributed accordingly. Though the government tried to acquire more vaccines after the domestic outbreak of COVID-19, vaccine availability was very limited in the global market. Accordingly, different vaccines inoculated and assembled in each body depend on vaccine availability, although they also reflect the relatively limited choices of individuals.

A significant portion of people did not trust AstraZeneca—which was considered "not safe enough" in many countries—so, they waited until the arrival of BNT in September 2021. As for domestically made Medigen, however, that is another story. As we can see here, the rationale for getting vaccinated varies notably among people. Even though the curves rise, the reasons for vaccination differ.

At the state level, the government defined priority groups, based on scientific evidence. At the city level, local governments distributed vaccines fairly to those in need, based on their physical and social-psychological conditions. At the community level, people sought neighbors, relatives, and friends' opinions to decide if they should get vaccinated. Different vaccination stations were also available: hospitals, clinics, public healthcare centers, and even collective vaccination stations. Though people had differing sources of information resulting in varying reasons for seeking out vaccination (i.e., scientific, administrative, social psychological, or social affective), they ultimately were vaccinated.

Heterogeneous Construction of the Social Body

Classifying people in the society according to their immunization priorities also distinguishes body values among the population. More precisely, those inoculated with AstraZeneca in early March 2021, at a time when vaccines were very limited in Taiwan, were very different from those who waited until late September to get vaccinated with BNT (the Pfizer-Biotech vaccine). The reasons for the former were more obligatory because most of them were healthcare providers, whereas the latter were voluntary.

As for those who chose Medigen, their reasons may be quite different. Just like in other countries where political leaders demonstrated how they were vaccinated to promote mass vaccination, President Tsai also received her vaccination with the Medigen vaccine on video on August 23, 2021. This act was partly to assuage disputes around the domestically made Medigen vaccine.

In the beginning, the Medigen vaccine was more popular among younger generations for at least two reasons. First, those who tended to support President Tsai constituted a much larger portion of these generations. They chose Medigen for political reasons. A young city councilor who received the Medigen vaccine said, "*Domestic vaccines are a part of our national strategic industry. When my country is in difficulty, I will contribute my tiny force to support her*" (Liberty Times, August 25, 2021). The second, more pragmatic, reason is that among these generations were students who worried about the coming semester on campus. As their priority was too low to get inoculated with imported vaccines, they had to accept Medigen.

Unfortunately for Medigen, BNT vaccines arrived in Taiwan in September 2021, just one month after the launch of the Medigen campaign. From then on, almost no one would take Medigen vaccines during the multiple campaigns shown in Zone 2. Medigen vaccines remained much less popular than other vaccines, including AstraZeneca's—acceptance of the latter climbed slightly during the same period.

From the cases of the Medigen and AstraZeneca vaccines, it is certain that vaccine acceptance due to "nationalism" is rare in Taiwan. Even though there is an affinity to vaccines for the social body constitution in Taiwan, it is not equally true for all vaccines. A similar situation transpired in the case of the 2009 H1N1 flu vaccine campaign. It was the first time that a Taiwanese producer was able to make flu vaccines. At that time, a few safety incidents occurred during the mass vaccination program with both imported- and domestically made vaccines. The domestically made vaccines were particularly criticized and alleged to cause the incidents despite the cases not necessarily involving domestically made vaccines.

In the pre-vaccination phase, the Taiwanese government launched a flu vaccination campaign in the autumn of 2020. This annual campaign was very popular, as shown in Figure 9.3. One year later, in October 2021, COVID-19 vaccination campaigns successively launched alongside other vaccination campaigns. At the community level, a community healthcare center switched the daily vaccination schedules between routine childhood, COVID-19, and flu vaccinations, as seen in Figure 9.5. This was not accidental. Similar to the vaccine-free strategies that can be regarded as responses to urgent demand based on decades of disease control experience, the systematic arrangement of weekly vaccination schedules is also the result of decades of mass vaccination experience.

Translation:

[Announcement of Chengda clinic (an outstation of Taipei municipal hospital)]

Following the policy of (Taipei) Public Health Bureau, outstations of each hospital will start inoculation for seasonal flu vaccines from October 1. Because currently there are other vaccination programs such as child routine vaccines and the COVID-19 campaign, and under the regulation of indoor capacity during the pandemic, our clinic arranges vaccination tasks in terms of types for each weekday.

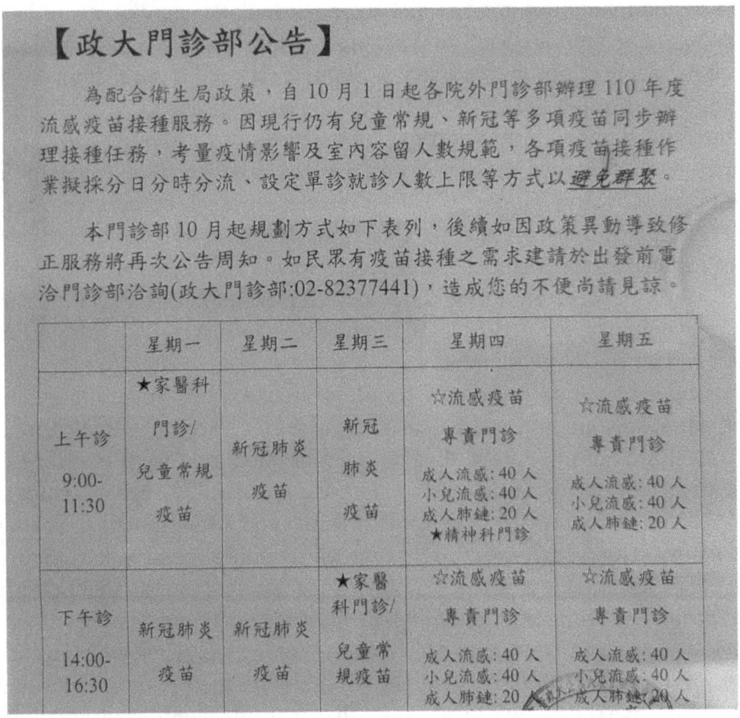

【政大門診部公告】

為配合衛生局政策，自 10 月 1 日起各院外門診部辦理 110 年度流感疫苗接種服務。因現行仍有兒童常規、新冠等多項疫苗同步辦理接種任務，考量疫情影響及室內容留人數規範，各項疫苗接種作業擬採分日分時分流、設定單診就診人數上限等方式以避免群聚。

本門診部 10 月起規劃方式如下表列，後續如因政策異動導致修正服務將再次公告周知。如民眾有疫苗接種之需求建請於出發前電洽門診部洽詢(政大門診部:02-82377441)，造成您的不便尚請見諒。

	星期一	星期二	星期三	星期四	星期五
上午診 9:00- 11:30	★家醫科門診/ 兒童常規疫苗	新冠肺炎疫苗	新冠肺炎疫苗	☆流感疫苗專責門診 成人流感: 40 人 小兒流感: 40 人 成人肺鏈: 20 人 ★精神科門診	☆流感疫苗專責門診 成人流感: 40 人 小兒流感: 40 人 成人肺鏈: 20 人
下午診 14:00- 16:30	新冠肺炎疫苗	新冠肺炎疫苗	★家醫科門診/ 兒童常規疫苗	☆流感疫苗專責門診 成人流感: 40 人 小兒流感: 40 人 成人肺鏈: 20 人	☆流感疫苗專責門診 成人流感: 40 人 小兒流感: 40 人 成人肺鏈: 20 人

Figure 9.5 Weekly Schedule for the Inoculation of Different Vaccines (Routine Vaccines for Children, Seasonal Flu, and COVID-19 Vaccines) of a Local Health Station in Taipei, from October 1, 2021 (Photo by the Author)

For each hour of each day only one type of vaccine will be distributed to a limited number of vaccines to prevent crowding.

From Monday to Friday (from left to right) and morning/afternoon (top/down), each half-day is arranged with certain types of vaccination including child regular vaccination, flu vaccination, adult pneumovaccine, and COVID-19 vaccination. (For example, Wednesday morning is limited to COVID-19 vaccination [40 persons], child regular vaccination [40 persons], and adult pneumovaccine [20 persons]).

The rapid reaction to meet the demand for COVID-19 vaccines among the community population was partly realized by the integration of the vaccines into the conventional vaccination system. Since vaccination practices are familiar to local healthcare providers, they were able to provide vaccinations once COVID-19 vaccines were available.

Reflection of Inner/Outer Worlds

Free vaccine strategies represent domestic configurations and simultaneously reflect the vaccine supply and distribution situations of the external world. This is especially true for Taiwan. As mentioned above, initial conditions in Taiwan included vaccination configurations that were particularly significant in the "adoption" rather than "production" of vaccines. Additionally, Taiwan lacks official international connections, particularly with the WHO. All these factors contributed to the unique pattern of the COVID-19 vaccine acquisition.

As mentioned above, different types of vaccines were imported into Taiwan at different times. Moreover, these vaccines were from different places with different platforms, as shown in Figure 9.6. Very limited amounts of vaccines were from the COVAX platform. Vaccines purchased by the government are still the most significant part, which includes domestically made Medigen. Furthermore, BNT vaccines were inaccessible to the Taiwanese government due to political reasons and were eventually donated by two Taiwanese enterprises, TSMC and Foxconn, and the Tzu Chi Buddhist foundation.

As a new vaccination program is implemented, experts generally evaluate the most effective spacing and number of vaccine doses, vaccine side-effects, and the rate of breakthrough infections, thus completing the circle from *normal* to *norme* based statistically on scientific reasons. However, obtaining such statistical data is technologically and ethically impossible in Taiwan, especially when vaccination is not obligatory. Third-party experience, that is, scientific research and reports from foreign countries, are the primary references for "*normal*" in the making of the domestic "*norme*" (vaccination guidelines). The domestic *norme* is possible because of people's long-term trust toward domestic medical experts who provide their scientific "judgments" to the government, rather than their own scientific research "results." It is social psychological rather than a solid scientific reason that drives the governmentality circle.

From the complicated context described above, it is clear that vaccination assembles the external position of Taiwan in the global society to the inner world

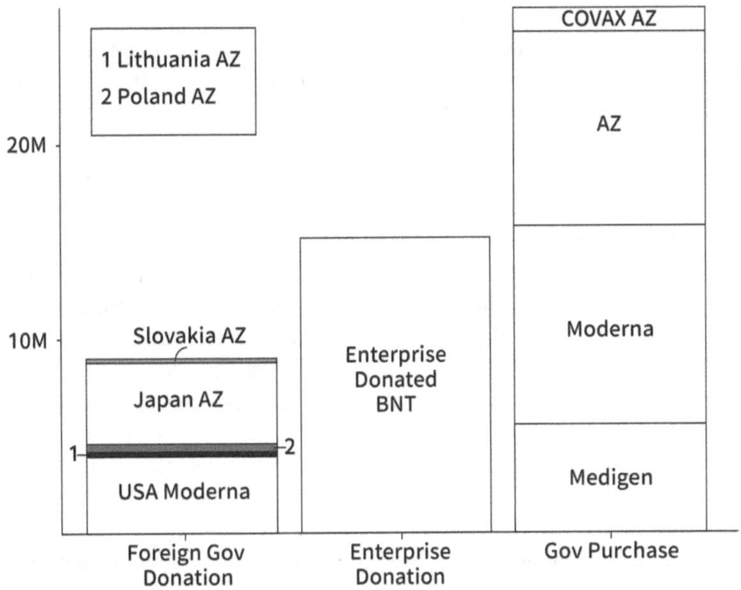

Figure 9.6 Profile of COVID-19 Vaccines in Taiwan before January 15, 2022

Source: TCDC.

inside the island. Similarly, the vaccination practices in the inner world of the local society reflect the external world, including the unfair situation of global vaccine distribution, as seen in Figure 9.6.

Free vaccine strategies initiate a process of body construction per the social body constitution. Taiwanese citizens received an AstraZeneca vaccine made in Thailand to induce immunity, an effect presumed by vaccine developers in Oxford, UK. The Thailand-made vaccine, recognized by the WHO, was distributed to Taiwan through the COVAX platform. Another vaccine, Moderna, using the mRNA technological platform, could be donated by the US government or purchased by the Taiwanese government and injected into another group of people. These vaccines reconstructed the social body with different kinds of individual bodies in the society.

The profile shown in Figure 9.6 also implies that vaccine nationalism had almost no effect in Taiwan: the vaccinated social body consists of a very small portion of domestically made vaccines, even smaller than that of those donated by small foreign countries. In fact, Medigen vaccines were gradually marginalized during the series of campaigns for COVID-19 vaccination.

Summary: Impossibility of Immunization Utopia

While herd immunity is impossible in the case of COVID-19 vaccination, and society was quasi-negative in early 2022, the vaccination rate is high enough. The reasons are complicated. However, the rapid rise in the vaccination rate is a consequence of piecemeal actions, realized by a series of campaigns that combine multi-layered governance of vaccines and vaccination. The multi-layered actions are comparable to the vaccine-free strategies as they are all outcomes of governmentality. It is impossible to end a pandemic through vaccination alone. In short, vaccine-only strategies cannot replace vaccine-free strategies. The problem with herd immunity is that the governmentality is too thin to prevent the virus.

A relatively high vaccination rate was not difficult to achieve in Taiwan, with the help of thick governmentality. The achievement comes from combined reasons such as people's fear of death, competition among local governments,[1] and the central government's credibility. Even in the pre-vaccination phase, non-COVID vaccines had been utilized in parallel with other vaccine-free strategies. Factors such as an insufficient domestic vaccine supply, relatively high uncertainty surrounding vaccine side effects, and particularly the miraculous success of "preemptive preparation" before the availability of vaccines, undermined the free vaccine strategy, which could not replace or even compete with vaccine-free strategies after the outbreak of the widespread local transmission in Taiwan.

However, one of the major issues that experts worried about with the promotion of vaccines like the HPV vaccination does not exist in the case of COVID-19 vaccines. That is, people inoculated with the HPV vaccines might consider themselves well protected and thus ignore self-protection and routine screening. With the strength of vaccine-free strategies in Taiwan, even vaccinated people infected with COVID-19 had to quarantine until they achieved a negative test result for most of the pandemic. Other restrictions, such as avoiding mass gatherings and mask-wearing still applied to those who have received up to three doses. In short, vaccination did not change much of what vaccine-free strategies imposed upon people's daily lives.

If vaccine-free strategies adopted by the government could be considered as "preemptive preparation," a free vaccine strategy as preventive action is already preparation in advance. However, the latter did not replace the former, even after achieving a high vaccination rate.

Thick Governmentality: Combining Vaccine-Free and Free Vaccine Strategies

"Neoliberal" Thick Governmentality

As Premier Su said:

> The budget for prevention, up to 73.4 billion, is primarily destinated for vaccine purchase, bonus commissions for preventive workers, increase of testing capacity, acquisition of preventive materials and medications, expansion of hospital facilities, fees for quarantine hotels, maintenance of collective quarantine sites, and financial support for preventive actions taken by local governments.
>
> (June 8, 2021, Legislative Yuan)

According to a monthly report from MOHW, until May 31, 2021, about 44 billion NT$ extra was designated for COVID-19 governance, of which 11.5 billion was budgeted for vaccine acquisition. However, only 5.1 billion (about 11%) had been utilized to buy vaccines. In the national budget of pandemic management, a very limited portion was attributed to vaccine purchases. Though vaccine acquisition was among the primary tasks, other unrelated tasks were more complicated, and were allocated more resources.

The situation changed slightly, as on April 30, 2022, MOHW had an accumulated budget of 154.3 billion NT$ for COVID-19, of which 44.4 billion (about 28.8%) was for vaccine acquisition. However, a significant portion of the budget was still allocated to subsidies for those who were obliged to quarantine. This means that vaccine-free strategies were still dominant despite mass vaccination being realized. The free vaccine strategy was built upon the base of various vaccine-free strategies that had been implicated before mid-May 2021.

In terms of resource allocation, strength of implementation, and degree of impact on daily lives, vaccine-free strategies were still dominant strategies in the late pandemic stage. In fact, just after the outbreak of COVID-19 in Taiwan, the government announced that within the National Specific Budget against COVID-19, a large portion was destinated for people experiencing financial difficulties:

> Budget for cash subsidies, up to 186.6 billion, is primarily destinated for families with children, disadvantaged people, laborers without insurance, self-employed, farmers and fishers, taxi drivers, rental car and shuttle bus drivers, tourist guides, and others who suffered from severe economic damages caused by the pandemic.
>
> (Premier Su, 8 June 2021, Legislative Yuan)

From May 31, 2021 to May 31, 2022, the total budget against COVID-19 was raised from 420 billion to 840 billion NT$. During this period, MOHW was allocated a percentage of the total budget climbing from 18% to 22%, while the share for the Ministry of Economic Affairs (MOEA) dropped 6%. Even so, MOEA, the ministry in charge of "productivity," still obtained 48% of the total budget. From the perspective of resource allocation, the money devoted to virus prevention, including vaccine acquisition, was much lower than the investment in economic promotion. As MOEA was always allocated around half of the total budget, the government's consistent preference for direct intervention in productivity is obvious.

Moreover, as shown in Figure 9.7, even though the funds allocated to MOHW increased rapidly after the outbreak, the share of vaccine-related expenses, including research and development, clinical trials, acquisition, quality control, and injury compensation, did not grow proportionally. The region between the two curves belongs to vaccine-free strategies. This means that vaccine-free strategies remained dominant tools against the pandemic.

The governmental actions reviewed by resource allocations reflect that protection of "productivity" precedes "health," a typical logic of neoliberal society. It is for this reason that the argument of thick governmentality is so applicable to this case.

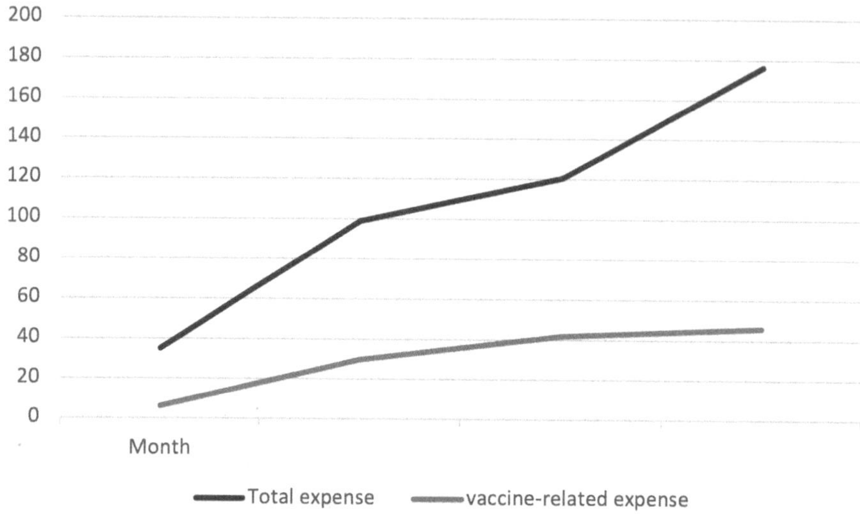

Figure 9.7 Evolution of Accumulative Expenses Within the National Specific Budget against COVID-19 Distributed to MOHW (Period: May 2021–September 2022; unit: Billion NT$)

Source: MOHW.

Thick Governmentality Reflects Body Constitution

It is impossible to strictly have vaccine-free strategies once vaccines become available. On the other hand, it is also hard to have free vaccine strategies without any other strategy. In other words, vaccine-free and free vaccine strategies can be considered as two components of thick governmentality. These two components with other actual factors constitute a real society and differentiate it from other societies.

Vaccine-free and free vaccine strategies can then be summarized, as shown in Table 9.2, by their concrete actions, major purposes, and dominant rationalities at four different levels. For example, Taiwan and South Korea utilized different concrete actions to achieve major purposes based on similar dominant rationalities. That is, thick governmentality can be realized by combining different concrete actions depending on the unique situations of a society and, at the same time, achieving major purposes that dominant rationalities aim at.

At the state level, a major purpose of governmentality is to protect the society. Even though the strategies are based on scientific or political rationalities, they could be concretized as enforcing strict border control or providing essential support to community and individual protection, depending on the initial conditions of vaccine-free strategies realized at different levels.

Moreover, since COVID-19 vaccines failed to prevent new variants such as Delta and Omicron, referred to as "breakthrough infections," the main reason for mass vaccination—to achieve herd immunity—seems impossible. However, with thick governmentality, the Taiwanese and South Korean societies still welcomed vaccines to avoid the potential disease burden. From this angle, the major personal

Table 9.2 Rationalities at Different Levels of Governance

Level of Governance	*Concrete Actions*		*Major Purposes*	*Dominant Rationalities*
	Vaccine-free	*Free Vaccine*		
State	General policy, border control, mask production	Vaccine acquisition, immunization policy	Protecting the society	Political, scientific
City	Regulation setting, space management, mask distribution	Vaccine distribution, vaccination reservation systems	City management	Economic, technological
Community	Mask distribution, entrance control	Vaccination practices, vaccination facilities, task forces	Community autonomy	Moral, sentimental
Individual	Mask-wearing, rapid screening	Vaccine acceptance	Self-protection	Egoistic

reasons for being vaccinated are very similar to those for wearing masks, as can be seen in the similarities between Figures 9.3 and 9.4.

From Figure 9.1, it is clear that the space inside the iterative circle is empty, which means only biopolitical actions and disciplinary actions are taking place in society and at individual levels. However, as we can observe from the pandemic governance and implications of vaccine-free and free vaccine strategies, there were different actions among the state, city, and community levels, and even the construction of collective housing. It means that the concept of thick governmentality can explain more in details of the pandemic governance as compared with the original version of Foucauldian governmentality. This particularly applies in East Asian societies such as Taiwan and South Korea, where modern capitalist institutions were considered "copies" of Western "advanced capitalist" societies and coexist with other social institutions and their related rationalities.

Since thick governmentality enters deep in the society, the cycle of governmentality also provides elements to construct daily life. To shorten the social distance to improve productivity, people are forced to adopt tools and adapt to a new form of daily life. By relinquishing a small part of their rights by wearing masks—a typical example of disciplinary power over individuals—the society can be protected.

Concluding Remarks

It is from the viewpoint of thick governmentality that we can observe how vaccine-free and free vaccine strategies were applied to produce effects in Taiwan during 2020–2022, the most severe period of the COVID-19 pandemic. These strategies function as heterogeneous components that are distributed among different parts of the social body, which is a complicated composition of segments or layers, from individual bodies to the state. Just as viruses cause different reactions in human bodies, the COVID-19 pandemic induced different reactions in societies, which can be regarded as differing social bodies in which thick governmentality is realized.

When vaccine-free strategies are applied, the social body is isolated from viruses. The multi-layered social body serves as a barrier preventing foreign viruses from entering the individual body and spreading within the social body. When free vaccine strategies are implemented, the social body imposes vaccines on each individual body to protect the social body. It is expected to produce a social immunity by immunizing individuals. Moreover, the vaccines may be from abroad, depending on the society's situation in the global context. Therefore, the social body acts as a lens, reflecting global situations inside the individual body.

Although the concept of a "resilient society" has been proposed to conceptualize a better public health strategy in a pandemic (Brunnermeier 2021), the case of Taiwan (and South Korea) reveals that the concept of thick governmentality can be more robust, especially for a society characterized by both neo-liberalism and traditionalism. A resilient society can be considered a part (or a kind) of thick governmentality. Additionally, when each strategy is implicated at the corresponding level, there are specific reasons for this strategy. There is no universal rationality for all strategies. Indeed, thick governmentality comprises diversified kinds of rationalities or even non-rationalities, coming from different governance layers. That is, there are diverse rationalities rather than just one rationality.

Note

1 See, for example, the headline of a media report: "Each day over 95% of attendance rate, the second dose vaccination rate reaches 5.5% in Tainan city which is higher than the national average rate." (Liberty Times, September 10, 2021).

References

Brunnermeier, Markus K., 2021, The Resilient Society: Endeavor Literary Press, Colorado Springs.

Chen, Tzung-wen, 2013, Technology of Power and Power of Technology: An Analysis of the History of Vaccine Adoption in Taiwan (in Chinese): Taiwanese Sociology, v. 25, p. 44–87.

Chen, Tzung-wen, 2014, Performing Health, Constructing Market-A Performativity Analysis of Pneumococcal Vaccine Markets in France (in Chinese): Taiwan: A Radical Quarterly in Social Studies, v. 95, p. 1–55.

Chen, Tzung-wen, 2015, Global Technology and Local Society: Developing a Taiwanese and Korean Bioeconomy Through the Vaccine Industry: East Asian Science, Technology and Society: An International Journal (EASTS), v. 9 (2), p. 167–186.

Chen, Tzung-wen, 2018, Three Metaphors of Vaccines (in Chinese), *in* Lin, Wen Yuan, Lin, Tzung-De, and Kuo, Wen Hwa eds., Science/Society/Human 3: National Chiao Tung University Press, Hsin Chu, p. 226–235.

Dean, Mitchell, 1999, Governmentality: Power and Rule in Modern Society: Sage, London.
Foucault, Michel, 1975, Surveiller et Punir: Naissance de la Prison: Gallimard, Paris.
Foucault, Michel, 1988, Technology of the Self, *in* Martin, Luther H., Gutman, Huck, and Hutton, Patrick H. eds., Technologies of the Self: A Seminar with Michel Foucault: Tavistock, London, p. 16–49.
Foucault, Michel, 1994, Histoire de la Sexualité I: la Volonté de Savoir: Gallimard, Paris.
Foucault, Michel, 1997, Il Faut Défendre la Société. Cours au Collège de France, 1976: Gallimard, Paris.
Foucault, Michel, 2004, Sécurité, Territoire, Population. Cours au Collège de France, 1977–1978: Gallimard, Paris.
Habermas, Jürgen, 1981, Theorie Kommunikativen Handelns. Bd. 1: Handlungsrationalität und Gesellschaftliche Rationalisierung: Suhrkamp, Frankfurt.
Horton, Richard, 2020, Offline: COVID-19—a Crisis of Power: The Lancet, v. 396 (10260), p. 1383.
Lemke, Thomas, 2011, Biopolitics: An Advanced Introduction: New York University Press, New York.
Rose, Nicolas, 2007, The Politics of Life Itself: Princeton University Press, Princeton.
Weber, Max, 1991, Die Wirtschaftsethik der Weltreligionen. Konfuzianismus und Taoismus: 1915–1920: Mohr Siebeck, Tübingen.

Part 4

Nationhood, Nationalism, and Global Health

10 The Return of NRICM101 to Taiwan

The Contributions of a Herbal Formula to Both COVID-19 Treatment and Nationalism

Po-Hsun Chen

Introduction

In this chapter, I illustrate the paradoxical situation that arose when Taiwanese-made COVID-19 herbal products that were inaccessible in Taiwan in 2020 were exported globally to much fanfare. I explore this topic by focusing on the Taiwanese herbal product "Taiwanese NRICM101" (臺灣清冠一號hereafter NRICM101) and on the vague and frequently disputed regulations governing the medical use of herbs in Taiwan. I also analyze traditional Chinese medicine (TCM) advocacy groups' nationalistic rhetoric (i.e., describing its development as what I call "a hero's journey") around NRICM101 to project Taiwan's anticipatory imaginary as a nation independent of China. A central point that I demonstrate is that, by granting NRICM101 emergency-use authorization (EUA), the Taiwanese government promoted Taiwanese nationalism both domestically and abroad while challenging Taiwan's biomedicine-dominated regulatory system and international organizations' ignorance, all within the context of the COVID-19 pandemic.

In early 2020, countries across the globe raced to develop and deploy public health resources, including traditional medicine, to reduce the spread and the severity of COVID-19. Many countries in East Asia have acknowledged the contribution of traditional medicines to national health systems and have regulated these medicines through national policies. During the COVID-19 pandemic, traditional medicines have contributed to disease prevention, control, and treatment, both domestically and overseas. In a top-down fashion, China's government collaborated with TCM technocrats in the development of TCMs tweaked specifically for COVID-19 treatment, and a result of this collaboration was the *TCM Diagnosis and Treatment Protocol for COVID-19*, which got underway in early 2020 (Chen, 2020). One function of the protocol was to strengthen Chinese nationalism (Liu, 2020). By contrast, South Korea exemplified a bottom-up approach to fighting COVID-19 with traditional medicines: young South Korean traditional medicine physicians deliberately bypassed government regulatory obstacles in order to treat confirmed COVID-19 cases with tailor-made herbal remedies (Flowers, 2021). In the case of Taiwan, official medicinal institutes and pharmaceutical companies have developed novel herbal drugs used in the fight against COVID-19. A central

DOI: 10.4324/9781003438380-15

question posed in the present study is how herbal medicine has contributed to prevention and control policies during the COVID-19 pandemic in Taiwan.

Since late March 2020, the Taiwanese government has invested in researching and developing herbal drugs in the fight against COVID-19. The herbal product NRICM101 was the country's first herbal drug granted an EUA for the treatment of COVID-19. However, the EUA was not issued until mid-May 2021 because of bureaucratic restrictions. Ironically, during this period of time, the Taiwanese government permitted the export of NRICM101 to countries around the world, attracting international attention and praise (*The Diplomat*, 2023). In this way, NRICM101 was deliberately used as a tool to support Taiwanese nationalism as part of President Ing-Wen Tsai's policy-based efforts to strengthen the global status of diplomatically isolated Taiwan (Office of the President, 2021a).

In describing the process by which NRICM101 expanded from being an export-only herbal remedy to a domestic one, I shine light on the disputed regulatory culture of Taiwan's two-track system, one track covering biomedicine and the other covering TCM. The second major point that I address is how NRICM101, by belonging to the category of drugs known as TCM, served to promote Taiwanese national identity during the pandemic. This curious marriage between innovative herbal technologies and nationalist discourse enabled NRICM101 to symbolize the glory of Taiwan and to showcase the island as a nation rather than a "renegade province" of China.

Taiwan's First Herbal Product Authorized for Emergency Use

In early 2020, the National Research Institute of Chinese Medicine (NRICM), one of the affiliated institutions of the Ministry of Health and Welfare (MOHW), developed a new herbal formulation, NRICM101, for the treatment of COVID-19.[1] Within months, NRICM101 became a symbol of Taiwanese nationalism, especially when the herbal product began being exported to multiple overseas markets in 2020 before obtaining an EUA for domestic use in mid-May 2021. Initially, the Taiwanese organization known as the National Union of Chinese Medical Doctors' Association, ROC (hereafter the NUCMDA) put together what it called a "national TCM team," adopting the widely disseminated nationalist slogan "Taiwan can help" and then modifying it to read "TCM can help" (NUCMDA, 2021a). In the winter of 2021, Ing-wen Tsai, the president of Taiwan, met with a NUCMDA chairman and expressed her appreciation for the pandemic-fighting contributions of both TCM physicians and NRICM101 (Office of the President, 2021b). At the 2021 Global Health and Welfare Forum in Taiwan, Vice President Ching-Te Lai, a professionally trained nephrologist, praised the export of NRICM101. He stated that NRICM101 benefits the diplomacy and international status of Taiwan (Office of the President, 2021c).

In mid-May 2021, Taiwan's MOHW granted an EUA to NRICM101 because the island was experiencing a sudden surge in COVID-19 cases. The NRICM had researched and developed this herbal formula as a treatment to reduce the severity of COVID-19. Once developed (around mid-2020), the NRICM granted

NRICM101 production rights to pharmaceutical companies that had been certified as having good manufacturing practices (GMP). Taiwanese media widely reported on this event, and legislators and the public voiced support for the treatment, the EUA, and the production scheme.

However, the EUA of NRICM101 immediately triggered numerous debates pitting proponents of the product against biomedical experts and even some TCM experts. Owing to the Taiwanese government's strict regulation of herbal medicine domestically, NRICM101 eventually obtained only an EUA, not a drug permit license. In 2022, Taiwan's *Temporary Guidelines for the Treatment of COVID-19* still rejected NRICM101 because the data surrounding its efficacy allegedly rested on unsound clinical trials. Hence, as of late 2022, neither the Taiwan Food and Drug Administration (TFDA) nor the Central Epidemic Command Center (CECC) had ever recognized NRICM101 as a formal treatment that physicians can prescribe for COVID-19. Even when the CECC was dissolved on May 1, 2023, NRICM101 remained unrecognized as a formal treatment. Without further regulatory action, NRICM101's EUA will expire in June 2024.

In brief, NRICM101 is Taiwan's first herbal drug granted an EUA, and its controversial journey has been entwined with a potent mix of Taiwanese nationalism and rigid governmental regulations. In this chapter, I employ the theoretical frameworks of classification and sociotechnical imagination to unpack and illustrate the paradox that NRICM101 was available overseas while remaining unavailable domestically during much of the COVID-19 crisis. I focus on the period from 2020 through 2023 (i.e., from the establishment to the dissolution of CECC), and I map out the layers of meaning behind the recent history of NRICM101 in Taiwan by analyzing such primary sources as the Legislative Yuan Gazette, newspapers, social media,[2] scientific reports, the statements of experts, the publications of professional associations, *Consumer Reports of Taiwan*, and official governmental announcements and publications.[3]

Innovations in Traditional Medicine and the Power of Nationalism

Innovation in traditional herbal medicine is a significant topic in history and in science and technology studies (STS). Among several well-known studies conceptualizing the modernization of herbal medicine is one by historian Sean Hsiang-Lin Lei (2014) concerning the antimalarial drug Changshan, a Chinese traditional herb, which serves as an example of the "re-networking" concept. Lei uses this STS concept to describe how interactions between experts, laborers, herbs, knowledge, and technology have led to pharmaceutical innovation.

The general backdrop for innovation as it relates to traditional medicine is the experience of non-Western countries pursuing modernity and promoting nationalism. The history of TCM in China, for example, is intimately linked to nationalism. Medical anthropologist Elisabeth Hsu (1999) and historian Kim Taylor (2005) insightfully note that efforts in the mid-20th century to re-structure the basic theories underlying TCM resulted in ideas that mirrored—and thus supported—Maoist ideology and biomedicine. Medical historians Bridie Andrews (2014) and Sean

Hsiang-Lin Lei (2014) examine the link between the modernization of TCM and the development of the Chinese nation-state in the modern period. The compelling and interesting arguments laid out in these and other studies have inspired other scholars, including me, to analyze the issue of TCM innovation relative to nationalism.

In tackling the related issues of nationalism and TCM innovation, I employ the STS concepts of sociotechnical imaginaries and classification to examine the role of NRICM101 in Taiwanese nationalism during the first two years of the COVID-19 pandemic.

The concept of sociotechnical imaginaries will enable us to analyze how the collective project to produce and distribute NRICM101 was also a collective project to strengthen both Taiwanese nationalism and global perceptions of Taiwan. Sheila Jasanoff, an STS scholar at Harvard University, proposes the idea that sociotechnical imaginaries can help explain complicated issues related to science, technology, nationalism, and politics, especially insofar as they concern national technology policies. The idea of sociotechnical imaginaries brings technological innovation, technology policies, and societal factors together into consideration. She defines "sociotechnical imaginaries" as goals that a society sets for itself on the basis of advances in science and technology (Jasanoff, 2015).

In other words, sociotechnical imaginaries are ideologies about the mediating role that science and technology play in national development for a desired future, including the development of nationalistic discourses and cultural identities. Herein, I apply the concept of sociotechnical imaginaries to analyze the tensions between COVID-19 governance, promoting nationalism, NRICM101 innovation, and the two-track regulatory system for biomedicine and TCM.

The second STS concept I use in the present study is, at least on the surface, a straight-forward one: classification. The classification of NRICM101 as a drug or a food has been an important topic in Taiwan. Thus, we can better understand the nationalistic trajectory of NRICM101 by examining how various stakeholders, ranging from medical scientists to pharmaceutical manufacturers to political leaders, have characterized and manipulated the classification of NRICM101. In particular, I emphasize the roles played by regulatory policy, herbal knowledge, and disease-control directives in this dynamic social construction process.

From an STS perspective, classification is not nearly as natural or neutral as is often assumed. Instead, as STS scholars Geoffrey Bowker and Susan Star (1999) argue, classification is a process not of mirroring the natural world perfectly but of organizing it accurately. STS research thus addresses the roles played by technologies, economics, political agendas, and moral orders in the production and evolution of classificatory systems.

Bowker and Star's conception of classification can shed considerable light on the history of herbal regulation in Taiwan. According to Michael Shi-Yung Liu's reminders in Chapter 1 and his previous remarkable works, we should recall that the Japanese empire, which colonized Taiwan from 1895 to 1945, implemented a medical policy in which biomedicine acted as a tool of the empire (Liu, 2009). Thus, in addition to treating and preventing diseases, biomedicine maintained social order in Japan's colonial possessions, including Taiwan. This perception may reflect, in part, the fact that the Japanese colonizers suppressed Chinese medicine throughout their 50-year rule over Taiwan. After the Second World War, the Republic of China assumed the reins of government in Taiwan. However, the Nationalist Party (Kuomintang, KMT), which governed the Republic of China, quickly suffered a string of military defeats at the hands of Chinese communist forces and was forced to retreat from mainland China to Taiwan. The island became the last bastion of the Republic of China but is today known around the world primarily as Taiwan. During the retreat of the KMT, Chinese medical personnel poured into Taiwan, and they brought with them a slew of Chinese medical regulations, enforced by the new KMT government (Soon, 2020). By and large, both the personnel and the regulations were steeped in the principles and practices of US-based biomedicine. Historian Ralph Croizier (1968) points out that, in 1950s Taiwan, biomedicine dominated medical policies, and biomedical physicians doubted the legitimacy of TCM physicians. Sociologist Yun-Wen Yeh (2013), in analyzing the relationship between biomedicine, TCM, and the KMT government in Taiwan, stated that TCM found itself once again pitted against biomedical groups in a struggle for political legitimacy, cultural acceptance, and economic security. The struggle wended its way into the early 21st century, when, over a period of several years, the Taiwanese government imposed many biomedicine-based regulations on the medical use of herbs (Huang, 2018).

This biomedical classification system has dominated drug regulations during the COVID-19 pandemic in Taiwan. On June 1, 2020, the Taiwan MOHW reviewed and authorized the *Guidelines for the TCM Treatment of COVID-19 by Clinical Stage* proposed by the NRICM, which included guidelines for NRICM101 use. However, Shan-Chwen Chang, a member of the advisory specialist panel of the CECC and a professor of internal medicine at National Taiwan University Hospital, objected to the inclusion of the TCM guidelines in the CECC's *Temporary Guidelines for the Treatment of COVID-19*, released on June 10, 2020. The reason for Chang's objection was that scientific data on TCM guidelines were insufficient. Clinical trials with randomized, double-blinded control and experimental groups were deemed necessary to confirm the clinical efficacy of NRICM101 (*United Daily News*, 2020). In other words, TCM treatments such as NRICM101 should submit to a sufficient number of sufficiently rigorous clinical trials before being integrated into COVID-19 prevention-and-control protocols.

However, because Taiwan's regulatory classification system rests chiefly on biomedical principles, it is ill-equipped, at least from a cultural perspective, to classify Chinese herbs as good, bad, or of indeterminate value. Sean Hsiang-Lin Lei (2002) insightfully observed that the assertion "TCM knowledge is based on experience" emerged from the polemic between biomedicine and TCM. This assertion and the discourse surrounding it have played a vital role in the challenges that TCM has encountered from biomedicine. The experience learned from clinical cases is critical in constructing TCM knowledge. Owing to the epistemic and cultural differences between biomedicine and TCM, biomedicine-based regulations concerning the TCM-based use of herbs are sometimes vague. Sociologist Chin-Chih An

(2010) pointed out that the biomedical regulation of herbal concoctions may generate insurmountable confusion concerning whether the concoctions are medicine or food—for example, is four-agent soup best classified as a herbal prescription or a functional food? The concept of functional food, which is most certainly a modern classification of herbal products, ignores the food-as-medicine belief widely held by both lay people and TCM experts.

Drawing on the theoretical frameworks of sociotechnical imaginaries and classification, I map the journey that NRICM101 has taken, tracking its interactions with technological innovation, herbal regulation, and Taiwanese nationalism. As my examination of NRICM101's journey unfolds, we will see that the herbal remedy has faced obstacles that go well beyond mere randomized controlled trials: it has undergone a cultural trial by fire against the backdrop of a biomedicine-dominated regulatory framework.

In what follows, I examine three stages in NRICM101's journey. The first stage concerns the technological innovations and the herbal regulations that have influenced NRICM101's recent journey in Taiwan. The second stage centers on how TCM supporters and practitioners strategically harnessed Taiwanese nationalism in their effort to overcome the challenges posed by clinical and cultural opposition to the herbal remedy. In the third stage, I discuss medical experts' objections to NRICM101. By analyzing the issues surrounding these three stages, I hope to reveal how public debates concerning the cultural, medical, and nationalistic merits of TCM shaped the high-profile role played by NRICM101 during the pandemic in Taiwan and globally.

Creating a COVID-19 Herbal Product via Re-networking Protocols

NRICM101 is more an innovative herbal formula than a TCM formula. According to an NRICM announcement, Director Yi-Chang Su assembled a draft of *Guidelines for the TCM Treatment of COVID-19 by Clinical Stage* on January 31, 2020, and then, on March 31, 2020, provided the finalized version of these guidelines to TCM departments in teaching hospitals, such as Tri-Service General Hospital and Taichung Veterans General Hospital. According to the guidelines, the targeted hospitals provide collaborative biomedicine and TCM consultations to treat patients with COVID-19. NRICM's guidelines recommended that COVID-19 patients presenting mild symptoms should be prescribed a standard formula made up of antiviral and immunoregulatory herbs that would help hospitals cope with the influx of COVID-19 patients. This formula was called "Taiwan NRICM101," or "NRICM101" for short (NRICM, 2021b).

According to Director Yi-Chang Su, NRICM101 has three hybrid features: it uses locally sourced raw materials, it is a standardized and quality-controlled formula, and it benefits from Su's personal experience in tackling ailments similar to the ones associated with COVID-19. First, Su asserted that all the herbal ingredients in NRICM101 can be cultivated in Taiwan andthus Taiwan can independently produce this new drug without having to rely on herbs imported from China (*AgriHarvest*, 2021).[4] Second, all the herbal materials in NRICM101 underwent strict quality control procedures. For example, all the herbs came from licensed herbal dispensaries and were thus permissible for use in TCM pharmacy departments in teaching hospitals. Su specifically guaranteed that the quality of each herb in the NRICM101 formula was assessed through a series of stringent bioactivity tests and fingerprint profile analyses, such as high-performance liquid chromatography fingerprint analysis (Tsai et al., 2021). Third, Su stated that his motivation for designing NRICM101 and other standardized infectious disease prescriptions stemmed from his experiences during the severe acute respiratory syndrome (SARS) epidemic in 2003. He recalled that a SARS-infected patient had recovered after being treated with Ching-Fang toxin-resolving powder, a basic TCM formula dating back to about 1550 CE during the Ming dynasty (*Initium Media*, 2022). Thus, as the COVID-19 pandemic took hold, Director Su set out to create the NRICM101 formula by analyzing the characteristics of the virus in relation to the foundational TCM principle that effective medicine must support right and dispel evil (NRICM, 2020). In addition, Su wanted to see the remedy used not just domestically but overseas, as well. While this objective potentially faced hurdles, as the European Union and the United States banned many medicinal herbs commonly used to treat infectious diseases in TCM, including ephedra, Manchurian wild ginger, and gypsum, none of these banned ingredients were included in the NRICM101 formula (New Southbound Policy Portal, 2022).

In early 2021, only one peer-reviewed article about NRICM101 was published. The article "A Traditional Chinese Medicine Formula NRICM101 to Target COVID-19 through Multiple Pathways: A Bedside-to-Bench Study" details the ingredients, mechanism, and preliminary clinical efficacy findings related to NRICM101. According to the article, the new formula consisted of ten herbs and three mechanisms that gave NRICM101 its antiviral and immunoregulatory properties (Tsai et al., 2021).

We can clearly identify the trademark signs of hybridity and re-networking in the research and development that went into NRICM101. Indeed, the journal article's subtitle contains the term "bedside-to-bench" (a reversal of "bench-to-bedside"), which obviously corresponds to the "reverse order protocol" in Sean Hsiang-lin Lei's historical study of how the KMT government invented the antimalarial drug Changshan during the Second World War. At that time, finding a replacement for quinine became a top priority for KMT troops as they retreated to southwest China, a region afflicted by endemic malaria. Lei mentions that the development of Changshan as a new antimalarial drug went through two main stages. In the first stage, developers reviewed traditional Chinese herbal medicines and selected the one that held the most promise in fighting malaria: the selected herb was Changshan, a tried-and-true herbal remedy with many centuries of use in TCM. The second stage, re-networking Changshan, was critical. Medical experts in the KMT government needed to use an array of hybrid methods ranging from laboratory experimentation to close readings of the TCM classic *Materia medica* in order to reconstruct Changshan's knowledge and strengthen its anti-malarial properties. These government scientists ended up reversing conventional biomedical protocols. Normally, the protocols require that experimentation (1) begin with effective molecules, (2) proceed to animal experimentation, and (3) conclude with research on human subjects. For Changshan, the protocol began with clinical findings (i.e., human subject research) and ended with pharmaceutical work in laboratories (i.e., molecular-level research and animal experimentation) (Lei, 2014).

In a similar way, Director Yi-Chang Su re-networked heterogeneous elements of biomedical and TCM methods in order to improve the medical properties of NRICM101 for treating COVID-19. This re-networking focused on the importance of locally cultivated herbs, the standardization of procedures, and the most critical part, the experiential relevance of Director Su's clinical work during the SARS epidemic. Many historians of TCM have noted that experience plays a crucial role in TCM education and clinical practice (Lei, 2002). Regarding NRICM101, clinical experience obtained from SARS inspired Su to design a herbal formulation targeting COVID-19. He then translated his experience into valuable medical knowledge that could be harnessed in the official institute's biomedical laboratory where the final version of NRICM101 took shape. He intended to sell this herbal product overseas, where COVID-19 was spreading rapidly. Finally, after following his "bedside-to-bench" protocol, Su tested the efficacy of NRICM101 in mass clinical trials.

Embedded in the innovations surrounding NRICM101 were two important factors: the scale of the global health crisis and Taiwanese nationalism. At the beginning of the COVID-19 pandemic, Director Su criticized China's COVID-19 herbal formulas, such as Lian-Hua-Qing-Wen-Jiao-Nang and Qing-Fei-Pai-Du-Tang. In a media interview conducted in the spring of 2020, Su argued that China's strategy had betrayed the TCM doctrine of tailor-made diagnoses and tailor-made prescriptions (Chen, 2020). Su was essentially arguing that Taiwan's TCM was more orthodox—and was thus more effective—than China's TCM. However, the development of NRICM101 was not based on pure TCM theory. To meet the demands of modern biomedical systems and mass disease control measures, the aforementioned Taiwanese teaching hospitals and Director Su's national research institute developed NRICM101 according to clinical biomedical procedures, not TCM procedures, which tend to involve such human subject practices as pulse taking and tongue examination. In fact, researchers working on NRICM101 were unable to personally access COVID-19 patients, as they were confined to isolation wards (NRICM, 2021b). Retrospectively speaking, Su's criticism of China's COVID-19 herbal formulas was based on not only professional standards but also Taiwanese nationalism.

Trapped in the Legal Gray Area between Drugs and Food

Although NRICM101 seemed promising and was being used in Taiwanese-teaching hospitals on a small scale during the first half year of 2020, governmental regulations restricted its development and use in the country. After the middle of 2020, ironically, NRICM101 was exported to Western countries but could not be marketed in Taiwan. This paradox was attributable mainly to the regulations and procedures governing the licensing of drugs in Taiwan (Legislative Yuan Gazette,

2021b). In the case of NRICM101, its developers understood that, in order for it to be classified as a new herbal drug, they had to satisfy a slew of biomedical protocols; if the protocols were not met, NRICM101 would be, at least in the eyes of the Taiwanese government, nothing more than a food supplement.

TCM groups initially expected NRICM101 to become a licensed herbal drug in Taiwan. However, according to *Guidelines on Examination and Registration of New Chinese Medicines* published by the Department of Chinese Medicine and Pharmacy (DCMP) MOHW, NRICM101 was a new formula, not a traditional one (Department of Chinese Medicine and Pharmacy, Ministry of Health and Welfare, N.d.). Thus, *Guidelines* stipulated that use of NRICM101 had to follow Taiwan's rules governing the authorization of new herbal drugs, including the requirement for a large clinical trial. This created a dilemma because Taiwan managed to control the spread of COVID-19, limiting the total number of confirmed cases to 823 in 2020 (Taiwan Centers for Disease Control, 2021). At the time, NRICM101 could not meet the regulatory threshold necessary to obtain governmental approval for therapeutic use, as the sample size of NRICM101's clinical trial (33 patients) was deemed to be too small and as the trial had involved a non-randomized distribution and a non-double-blinded model (Tsai et al., 2021). In short, the developers of NRICM101 faced steep hurdles in getting Taiwanese authorities to classify their herbal formula as a new herbal drug.

Curiously, NRICM101 cannot be approved as a food supplement in Taiwan. The island's TCM community has long subscribed to the "medicine–food homology" concept (藥食同源), which holds that some medicinal herbs are also appropriate for daily diets. Thus, TCM physicians can treat diseases and promote health by prescribing medicinal herbs as food ingredients (Li and Shih, 2018). According to sociologist Chin-Chih An (2010), the common belief that food is medicine generates a legal gray area in governments' regulation of biomedical drugs, herbal drugs, and food ingredients. Thus, the chasm between biomedicine and TCM regarding the classification of drugs and foods has resulted in a two-track regulatory system that generates no small amount of legal gray area for herbs that are thought to be simultaneously dietary and medicinal. In the case of NRICM101, the "food as medicine" concept and its corresponding legal gray area erected a governmental barrier that prevented the newly innovated medicinal herb from being officially labeled a food supplement.

The legal gray area in which NRICM101 found itself trapped can be traced back to the year 2000. In that year, the DCMP at the MOHW issued *A Listing of Edible Chinese Medicinal Ingredients* which explicitly categorized these herbs as food products that could be sold freely by food producers. The initial list included 12 items, but that number had increased to 215 items by 2012. Much of this increase occurred in the year 2008, when the list was augmented with 161 edible items taken from perhaps the most renowned Chinese medical work, *Materia medica*, written by Shi-Zhen Li and first printed in the late 16th century. Interestingly, however, the list was greatly streamlined to include just 37 edible items in 2018 because the advisory board of the DCMP considered the 2012 version inappropriate for regulation (Li and Shih, 2018). The shorter list of edible herbs means food industry leaders have less right to sell food supplements made from herbs. The reduction of items in 2018 makes it more necessary to visit TCM physicians to access herbal products.

In 2005, the TFDA issued another publication, *The Reference List of Food Ingredients*. Essentially, the publication listed items that the TFDA had certified as food ingredients: in 2005, the list had 673 items; in 2018, there were 752 items; and in late 2021, there were 761 items. Of these 761 items, 32 overlapped with items on the list compiled by the DCMP (Du, 2022). All food supplements should be produced with ingredients on this list. Even though the TFDA list highly overlapped with the DCMP items, of the ten herbal ingredients in NRICM101, only three (mulberry leaf, peppermint, and fishwort) are on the most recent iteration of *The Reference List of Food Ingredients* published by the TFDA, while only the peppermint is on the DCMP's list. Both lists hindered NRICM101 from being marketed as a food supplement.

In brief, the certification dilemmas that the NRICM101 encountered were rooted not only in scientific objections but in cultural ones, as well. In Taiwan's drug regulation apparatus, NRICM101 needed to overcome a high scientific threshold set by the biomedical community. However, in the Taiwanese governmental apparatus overseeing the regulation of food supplements, NRICM101 was trapped in a gray area mutually constructed by the food industry and TCM groups. The gray area has given rise to a series of dilemmas that left the NRICM101 in a kind of limbo: the formula was neither Chinese medicine nor biomedicine, neither a food nor a drug.

A Hero's Journey, NRICM101, and the Nationalistic Rhetoric

To break through the regulatory limits blocking NRICM101's domestic use as a herbal treatment for COVID-19, TCM groups decided to intervene. We know from multiple studies (e.g., Anderson, 1983[2006]) that media and language can powerfully bolster nation-building, which includes citizens' sense of belonging to an imagined community. In Chapter 11, Yu-hui Tai also demonstrated that China's media propaganda was crucial in promoting Chinese nationalism internally and externally during the pandemic. Aware of this power of media and language, Taiwan's TCM groups articulated the new herbal product in the language of Taiwanese nationalism, "Taiwan can help," and constructed a "hero's journey" narrative that would firmly and positively link NRICM101 to the image of a powerful Taiwan.

On July 5, 2020, the president of the Legislative Yuan, Si-Kun You, gave a speech at the 90th Chinese Medical Festival. He proposed that "traditional Chinese medicine (中醫)" ought to be distinguished from "traditional Taiwanese medicine (臺醫)." The proposal was not entirely original, as Japan, South Korea, and Vietnam had already distanced themselves onomastically from China by naming their traditional national medicines Kampo medicine, Korean medicine, and traditional Vietnamese medicine, respectively. Given the spread of Taiwanese nationalist sentiment and given the Chinese state's insistence that Taiwan rightfully belongs to China, it was thought that a movement to substitute the term "traditional Taiwanese medicine" for the common term "traditional Chinese medicine" in reference to traditional medicine practiced in Taiwan might appeal to nationalist sentiment while countering the Chinese state's efforts to suppress this sentiment. However, on July 6, 2020, the NUCMDA issued a press release expressing opposition to Si-Kun You's proposal. Ironically, the press release—despite its rejection of the term "traditional Taiwanese medicine"—used the term "Taiwanese Chinese medicine" (臺灣中醫藥) rather than the term "Chinese medicine" (中醫藥) (NUCMDA, 2020). Although TCM groups felt a little uneasy with the explicit nationalist rhetoric (NUCMDA, 2020), they gradually became aware of the value in distinguishing Taiwan's TCM from China's TCM during the COVID-19 pandemic.

In June 2020, the number of COVID-19 infections had stabilized in Taiwan. Therefore, the NRICM decided to export NRICM101 overseas as a food supplement. In a Legislative Yuan interpellation, Democratic Progressive Party legislator Ying Chen asked the MOHW to appropriate funds to NRICM for NRICM101 innovation in the first half of 2020. Director Yi-Chang Su's strategy was to export NRICM101 overseas, where clinical trials would accumulate enough data to meet the requirements for herbal drug certification laid out by Taiwanese regulators (Legislative Yuan Gazette, 2020). In May 2020, the NRICM transferred some of its production technology to Taiwanese GMP pharmaceutical companies and authorized them to mass manufacture NRICM101. In October 2020, Sun Ten Pharmaceutical Company became the first company to export the commodified NRICM101 (NRICM, 2021a). The Taiwanese government, including the Bureau of Foreign Trade, facilitated this process (Legislative Yuan Gazette, 2021b), and in January 2021, Singapore became the first country to approve NRICM101 for use as a Chinese proprietary medicine (Brand name: RespireAid, 天冠10 approved by the Singapore Health Sciences Authority). NRICM101 became available in the United States, United Kingdom, Australia, and Europe countries. These achievements seemed promising, and the NRICM and Taiwanese legislators doubled their efforts to promote this new herbal product, referring to it as "the glory of Taiwan" (Legislative Yuan Gazette, 2021a).

However, along its journey, NRICM101 continued to encounter obstacles. Once Sun Ten began exporting NRICM101, the company encouraged COVID-19 positive individuals taking the herbal formula to report their health data as evidence of the formula's efficacy. Sun Ten hoped to collect this information "And pass it on to physicians so that certification advisory committees would be unable to criticize [NRICM101]" (*CommonWealth Magazine*, 2021). This strategy was unsuccessful. Director Yi-Chang Su discovered that both this business strategy and this collected data lacked reliability. Su admitted as much in a public comment: "The data collected by these companies are only for business use [not for clinical studies]." Furthermore, Su said that "for collecting the reliable data, the Tri-Service General Hospital research team will apply for Institutional Review Board certification through *ClinicalTrials.gov*" (Legislative Yuan Gazette, 2021b; ClinicalTrials.gov, 2020).

The journey that NRICM101 embarked upon overseas has parallels to the fabled hero's journeys in famous stories, such as *The Odyssey*. In a hero's journey, a courageous traveler leaves home in order to accomplish a great task, and throughout this journey, the traveler encounters and overcomes many formidable challenges.

NRICM101 overcame regulatory and cultural obstacles around the world. And just as Odysseus returned home to Ithaca, where he righted many wrongs, so too did NRICM101, after extensive encounters around the world, return to Taiwan, where the herbal remedy achieved the previously unachievable: regulatory approval for use (temporarily) as a herbal medicine in the treatment of COVID-19. The core challenge that NRICM101 faced at home was the ironic inaccessibility of Taiwanese-made NRICM101 in Taiwan. Although, in March 2021, only 20–30 foreign COVID-19 cases involving NRICM101 treatment reported their conditions to Taiwanese GMP pharmaceutical companies (Legislative Yuan Gazette, 2021b), TCM advocacy groups in Taiwan promoted NRICM101's "heroic" achievements to the public. These groups specifically lauded the contributions of NRICM101 in a way that channeled the Taiwanese government's propagation of a certain nationalistic sentiment. For example, at the 2021 Taipei Traditional Chinese Medicine International Forum (the 91st Chinese Medical Festival), the NUCMDA boasted about the ingredients of NRICM101 and celebrated Taiwan's successful export of the formula (*Public Television Service*, 2021). Indeed, in attendance at the forum was Taiwanese President Ing-Wen Tsai, who openly endorsed NRICM101:

> Taiwanese GMP pharmaceutical companies obtained authorization from Euro-American countries to sell NRICM101 there [...] this herbal commodity is the best-seller in Euro-American countries and has put Taiwan in the global spotlight.
>
> (Office of the President, 2021a)

The president's speech was full of explicit nationalist rhetoric, which perhaps helps explain why, soon afterward, TCM advocacy groups in Taiwan were couching their discussion of NRICM101 in nationalistic terms: the groups praised the "national TCM team" and, when a resurgence of COVID-19 struck Taiwan in May 2021, proudly declared that "TCM can help," imitating the nationalistic government slogan "Taiwan can help" (NUCMDA, 2021a).

Taiwanese TCM advocacy groups, official Taiwanese research institutes, and Taiwanese pharmaceutical companies looked forward to breaking through the Taiwanese government's regulatory gridlock blocking the entrance of new drugs such as NRICM101. Each of these stakeholders constructed a "hero's journey" narrative portraying NRICM101's travels outside Taiwan as a series of glorious overseas achievements, the apex of which was NRICM101's status as a bestselling food supplement in these foreign countries.

Taiwanese Nationalism, the NRICM, and Emergency-Use Authorization

In mid-May 2021, COVID-19 was surging again in Taiwan, but vaccines were in short supply for everyone. In these troubling circumstances, the Taiwanese MOHW granted EUA to NRICM101 in an act of strategic expediency, with the aim of at least mitigating panic in Taiwanese society, even though NRICM101's clinical study in Taiwan was not rigorous due to the lack of community transmission in 2020. NRICM101 obtained the EUA on May 18, 2021. According to regulations contained within the *Pharmaceutical Affairs Act* (Laws and Regulations Database of the Republic of China, 2018 [1993]), this authorization meant that, in treating COVID-19 symptoms, NRICM101 would be used as a pharmaceutical drug rather than as a food supplement.

There was an important limitation to this authorization: it was temporary. The EUA would be withdrawn once the government lifted its nationwide COVID-19 restrictions. Thus, even though the EUA provided the NRICM101 with a new classificatory status and a certification for medical use, the formula's journey remained—and still remains—uncertain.

Media-based promotion of NRICM101 was an important strategy in Taiwan. As a point in fact, NRICM Director Yi-Chang Su introduced NRICM101 to the public right after the EUA was approved, when he appeared on talk shows singing the praises of his new medicinal concoction (e.g., *Sanlih E-Television*, 2021). When promoting NRICM101, TCM advocacy groups relied heavily on the testimony of COVID-19 patients who had taken the formula to combat the virus' symptoms. Even after NRICM101 obtained an EUA from Taiwanese regulatory authorities, many TCM departments in Taiwanese medical centers voluntarily reported evidence of the benefits of NRICM101. The chairman of the NUCMDA wrote a published article in the publication of the Consumers' Foundation, in which he mentioned two recovery cases in Taiwanese medical centers. The case reports attracted widespread public interest as they included testimonials from celebrities (Ko, 2021). This kind of news was more "human interest" news than "hard news," and partly for this reason, it went far in promoting NRICM101 to the Taiwanese public. At the same time, TCM advocacy groups made a point of marketing NRICM101 as a serious, rigorously vetted TCM pharmaceutical (NUCMDA, 2021b).

Although no sound data from randomized controlled trials became available with respect to the efficacy of NRICM101, TCM advocacy groups repeatedly cited patient testimonials when trying to broaden the use of NRICM101. One instance of this reliance on testimonials came from the Taiwanese legislator Ying Chen, who, on October 21, 2021, interpellated the minister of the MOHW, Shih-Chung Chen, to discuss a recent close call involving NRICM101: a mother suffering from a COVID-19 infection was unable to immediately take NRICM101 because the results of her COVID-19 PCR test and other tests were issued late. Fortunately, after numerous interventions, the patient received NRICM101 from a TCM physician—and she recovered. Legislator Chen used this case to convince the minister to loosen the standards governing patients' acquisition of NRICM: specifically, Ying Chen asked that the MOHW no longer require physicians to obtain a positive PCR test before they prescribe NRICM101. Minister Chen, for his part, insisted that any policy decision regarding NRICM101 should rest partly on clinical trial data so as to avoid unnecessary risks to the public's health (Legislative Yuan Gazette, 2021c).

The EUA brought NRICM101 back to Taiwan, launched the medical community's widespread use of the formula, and, in doing so, rescued the formula from the gray area between certified pharmaceutical drugs and everyday food ingredients.

But the story did not end there, because TCM advocacy groups in Taiwan treated the newly classified formula as a pillar of Taiwanese nationalism—an imaginary that helped the formula skirt the biomedicine-dominated regulatory culture of Taiwan.

Criticism of NRICM101's Return Journey

The EUA granted NRICM101 not only temporary legal status as a prescribable drug but also a veneer of nationalism. However, the hero's journey of NRICM101 continued to draw criticism from medical experts. In this section, I will briefly explore this criticism and then discuss how it may have contributed to systemic shortages of NRICM101.

Of all the criticism leveled at NRICM101, the lack of randomized controlled trials was the Achilles' heel for the formula. Ching-Shwun Lin, a professor at the Department of Urology, University of California San Francisco, argued that only one peer-reviewed journal article had ever been written about NRICM101 in 2021. In that article, the discharge criterion was three consecutive negative tests. This standard was not indicative of a complete recovery from COVID-19 because some patients can test negative but still suffer from severe symptoms. Cheng-Chung Wei, the director of the Center of Clinical Trials at Chung Shan Medical University Hospital in Taiwan, criticized NRICM101's clinical trial for its mere 12 case reports and for not being a randomized controlled trial. Thus, in Wei's view, the efficacy of NRICM101 was questionable, and the so-called clinical trial was insufficiently rigorous (*Initium Media*, 2022). Some scholars at China Medical University also pointed out that most TCM studies of COVID-19 involved only cell- and animal-based experiments. Higher-level research designs, such as randomized double blind-controlled trials involving humans, were needed to prove the actual efficacy of a TCM formula (Chang and Hsieh, 2021).

An implication of this criticism is that there has been a systemic lack of development of TCM in Taiwan. We, of course, can criticize the country's biomedicine-dominated regulatory culture for some of the obstacles that NRICM101 had to overcome. Nevertheless, the successful return of NRICM101 to its home country ironically demonstrated that the herbal drug system in Taiwan was incapable of coping, at least in the short term, with the emerging pandemic even though the NRICM had already collaborated with Taiwanese medical centers and GMP-certified pharmaceutical companies to conduct clinical trials. Director of the DCMP Yi-Tsau Huang explained that the low rate of COVID-19 in Taiwan in 2020 had, in fact, hindered patient recruitment for clinical trials. Although the NRICM was planning to conduct randomized controlled trials in foreign countries, the pioneering research in these countries ended up relying on only 20–30 cases in half a year (Legislative Yuan Gazette, 2021b). In mid-2022, the second peer-reviewed article was published in an international journal (Tseng et al., 2022). Unfortunately, although this multicenter study recruited 345 patients and provided real-world evidence of NRICM101 from their medical records, the TFDA and the CECC still disapproved of NRICM101's drug permit license because this retrospective study could not replace randomized-controlled trials. Furthermore, with the rapid spread of the Omicron variant in mid-2022, herbal ingredients critical to the production of NRICM101 were in short supply in Taiwan (Legislative Yuan Gazette, 2022a). In other words, although the EUA obtained by NRICM101 exempted it from the regulatory restrictions imposed on new herbal formulas, and although the nationalistic rhetoric surrounding NRICM101 satisfied the national imaginaries of many proud Taiwanese, the barriers that blocked the return of NRICM101 to Taiwan reflected systemic problems within Taiwan's TCM advocacy network, regulatory framework, and industry.

Additional criticism regarding NRICM101 came from within the TCM community—namely, from senior TCM physicians. In the hero's journey taken by NRICM101, although the NUCMDA strongly supported the innovation of the formula, senior TCM physicians expressed diverse opinions on the overall process. For example, senior TCM physician Miao-Ho Chen stated that the treatment of NRICM101 deviated from TCM principles. Conventional TCM theory privileges tailor-made diagnoses and prescriptions. In some TCM quarters, criticism was leveled at the ingredients of NRICM101, which, being "cold-natured herbs," are harmful to patients in the cold constitution with experiencing symptoms such as chronic diarrhea and an unhealthy aversion to cold (*Initium Media*, 2022). By openly complaining about the unorthodox formulation of NRICM101, TCM physicians exhibited their profound concern that NRICM101 had deviated from conventional TCM theory.

We should also take note of the criticism that knowledgeable TCM physicians leveled against NRICM101. Their central objection was that NRICM101 transgressed the principles of TCM and that its use might distort these principles at both epistemological and practical levels. Specifically, NRICM101, a government-endorsed and standardized formulation, could replace TCM physicians' experience-based practices and tailor-made prescriptions. In fact, NRICM101 has already changed certain governmental regulations pertaining to TCM clinical practices and TCM business health insurance offerings. For example, in mid-2022, a prescription for NRICM101 became the required document for pandemic payouts in private COVID-19 insurance (Legislative Yuan Gazette, 2022b).

Discussion: The Shift from Traditional Chinese Medicine to Taiwanese Chinese Medicine

As Taiwan's first EUA herbal product, NRICM101 has come to symbolize progress in the country's TCM innovations and regulations. The process by which NRICM101 was socially constructed in Taiwan during the first two years of the pandemic reflects the various systemic obstacles that herbal formulas have faced domestically and abroad. Furthermore, the "hero's journey" narrative surrounding the NRICM101's travels abroad reflected the collective desire of the Taiwanese people to combat the pandemic. All of these strategic efforts on the part of NRICM101 supporters to get the formula certified for prescription domestically transformed NRICM101 into a metaphoric symbol of Taiwanese nationalist imaginaries. In this section, I revisit the issues of classification, nationalism, and sociotechnical imaginaries as they relate to the hero's journey of NRICM101.

At first glance, it would appear that in order to obtain certification as a prescribable medicine, NRICM101 needed to combat the biomedicine-dominated culture of Taiwan. From the STS perspective, classification is a dynamic process reflecting such "non-scientific" factors as political power and stakeholder interests (Star and Griesemer, 1989; Bowker and Star, 1999). In the first stage of NRICM101's journey, the formula encountered obstacles in the form of an asymmetrical regulatory culture in which a two-track system prioritized biomedicine yet attempted to appease TCM. Even though NRICM101 was an innovative re-networking of locally cultivated herbs, scientific standardization, and clinical data, the formula, without data from randomized controlled trials, still struggled to satisfy Taiwan's stringent drug approval criteria. The Taiwanese government's decision to grant EUA to NRICM101 was the event that brought the exiled formula back to Taiwan after a long and lauded journey overseas. In terms of classification, the EUA reflected the new—though temporary—status of NRICM101. NRICM101 seemed to be painted into a corner by overly rigid and explicit regulations in Taiwan before obtaining the EUA. This temporary classification exempted NRICM101 from the biomedical barriers of new drug regulations and freed NRICM101 from the corner where a thing's status as a drug or a food is indeterminate.

Upon second glance, it appears that the hero's journey of NRICM101 reflected and even projected the national and international aspirations of many Taiwanese. TCM advocacy groups, although initially uncomfortable with efforts to distinguish between traditional Chinese medicine and traditional Taiwanese medicine, gradually realized that nationalism could play a critical role in challenging the regulatory barriers faced by NRICM101. A major turning point in this evolution was Director Yi-Chang Su's criticism of China's COVID-19 herbal formulas that betrayed conventional TCM theory. Director Su was appealing to Taiwanese nationalistic sentiment when he implied that Taiwanese TCM was more orthodox than Chinese TCM. In essence, Taiwan was not just different from China but better than it.

The "hero's journey" narrative that began when "the glory of Taiwan"—NRICM101—was exported for use in overseas markets fed into the nationalistic imaginaries embraced by a wide and growing swath of the Taiwanese public. Even though the NUCMDA politely rejected proposals to replace the conventional term "traditional Chinese medicine" with the overtly nationalistic term "traditional Taiwanese medicine," TCM-friendly legislators, NUCMDA members, and NRICM members framed the export of NRICM101 as a hero's long journey for the greater glory of Taiwan. TCM advocacy groups also adapted the government slogan "Taiwan can help" into "TCM can help." In the diplomatic article on the Southeast policy website, furthermore, the Ministry of Foreign Affairs highlighted Taiwan and otherized China by exaggeratedly claiming that Taiwan's NRICM101 "has the potential to be a Covid remedy for the whole planet" (New Southbound Policy Portal, 2022). In these ways, NRICM101 came to symbolize a shift from traditional Chinese medicine to Taiwanese Chinese medicine.

Upon a third and final glance, it is also noteworthy that nationalistic narratives of NRICM101 not only serve the public health demands for disease control but also meet Taiwanese desires for a better geopolitical situation. The name "Taiwan NRICM101" implies Taiwanese sociotechnical imaginaries in the COVID-19 pandemic. Taiwan NRICM101's trials in the biomedicine-dominated regulatory apparatus symbolically intertwine with the ordeals of the Taiwanese government in geopolitics. Thus, NRICM101 significantly mediates the psychological projection with its spin on the nationalist slogan "Taiwan can help": "TCM can help."

NRICM101's heroic construction as a product for "the glory of Taiwan" not only indicates that NRICM101 is a Taiwanese-made formula but also showcases the island as a nation independent of China. In this worldwide pandemic, this nationalistic NRICM101 mediates and reflects Taiwan's desired future as a country recognized by other countries, as Yu-Yueh Tsai mentioned in Chapter 12 on the long-sought recognition of the nation-state by the World Health Organization. Therefore, NRICM101 is both a herbal formula for treating COVID-19 and a tonic for boosting Taiwan's nationalism.

Conclusion

In this chapter, I have provided a pioneering analysis of the co-production between COVID-19 governance, herbal regulation, NRICM101, and Taiwan's nationalism during the pandemic. I have analyzed the official development, export, and temporary certification of NRICM101, a Taiwanese-made herbal remedy used to treat COVID-19 patients. I have examined why Taiwanese-made NRICM101 was initially inaccessible in Taiwan, and I then described how NRICM101, after a nationalistic "hero's journey" narrative overseas, obtained domestic EUA from the Taiwanese government. I have also shown how classificatory and nationalistic imaginaries in Taiwan turned NRICM101 into something more than just a herbal formula.

Historians of TCM have already illustrated the close connection between TCM innovations and nationalism. NRICM101, the first herbal product to obtain an EUA in Taiwan, further illustrates this connection. However, the collective decision of many TCM advocates in Taiwan to merge this herbal product with the rhetoric of Taiwanese nationalism challenged both Taiwan's biomedicine-dominated regulatory apparatus and Taiwan's status as a "renegade province" that rightfully belongs to China. The makers of NRICM101, together with TCM advocacy groups, strategically appropriated Taiwanese nationalism and painted NRICM101 as "the glory of Taiwan" to assert Taiwan as a nation independent of China. This process forged a new imaginary, as the concept of traditional Chinese medicine in Taiwan ceded its place to the concept of Taiwanese Chinese medicine.

Notes

1 Descriptions and critiques of this new herbal drug can be found on the internet, but systematic analyses are scarce, especially from the "science, technology, and society" perspective (Editorial Office, 2021; Chen, 2021a; 2021b).

2 The social media platforms that I used include primarily online newspapers, online magazines, and YouTube videos.
3 The journal *Consumer Reports of Taiwan* is published by Consumers Foundation Chinese Taipei, which is an independent, non-profit organization that was founded in 1980 and that aims to protect the rights of consumers through popular activism and policy advocacy.
4 *AgriHarvest* is published in Taiwan by the Harvest Publishing Group, which was previously known as the Sino-American Joint Commission on Rural Reconstruction. The Harvest Publishing Group is now funded by the Council of Agriculture, Executive Yuan, Taiwan.

References

AgriHarvest. 2021. "All of the Herbs in NRICM101 Can Be Cultivated Domestically." May 28. Accessed December 16, 2021, https://www.agriharvest.tw/archives/60587.

An, Chin-Chih. 2010. "From Chinese Herbs to Functional Food: A Study of the Category Revolution of Food and Drug by a Biography of Four-agent Soup." *Taiwanese Journal for Studies of Science, Technology and Medicine* 11: 89–148.

Anderson, Benedict. 1983 [2006]. *Imagined Communities: Reflections on the Origin and Spread of Nationalism*. London: Verso.

Andrews, Bridie. 2014. *The Making of Modern Chinese Medicine, 1850–1960*. Vancouver: University of British Columbia Press.

Bowker, Geoffrey C., and Star, Susan L. 1999. *Sorting Things Out: Classification and its Consequences*. Cambridge: MIT Press.

Chang, Qwang-Yuen, and Hsieh, Ching-Liang. 2021. "The Possibility of Using Traditional Chinese Medicine for the Treatment of COVID-19: A Narrative Review." *Journal of Internal Medicine of Taiwan* 32(4): 281–288.

Chen, Po-Hsun. 2020. "Guideline and Knowledge Space of Traditional Chinese Medicine in Epidemic Prevention and Control." *Taiwanese Journal for Studies of Science, Technology and Medicine* 30: 243–255.

Chen, Po-Hsun. 2021a. "The Evidential Culture and Risk Management Surrounding an Anti-COVID-19 Herbal Formula." *HashtagCOVID*, May 29. Accessed May 29, 2021, https://vocus.cc/article/60b209f0fd897800012d88df.

Chen, Po-Hsun. 2021b. "The Inescapable Ambiguity of NRICM101." *COVID-19*, May 29. Accessed May 29, 2021, https://covid19.nctu.edu.tw/article/8320.

ClinicalTrials.gov. 2020. "The Outcomes of NRICM101 on SARS-COV-2 (COVID-19) Infection." Accessed May 24, 2021, https://clinicaltrials.gov/ct2/keydates/NCT04664049.

CommonWealth Magazine. 2021. "This Chinese Prescription Can Protect Us from the Pandemic!" February 1. Accessed May 24, 2021, https://www.cw.com.tw/article/5107785?utm_campaign=fb_cw-social-daily-210202-5107785&utm_medium=social&utm_source=fb_cw&fbclid=IwAR0s6w4UcFW4TRfV1APHx_kkPqDDjOx_bJ2KeE0GJ_DzJXTe-nbIa_jNo-4.

Croizier, Ralph C. 1968. *Traditional Medicine in Modern China: Science, Nationalism and the Tensions of Cultural Change*. Cambridge, MA: Harvard University Press.

Department of Chinese Medicine and Pharmacy, Ministry of Health and Welfare. N.d. "Guidelines on the Examination and Registration of New Chinese Medicines." Accessed May 24, 2021, https://dep.mohw.gov.tw/docmap/cp-701-4762-108.html.

Du, Ying-Chun. 2022. "Can You Clearly Differentiate Chinese Medical Materials from Foods?" *Consumer Reports of Taiwan* 489: 68–70.

Editorial Office. 2021. "NRICM101 and the Governance of Traditional Chinese Medicine." *HashtagCOVID*, May 27. Accessed May 27, 2021, https://vocus.cc/article/60af418bfd897800011fdcf7.

Flowers, James. 2021. "Bypassing the Technocratic State in South Korea." *Asian Medicine* 16(1): 36–57.

Hsu, Elisabeth. 1999. *The Transmission of Chinese Medicine.* Cambridge: Cambridge University Press.

Huang, Yi-Tsau. 2018. *The Development of Traditional Chinese Medicine in Taiwan*, Third Edition. Taipei City: Ministry of Health and Welfare.

Initium Media. 2022. "NRICM101 Puts Spotlight on Taiwan, but Does the Formula Have a Curative Effect?" June 16. Accessed August 13, 2022, https://theinitium.com/article/20220616-taiwan-nricm101/.

Jasanoff, Sheila. 2015. "Future Imperfect: Science, Technology, and the Imaginations of Modernity." In *Dreamscapes of Modernity: Sociotechnical Imaginaries and the Fabrication of Power*, edited by Sheila Jasanoff and Sang-Hyun Kim, 1–33. Chicago and London: University of Chicago Press.

Ko, Fu-Yang. 2021. "There are No Outsiders in the War against COVID-19." *Consumer Reports of Taiwan* 484: 32–35.

Laws and Regulations Database of the Republic of China. 2018 [1993]. *Pharmaceutical Affairs Act.*

Legislative Yuan Gazette. 2020. *Committee Records, LCIDC01_1095801_00004* 109(58). September 23.

Legislative Yuan Gazette. 2021a. *Committee Records, LCIDC01_1103301_00004* 110(33). March 18.

Legislative Yuan Gazette. 2021b. *Committee Records, LCIDC01_1103701_00003#* 110(37). March 25.

Legislative Yuan Gazette. 2021c. *Committee Records, LCIDC01_1109401_00002.* 110(94). October 25.

Legislative Yuan Gazette. 2022a. *Committee Records, LCIDC01_1117601_00001.* 111(76). May 9.

Legislative Yuan Gazette. 2022b. *Committee Records, LCIDC01_1118201_00004.* 111(82). May 19.

Lei, Sean Hsiang-Lin. 2002, "How did Chinese Medicine Become Experiential? The Political Epistemology of Jingyan." *Positions: East Asian Cultures Critique* 10(2): 333–364.

Lei, Sean Hsiang-Lin. 2014. *Neither Donkey nor Horse: Medicine in the Struggle over China's Modernity.* Chicago: University of Chicago Press.

Li, Ai-Lun and Shih, Chun-Chuan. 2018. "Analyzing the Controversies Surrounding the Management of Edible Chinese Medicinal Materials." *Taiwan Bar Journal* 22(5): 16–32.

Liu, Michael Shi-Yung. 2009. *Prescribing Colonization: The Role of Medical Practice and Policy in Japan-Ruled Taiwan*, Ann Arbor, MI: Association for Asian Studies.

Liu, Shao-Hua. 2020. "Traditional Medicine." In *Disease x society 10 keywords*, edited by Liu, Shao-Hua, 113–131. Taipei: SpringHill Publishing.

National Research Institute of Chinese Medicine. 2020. "Announcement: TCM Diagnosis and Treatment Protocol for COVID-19." *Journal of Chinese Medicine* 31(1): 1–3.

National Research Institute of Chinese Medicine. 2021a. "Clarifications about NRICM101 from the National Research Institute of Chinese Medicine (NRICM)." May 30. Accessed May 31, 2021, https://www.nricm.edu.tw/p/406-1000-6504,r61.php?Lang=zh-tw.

National Research Institute of Chinese Medicine. 2021b. "FAQs on NRICM101." February 18. Accessed May 24, 2021, https://www.nricm.edu.tw/p/406-1000-6387,r51.php?Lang=zh-tw.

National Union of Chinese Medical Doctors' Association, ROC. 2020. "'Chinese Medicine' and 'Chinese Herb' are Official Terms of Great Historical Value." July 6. Accessed July 11, 2022, http://www.twtm.tw/new.php?cat=16&id=1865.

National Union of Chinese Medical Doctors' Association, ROC. 2021a. "The Emergency Mobilization of the Taiwanese National TCM Team for Epidemic Prevention." May 31. Accessed May 31, 2021, http://www.twtm.tw/new.php?cat=16&id=2191.

National Union of Chinese Medical Doctors' Association, ROC. 2021b. "NRICM101 is a Prescription Medicine and Cannot Be Sold Over the Counter." May 18. Accessed May 24, 2021, http://www.twtm.tw/new.php?cat=16&id=2174.

New Southbound Policy Portal. 2022. "A TCM Prescription for Covid: Taiwan's NRICM101." *Ministry of Foreign Affairs*, April 25. Accessed August 10, 2022, https://nspp.mofa.gov.tw/nsppe/news.php?post=217952&unit=410&unitname=Stories&postname=A-TCM-Prescription-for-Covid:-Taiwan%E2%80%99s-NRICM101.

Office of the President, Republic of China (Taiwan). 2021a. "President: In the Post-COVID-19 Era, Appreciation for Traditional Medicine Will Grow Worldwide." March 14. Accessed May 24, 2021, https://www.president.gov.tw/NEWS/25966.

Office of the President, Republic of China (Taiwan). 2021b. "Meeting with the Representative of the National Union of Chinese Medical Doctors Association." November 11. Accessed December 5, 2021, https://www.president.gov.tw/News/26338.

Office of the President, Republic of China (Taiwan). 2021c. "The 2021 Global Health and Welfare Forum in Taiwan." October 31. Accessed December 5, 2021, https://www.president.gov.tw/News/26308.

Public Television Service NEWS. 2021. "The National Research Institute of Chinese Medicine's NRICM101 Could Confront COVID-19." March 13. Accessed May 24, 2021, https://news.pts.org.tw/article/517040?fbclid=IwAR3qIwObj0nVn4-P9Pn3tZjIX7aEV72OzQa882nFFdalQHPZSyoUh2k4JiY.

Sanlih E-Television. 2021. "Timely Assistance in Confronting COVID-19!" May 19. Accessed May 24, 2021, https://youtu.be/-AFTYnT290Q.

Singapore Health Sciences Authority. PZ4972 INFOSEARCH: Chinese Proprietary Medicine. Accessed May 24, 2021, https://eservice.hsa.gov.sg/prism/common/enquirepublic/SearchCPProduct.do?action=getCPProductDetails.

Soon, Wayne. 2020. *Global Medicine in China: A Diasporic History*. CA: Stanford University Press.

Star, Susan L., and Griesemer, James. 1989. "Ecology, 'Translations' and Boundary Objects: Amateurs and Professionals in Berkeley's Museum of Vertebrate Zoology, 1907–39." *Social Studies of Science* 19(3): 387–420.

Taiwan Centers for Disease Control. 2021. "Statistics for Confirmed Local and Overseas COVID-19 Cases." Accessed December 28, 2021, https://nidss.cdc.gov.tw/nndss/disease?id=19CoV.

Taiwan Food and Drug Administration, Ministry of Health and Welfare. "The Reference List of Food Ingredients." Accessed May 24, 2021, https://consumer.fda.gov.tw/Food/Material.aspx?nodeID=160.

Taylor, Kim. 2005. *Chinese Medicine in Early Communist China, 1945–1963: A Medicine of Revolution*. London: Routledge.

The Diplomat. 2023. "Sustainable Health Development in the Post-pandemic Era: Taiwan Can Help." April 26. Accessed May 23, 2023, https://thediplomat.com/2023/04/sustainable-health-development-in-the-post-pandemic-era-taiwan-can-help/.

Tsai, Keng-Chang, Huang, Yi-Chia, Liaw, Chia-Ching, et al. 2021. "A Traditional Chinese Medicine Formula NRICM101 to Target COVID-19 through Multiple Pathways: A Bedside-to-Bench Study." *Biomedicine & Pharmacotherapy* 133: 111037.

Tseng, Yu-Hwei., Lin, Sunny Jui-Shan., Hou, Sheng-Mou., et al. 2022. "Curbing COVID-19 Progression and Mortality with Traditional Chinese Medicine among Hospitalized Patients with COVID-19: A Propensity Score-matched Analysis." *Pharmacological Research* 184: 106412.

United Daily News. 2020. "Not Currently Recognized in the *Guidelines for the TCM Treatment of COVID-19 by Clinical Stage*." June 10. Accessed May 24, 2021, https://udn.com/news/story/120940/4626628.

Yeh, Yun-Wen. 2013. *The History of Traditional Chinese Medicine in Taiwan: The Relationship between Medicine and Politics*. Taipei: Wunan Book.

11 Which Is More Toxic—A Virus or Hostility? Discourse and Sentiment Analysis of the Chinese Government and Media's Statements on Taiwan during the COVID-19 Period

Yu-Hui Tai

Introduction

The Economist's cover story on March 11, 2023, titled "The Struggle for Taiwan", illustrates the intense global concern over whether China and Taiwan will go to war, and how cross-strait relations and the related geopolitics have become highly tense. Since Xi Jinping came to power in 2012, he has promoted his concepts of the Chinese Dream (中國夢) and the great rejuvenation of the Chinese nation(中華民族的偉大復興). With China's recent economic decline, nationalism has become a source of legitimacy for the Chinese Communist Party's rule. Unifying Taiwan has become Xi's policy goal, and in February 2019, he proposed the "One Country, Two Systems, Taiwan Plan" policy, adopting a more aggressive stance toward Taiwan and aiming to unify Taiwan through China's hard power.

In this context, almost every aspect of Taiwan's politics, society, economy, and culture has been influenced by Chinese factors, including Taiwan's pandemic governance. Therefore, to understand Taiwan's pandemic governance, it is necessary to analyze China's influence in addition to internal factors in Taiwan.

Since Xi Jinping came to power, there has been an ideological turn in China's government leading to an emphasis on propaganda work. At the end of 2022, China experienced the anti-lockdown White Paper Movement, which forced the Xi regime to abandon its zero-COVID policy. However, Xi Jinping did not admit failure. On the contrary, he claimed that China's pandemic governance was a great victory. The Xi regime proclaimed a significant victory in the prevention and control of the pandemic during the Communist Party's Politburo Standing Committee meeting on February 16, 2023. The regime claimed that China's COVID-19 death rate remained the lowest globally and described China's emergence from the pandemic as "a miraculous event in the history of human civilization for a populous country" (Xinhua News Agency 2023). This assertion appears to reflect the regime's heavy reliance on its propaganda machinery to rebrand the image of China's COVID-19 response from that of a perpetrator of a cover-up to that of a successful prevention model.

DOI: 10.4324/9781003438380-16

The extensive use of propaganda by Xi Jinping during the COVID-19 pandemic highlights the significance of exploring how the Chinese government employed propaganda. Prior research has revealed that the Chinese government utilized two strategies to accentuate the superiority of China's governance model during the pandemic. The first strategy entailed projecting a positive and optimistic portrayal of China's pandemic response by emphasizing elements such as low death rates, an efficient government, and "social unity through positive energy" (zheng nengliang 正能量). The second strategy involved repeatedly emphasizing the high casualty rates, politicians' self-interest, and social chaos in Western countries during the pandemic, thereby highlighting the superiority of China's governance model over the Western system of representative democracy.

While there is a significant body of literature on China's propaganda practices during the COVID-19 pandemic, much of it has focused on comparisons between China and the United States. However, China's propaganda strategy in relation to another competitor, Taiwan, has not received much attention. Taiwan's successful pandemic governance, characterized by representative democracy and coexistence with the virus, has avoided high casualty rates and social chaos, and is widely considered a global model. Given China's claim that Taiwan is part of the country, the Chinese government faces a dilemma in explaining how Taiwan's performance is consistent with its narrative of the superiority of the Chinese governance model. The pandemic governance in Taiwan has challenged the superiority of the Chinese model. Consequently, the CCP must employ cognitive warfare and ideological propaganda to uphold its legitimacy.

This elucidates the imperative to investigate how the Chinese government and media portrayed Taiwan during the COVID-19 pandemic, and its impact on Taiwan's pandemic governance. It is worth noting that much propaganda research on the Chinese government during the pandemic has focused on the early stages of the outbreak in 2020. However, following the initial outbreak and lockdown in Wuhan, this period was characterized by China's effective pandemic control policies, resulting in a gross domestic product (GDP) growth rate of 2.3%, while many other countries were facing chaos and recession. Studies have highlighted the effectiveness of China's "positive energy" propaganda narrative during this period, particularly in highlighting the perceived shortcomings of Western countries and promoting the superiority of the Chinese model. Nevertheless, subsequent waves of outbreaks in 2021, social controversies surrounding the lockdown of Shanghai in 2022, and the nationwide protest movement in November 2022 challenged this narrative, leading the Xi Jinping regime to abandon its zero-COVID policy in December 2022. These distinct phases of the pandemic in China highlight the need to cover a longer period in order to understand China's evolving pandemic propaganda. Examining a longer time period is also crucial to understand Chinese propaganda's influence on Taiwan's pandemic governance throughout the pandemic.

By taking a long-term perspective spanning 2.5 years from January 2020, when the pandemic began, to the end of the Shanghai lockdown in May 2022, this study aims to provide a more comprehensive understanding of the Chinese government's propaganda policies during the pandemic, including its portrayal of Taiwan, and its impact on Taiwan's pandemic governance.

Prior research has focused mainly on analyzing the Chinese government's propaganda efforts through a single official media outlet, such as the *People's Daily* or its English-language version, *China Daily*. However, the Chinese government's propaganda machines operate across multiple platforms including government spokespersons, official media outlets, subsidiaries of official outlets, and private media platforms. To achieve a more comprehensive understanding of how the Xi Jinping regime used propaganda during the pandemic, particularly with regard to Taiwan, this study examines news reporting on Taiwan across six different sources over a prolonged period.

Given the complexity of the research topic, this study adopts a mixed methods approach that combines quantitative and qualitative methods to analyze news reporting on Taiwan during the COVID-19 pandemic. Each news article is scored for emotional sentiment. Discourse analysis is conducted regarding significant events, such as the lockdown of Wuhan (January 23–April 8, 2020), the lockdown of Shanghai (March 27–May 30, 2022), and the period of rising COVID-19 cases in Taiwan (May–June 2021). By comparing the reporting perspectives of six different sources during these events, the study aims to provide a comprehensive understanding of how the CCP employed propaganda to undermine Taiwan's pandemic governance and strengthen its own pandemic governance. By analyzing the operations of the CCP's propaganda machine during the pandemic, as well as how China conducted internal propaganda toward its own people, collaborated with external propaganda to launch a cognitive war against Taiwan, and influenced Taiwan's pandemic governance, we can gain valuable insights into cross-strait policies and potential shifts in the global geopolitical landscape. This research can also help Taiwan and the rest of the world develop new governance strategies to address the challenges of hostile propaganda and misinformation in the post-pandemic era.

Literature Review

The Chinese Communist Party (CCP) and Governance Ideology Research

While the operation of the CCP regime has certain particularities, it is overall a typical party-state system where the party is the core of the political system. Their functions are fused, but the party leads the government. In general, the party decides the key national policy guidelines and the appointment and dismissal of officials.

After China adopted the Reforms and Opening Up Policy in 1978, most Western countries believed that China would gradually adopt the Western representative democratic system due to economic growth and an increase in the size of the middle class. Under this premise, various countries adopted an "Engagement Policy" with China to incorporate it into the world capitalist system and continued to follow such a policy for decades (Ding 2002; G. Yang 2009; Gilley 2004; Goldman 2005; O'Brien and Li 2006; Ogden 2002).

However, after more than 40 years, the CCP's authoritarian rule has persisted and shattered the fantasy that a market economy would lead to political changes. As the CCP regime continued to maintain firm control of society and its attitude toward the international community changed from Deng Xiaoping's "keep a low profile and gain strength" (taoguangyanghui韜光養晦) to Xi Jinping's "striving for achievement" (fenfayouwei奮發有為), territorial conflicts with neighboring countries arose, causing a variety of countries to readjust their foreign policies with China. The outbreak of the China-US trade war in 2018 marks a change in course from the "Engagement Policy" adopted by Western countries after Nixon's visit to China in 1972.

Academic research has also reflected these changing perceptions of China. Many researchers have shifted from studying the democratization of China to studying how China's authoritarian government has survived (Perry 2015). For example, a well-known China studies researcher, Andrew J. Nathan, proposed the concept of "authoritarian resilience" in 2003 to analyze the CCP's ability to adapt to the times (Nathan 2003), and Shambaugh and Dickson have also explored the CCP's capacity for adaptation (Dickson 2003, 2008, 2010; Shambaugh 2008). Some scholars have also analyzed the CCP's governance technologies (Heilmann and Perry 2011; K. Tsai 2007; L. Tsai 2007; Perry 2015; Reilly 2012; Whyte 2010).

Scholar Rongbin Han noted that many studies of the CCP's authoritarianism focus on the dualistic notion of control and resistance (Han 2018). However, the regime cannot rely solely on repression to maintain power. Studies by Marx on the superstructure, Althusser on ideological state apparatuses, and Gramsci on hegemony all state that a ruling regime requires an ideology to achieve standard governance (Althusser 1971; Gramsci 1971; Marx and Engels 1974). Some scholars believe that the CCP has been able to remain in power because of its successful ideological framework. Brady and Wang (2009) believe that scholars claiming that the CCP is either implementing political reforms or heading toward collapse have ignored the actual operations of the CCP's ruling machine. They believe that after the Tiananmen Square Incident in 1989, the CCP modernized its propaganda system to create a new order of populist authoritarianism. This has enabled the CCP's one-party dictatorship system to gain social support. Frank Pieke noted that the role of ideology today is not to make people believe in the CCP but to build proactive and autonomous subjects to form a governable society (Pieke 2012). For example, some people are willing to voluntarily post online comments to help the CCP maintain its hegemony (Han 2018). Recent studies of the CCP ideology have mostly focused on how this ideological work legitimizes the CCP regime (Bondes and Heep 2013; Brown 2012; Gilley and Holbig 2010; Holbig 2009, 2011, 2013; Sandby-Thomas 2011; Sausmikat 2006; Su 2011; Tai 2019) or on the purging of political enemies through ideological struggle (Bo 2004; Fewsmith 2003; Lieber 2013; Shih 2008; Zheng and Lye 2003).

Kuo and Hung (2007) combined the CCP's propaganda work with psychological warfare research, suggesting that the CCP began to develop such strategies after the two Gulf Wars. Psychological warfare refers to

> the application of psychological principles to stimulate and influence people's cognition, will, and emotions through propaganda and other means, so that they change and develop in a direction favorable to their side and unfavorable to the enemy, thereby strengthening their front and disrupting the enemy.
>
> (Kuo and Hung 2007)

Chen (2022) argues that China's digital propaganda and information control techniques—the monopolistic exercise of market authoritarianism—have empowered the Xi regime to manipulate public discourse and shape public opinion via social media. Chen argues that these techniques forge a sense of community and unite the general public under the Chinese government, legitimizing autocratic rule. Because of China's current status as a major power, some researchers have focused on the influence of China's propaganda work on other countries and not just the Chinese people, such as the development of the "Go Global Policy" and its impact on other countries (Tai 2018). Shen (2021) analyzed the cognitive war in China and how the CCP used it to attack Taiwan. He points out that it is now a hybrid war in which disinformation plays an important role in creating social confusion within other countries.

Chinese Government and Media Coverage during the Pandemic

The pandemic first broke out in Wuhan and then spread worldwide. The Chinese government initially concealed the outbreak from the public and punished whistleblowers like Dr. Wenliang Li. Meanwhile, the pandemic spread worldwide. By March 6, 2023, a total of 671,615,640 confirmed cases and 6,879,856 deaths had been reported worldwide.

The Chinese Communist Party's concealment of the pandemic initially aroused public anger both domestically and abroad. However, the Party has since actively sought to improve its image through propaganda efforts. As a result, there have been numerous studies that have analyzed the Chinese government's press releases and media coverage during the pandemic and explored the strategies employed by the CCP to rehabilitate its image. Gui (2021) analyzed nine weeks of news reports from *Xinwen Lianbo*, China's most important news program, from January to March 2020, and discovered that the metaphorical war frame dominated throughout the corpus (Gui 2021). Keywords like "battle" (戰鬥), "frontline" (一線), "weapon" (武器), and "victory" (勝利) permeate the discourse and establish the dominant metaphor of war. On February 3, President Xi gave a speech at a working conference saying that the type of war had expanded into a people's war and total war. The people's war frame means that all Chinese people should serve as soldiers, and that the public should join efforts to fight against their common enemy, COVID-19, and be willing to sacrifice their rights and accept policies like travel bans and lockdowns. "The total war frame defines that the range of war is much larger than military actions, implying that at this stage, apart from pandemic prevention and control, it was also very important to maintain economic, political and social stability" (Gui 2021, 968).

Another strategy involves creating a contrast between China's well-controlled pandemic situation and the social disorder and heavy death toll in the United States. This is achieved through emphasizing China's societal order and stability, thus fostering the perception of the CCP's successful pandemic governance. Gong and Firdaus (2022, 13) analyzed 308 articles from *China Daily*, finding that "although *China Daily* initially depicted COVID-19 as a bane, it has since been portrayed as a relative boon by applying positive themes such as cooperation, pandemic recovery, and informativeness, while themes of political tension emerged, like Occidentalism". This research points out that *China Daily* has worked to gradually improve the CCP's image by creating the impression that the CCP's pandemic strategy is better than those of Western countries, and thus that the China model is superior to that of the West.

Meadows, Tang, and Zou (2022) examined the Sina Weibo posts published by three leading state-run media entities (CCTV, *People's Daily*, and Xinhua News Agency) during the first wave of the COVID-19 outbreak. The study found the use of information and bolstering strategies to maintain and increase government legitimacy. Cindy Sing Bik Ngai, Le Yao, and Rita Gill Singh (2022) compared the coverage of coping strategies and emotions in stories about COVID-19 in the *New York Times* in the United States and China's *People's Daily*. In the news coverage analyzed, negative emotions in the form of fears and anxiety were predominant in the *New York Times*, whereas positive emotions such as gratitude, cheer, and good wishes prevailed in *People's Daily*. Han, Xu, and Huang (2022) found that a reliance on such upbeat official news sources and a collectivist cultural orientation can explain positive government evaluations in China. This research demonstrates the significance and validity of using media propaganda to maintain the government's legitimacy.

In the face of international backlash, the CCP has utilized its external propaganda machinery to vigorously deflect responsibility for initially concealing the pandemic. The Chinese government has adopted a "media going global" policy to expand its world influence and a "tell China's stories well" framework (Huang and Wang 2019; S. Yang 2018). Yu (2022) analyzed 63 reports in China's English-language news media and found that the Chinese media developed three main strategies: enemification, victimization, and heroization. First, the enemification strategy aims to tell the world that the enemy is not China but COVID-19. It also adopts metaphors suggesting "a war-time rhetoric that implicitly treated the United States and China as enemies, evoking a sense of nationalism during a time of war" (Yu 2022, 261). Second, the victimization strategy means that the Chinese people are pandemic victims who hence should not be blamed and required to pay compensation to other countries. (Yu 2022, 262). Third, the heroization strategy "amplified China's heroic role in managing to contain COVID-19 and assisting other countries in combatting the pandemic on humanitarian grounds, which thereby delegitimized hostility toward China or charges brought against China" (Yu 2022, 264).

These studies mainly focused on the first half of 2020 and provided timely contributions on how the CCP used media propaganda to reverse its image and maintain legitimacy early in the pandemic. These strategies include using war framing to battle the virus and foreign enemies (such as the United States) and to urge the Chinese people to take responsibility in this total war to maintain a stable society. They adopt affirmative content full of positive energy to praise the CCP's efforts while using negative content to provoke anti-US emotion and nationalism.

However, previous studies mainly focused on the first half of 2020 and ignored the repeated outbreaks that occurred later or the significant complaints over Shanghai's lockdown in 2022 and the nationwide White Paper Movement in November 2022. The data collected in this research covers the period from January 1, 2020, to May 31, 2022, and thus are more comprehensive than former research.

Second, these other studies indicate that in addition to positive publicity about the CCP, there was a strong emphasis on external enemies and patriotism. However, the only external enemy mentioned in the existing research was the United States and there is no mention of Taiwan, a key player in the Sino-American conflict. Taiwan is particularly relevant to China's COVID-19 propaganda because it is a Chinese society that has adopted representative democracy and has been widely commended for its pandemic governance. The performance of the Taiwanese government in managing the COVID-19 pandemic could affect Xi Jinping's propaganda work and challenge his claim of the superiority of the Chinese model. Thus, how the Chinese government and media outlets reported on Taiwan during the pandemic is a key issue in understanding its COVID-19 propaganda.

Third, the CCP actively intervenes to exert influence on various facets of Taiwan, encompassing politics, economy, society, culture, and even leveraging the pandemic to affect Taiwan. To comprehend how the CCP influences Taiwan's pandemic governance, it is essential to gain an understanding of how they report on Taiwan's pandemic and the subsequent impact of such reporting on the Taiwanese government and society. Simultaneously, we can also comprehend how the CCP, through reporting on "others", reinforces its own nationalism to sustain the legitimacy of its regime.

Research Methodology

I investigated six sources of information in this study to explore China's sentiment and discourse toward Taiwan during the COVID-19 period. Unlike existing research that only examined China's national media, I also chose major state institutions and media outlets related to Taiwan. Taiwan is a frequent target of these sites. It is significant and necessary to analyze the delicate interactions and subtle relationships between these platforms to grasp the dialectical operation of the propaganda machine. These institutions are listed below:

The Taiwan Affairs Office of the State Council

The Taiwan Work Office of the CCP Central Committee and the Taiwan Affairs Office of the State Council are two titles for the same agency. It is the administrative agency under the State Council of Mainland China responsible for setting and implementing guidelines and policies related to Taiwan.

Taiwan.cn

Taiwan.cn is a website managed by the Taiwan Affairs Office of the State Council. It was founded in July 1999 and organized by the Beijing Strait Culture Exchange Limited Company.

Ministry of Foreign Affairs of the People's Republic of China (MOFA)

One of the "Leading Group of the CCP Central Committee for Novel Coronavirus Prevention and Control" members is Minister Wang Yi of the MOFA. The membership of this diplomat makes it apparent that China attaches great importance to international relations in the battle against COVID-19.

People's Daily

The members of the "Leading Group of the CCP Central Committee for Novel Coronavirus Prevention and Control" also include Huang Kunming (member of the Politburo and Minister of the CCP Propaganda Department). *People's Daily* is the most senior party media outlet under the Publicity Department, and it is the official newspaper of the CCP Central Committee. It is the party and the government's mouthpiece and a key window for China's foreign cultural exchanges.

Global Times

The *Global Times* is an international newspaper sponsored by the *People's Daily* headquarters. *Global Times* is a strong proponent of Chinese nationalism and official ideology; its language style is more colloquial, straightforward, and radical than other official media and it has considerable influence in mainland China. The *Global Times* is also considered by outsiders to reflect the position of Chinese government organs such as the MOFA and the Ministry of State Security regarding issues they support but are not allowed to discuss publicly.

Guancha.cn

Guancha.cn's founder, Li Shimo, was born in Shanghai. He received a bachelor's degree in economics from the University of California, Berkeley, an MBA from the Graduate School of Business at Stanford University, and a PhD in political science from Shanghai's Fudan University. Li Shimo lived in the United States for an extended period and founded Chengwei Capital in 1999. In the same year, he returned to Shanghai and co-founded Chengwei Capital China with Feng Bo, the husband of Deng Xiaoping's granddaughter Deng Zhuoyue. Li Shimo founded Guancha.cn in November 2012. Li Shimo has given numerous speeches and written articles supporting the CCP regime and the Chinese model. He believes that "the regime's legitimacy is deeply rooted in the people's hearts" (HKEJ 2017) and considers himself a fan of Xi Jinping (Rachman 2020).

Research Period

The articles analyzed were dated between January 1, 2020, and May 31, 2022. The purpose is to investigate China's attitudes and discourses toward Taiwan since the start of the COVID-19 pandemic.

Data Acquisition

1 I used web crawler technology to obtain news articles from the Internet and convert them into text for storage.
2 I used dynamic browser simulations such as selenium and requests, urllib, and other program libraries to obtain webpages.

Data Filtering

1 I used a keyword search method to find texts related to the topics of interest and set the following keywords based on words commonly used on Chinese platforms. (Since the articles originated from China, the keywords used for filtering are simplified Chinese.)
2 Taiwan-related keywords: Taiwan, wanwan (Chinese netizens' nickname for Taiwan), Democratic Progressive Party, Kuomintang, deep green, Taiwan independence, the Island, Tsai Ing-Wen.
3 Epidemic-related keywords: epidemic, COVID-19.

Text Scoring—Sentiment Vocabulary Database

Understanding China's attitude toward COVID-19 prevention in Taiwan requires analyzing the degree of intensity of the words.

Each news article was first segmented into sentences using punctuation marks and then further divided into words using the Jieba word segmentation system in Python. The emotional sentiment of each sentence was then scored based on a sentiment vocabulary database to indicate the intensity of the positive or negative sentiments. Finally, the average emotional score of the entire text was obtained by averaging the scores of all sentences. To prevent the length of the article from affecting the emotional score, the total score was calculated by summing the scores of each sentence before averaging.

Text Analysis

To gain a deeper understanding, I combined the text corpus analysis with a sentiment vocabulary database analysis to quantify the sentiment scores from each platform. This process allows comparison of the emotional sentiments toward Taiwan contained in articles published in various platforms during the COVID-19 pandemic. Next, I conducted a qualitative text analysis via critical discourse analysis (CDA) to learn more about the differences between platforms. This method of combining text corpus and CDA is called corpus-assisted discourse studies (CADS). The textual analysis of the articles primarily focused on three periods: the Wuhan lockdown, Taiwan's increasing community transmission from May to June 2021, and the Shanghai lockdown.

Research Findings

Taiwan-Related News Reports Dominated by Chinese Nationalism

From January 2020, when the pandemic began, to May 30, 2022, when the Shanghai lockdown ended, the six major platforms comprising governmental bodies, state-sponsored media, and private media outlets reported a total of 3,940 articles related to Taiwan's COVID-19 pandemic. *People's Daily Online* had the highest number of reports, accounting for 30.81% with 1,214 pieces. *Guancha.cn* ranked second with 1,005 articles, accounting for 25.51% of the total. *Taiwan.cn* followed closely with 935 articles, accounting for 23.73%, while *Global Times* had 346 articles, accounting for 8.78% (Table 11.1).

Compared with official media and government departments, the non-official media outlet *Guancha.cn* reported an unexpectedly high number of COVID-19-related articles that mentioned Taiwan, with 1,005 articles accounting for 25.51% of the total reports, ranking second. This was a significant finding. *Guancha.cn* is known to promote Chinese nationalism and to assume a hawkish position on Taiwan. Its founder is also known to admire Xi Jinping. Additionally, *Global Times*, which stimulates Chinese nationalism with extreme rhetoric, ranked fourth in the number of reports on Taiwan's pandemic with 346. The high volume of reports on Taiwan's pandemic response in these popular media outlets suggests that Taiwan

Table 11.1 Number of Taiwan-related News Articles from Platforms during the Pandemic

	People's Daily Online	*Guancha.cn*	*Taiwan.cn*	*Global Times*	*Ministry of Foreign Affairs*	*Taiwan Affairs Office*
Total pieces	1214	1005	935	346	261	179
Percentage	30.81%	25.51%	23.73%	8.78%	6.62%	4.54%
Ranking	1	2	3	4	5	6

Data source: Prepared by the author.

Table 11.2 Sentiment Scores of Taiwan-related Reporting by the Six Platforms

	Global Times	*Taiwan Affairs Office*	*Guancha.cn*	*Ministry of Foreign Affairs*	*Taiwan.cn*	*People's Daily Online*
Overall average	−0.8099550669	1.488178979	1.569649553	2.044712094	3.07331966	4.528465037
Ranking	1	2	3	4	5	6

Data source: Prepared by the author.

played a significant role in China's domestic propaganda during the COVID-19 pandemic.

Most of these news reports were dominated by negative sentiments. Our study found that, among the six major platforms, *Global Times* had the highest negative sentiment score in reporting on Taiwan's pandemic, followed by the Taiwan Affairs Office and *Guancha.cn*. Despite being responsible for cross-strait policies, the Taiwan Affairs Office had the second-most negative attitude toward Taiwan in its pandemic reporting. This suggests that the CCP's official Taiwan policy is characterized by a hostile attitude. Furthermore, the Taiwan Affairs Office, along with the nationalistic media outlets *Global Times* and *Guancha.cn* ranked in the top three in adopting a negative attitude toward Taiwan during the pandemic, shaping a negative image of Taiwan and stirring up hostility toward Taiwan in Chinese society. This hostility may continue to extend into official policies and civil society after the pandemic, leading to the formulation of hardline cross-strait policies and an increase in the tension between the two sides (Table 11.2).

These reports also stimulated animosity toward Taiwan among the Chinese people. The first method employed by the CCP is to create a perception among Chinese society that Taiwan is collaborating with hostile foreign countries, and thus that Taiwan is a traitor that is obstructing the reunification of the country, China's rise, and the rejuvenation of the Chinese nation. The second approach is to create a perception among the Chinese people that Taiwan discriminates against China, thus triggering their resentment and hostility toward Taiwan.

Taiwan's exclusion from the WHO meant that it could not obtain complete and timely information on the pandemic and not allowed to join professional meetings. While other countries supported Taiwan's inclusion in the organization, the Chinese government claimed that it had provided Taiwan with adequate information and regarded such calls as a gross violation of China's sovereignty. Similarly, when Western countries planned a human rights conference on Xinjiang, the Chinese government accused them of attempting to undermine China from within and asserted that they supported Taiwan based on the same rationale (Liu 2021).

The second way in which China stimulated nationalist sentiment was describing Taiwan's perceived discrimination against China, which fueled anger among the Chinese people. The first instance occurred in 2020 when the Taiwanese government, facing a shortage of masks, banned exports. The *Global Times* published several anonymous WeChat articles accusing Taiwan of a heartless pandemic prevention policy. They also quoted Taiwanese political talk show commentators, Kuomintang legislators, and Taiwanese celebrities to prove that Taiwanese people were dissatisfied with the policy. For instance, Huang Zhi-xian, a commentator on a Taiwanese political talk show, called the government "an inhumane and conscienceless regime", while KMT legislator Cai Zheng-yuan claimed that "banning mask exports meant losing international public opinion support". Taiwanese entertainer Christine Fan condemned this measure on her Facebook page, writing "the ban is vulgar, immoral, and thuggish behavior" (Bu Yi Dao 2020). Other articles continued to emphasize that Taiwan harbored resentment due to China's economic growth and that the Taiwanese government's constant promotion of Taiwanese independence resulted in animosity toward China (You Li Er You Mian 2020a). These articles, whose sources were unclear, suggested to Chinese readers that Taiwan's social mentality was distorted and that it harbored a grudge against China. Consequently, Taiwan's pandemic prevention policy was not based on scientific judgment but rather on political conspiracy.

On February 25, 2020, Guancha.cn publicly accused the Taiwanese channel *Era News* of referring to China as a "sick man" (Tong 2020). The article deliberately evoked memories of the late Qing dynasty, the times when China faced aggression from Western and Japanese imperialists and when China was demeaningly referred to as the "sick man of Asia". China's patriotic education constantly emphasizes its century of humiliation and how the CCP has saved the Chinese nation. Drawing on these long-standing narratives, these articles again portrayed Taiwan as a traitorous enemy that abetted Western imperialism.

China's media portrayed Xinjiang, Taiwan, and Hong Kong as traitors within China that colluded with the United States, Japan, Europe, and Britain to undermine China's rise and spread false information regarding its pandemic situation. However, these reports also emphasized the internal conflicts within this alliance, attempting to persuade the Chinese people that this alliance is based only on the expedient self-interest of the participants, and that it is thus full of conflicts and contradictions, what Mao Zedong once called a "paper tiger". Otherwise, Chinese readers might question why these countries support Xinjiang, Hong Kong, and Taiwan and believe in their legitimacy, or why this alliance is so powerful. Accordingly, these reports portrayed the US Speaker of the House Nancy Pelosi's visit to Taiwan as a cynical attempt to boost her own reputation (*Global Times* 2022a) and falsely claimed that Japan donated vaccines to Taiwan that had actually already expired.

Cognitive Warfare and Fake News about Taiwan

Taiwan fared well during the pandemic, with a low death rate compared to most other countries. This meant China was unable to utilize its previous COVID-19 propaganda narrative, which depicted Western democratic countries as selfish and chaotic with high death rates in contrast to the superior Chinese approach.

Instead, reports on Taiwan mainly focused on May and June 2021, when Taiwan's pandemic situation began to worsen and entered the stage of community transmission. These reports, which accounted for 16.6% of all reports, did not claim that Taiwan had a high mortality rate. Instead, they emphasized supposed signs of government mismanagement and growing chaos, such as portraying two brief power outages as sign of systemic electricity shortages and presenting Taiwan descending into chaos due to a lack of water and vaccines. Later when there were reports of unusual cases of meningitis among Taiwanese children with COVID-19, the Chinese propaganda machine portrayed this as evidence that Taiwan's policy of coexisting with the virus was cruel and had caused the deaths of many children. This attempt to portray the supposed dangers of policies of coexisting with the virus in Taiwan and other countries was clearly an attempt to bolster support for China's zero-COVID policy as events such as the protracted and chaotic Shanghai lockdown caused many Chinese people to become unhappy with their government's harsh pandemic policies (*Global Times* 2022b).

Reports on Taiwan's pandemic situation also repeatedly emphasized that the Democratic Progressive Party government planned to exploit the pandemic to inflame cross-strait tensions as part of a strategy to achieve Taiwan's independence. For instance, there were reports that claimed the Taiwanese government deliberately delayed the coordination of cross-strait charter flights during the Wuhan lockdown to provoke fear of China among Taiwanese. Other reports cited the views of Taiwanese individuals who criticized the character and ability of Taiwan's officials, leading Chinese readers to believe that Taiwanese people generally hoped that these officials would step down. Such reports obscured the fact that liberal democracies like Taiwan necessarily grant citizens the freedom to debate policies and criticize government officials.

The primary sources of information in these news reports can be categorized into three types.

1 Main Chinese state media outlets (such as Xinhua News and *People's Daily*).
2 Anonymous sources (such as WeChat official accounts, independent writers, and Taiwanese netizens). These sources were primarily found in sensationalist media outlets (such as *Global Times* and Guancha.cn).
3 Overseas external propaganda, including a large number of quotes from pro-CCP Taiwanese media and individuals (politicians, media figures, and entertainers) and overseas Chinese organizations.

The dissemination of news is organized according to a division of labor. Typically, official media such as the *Xinhua News Agency* releases straightforward news reports, while *Guancha.cn* and *Global Times* are entrusted with producing exaggerated and provocative reports. These outlets frequently cite anonymous sources, such as WeChat discussions, independent writers, and Taiwanese netizens.

Reports also often feature statements from anti-DPP Taiwanese, including politicians, political commentators, and entertainers and news channels on YouTube. By quoting the remarks of these Taiwanese figures, the Chinese outlets seek to portray Taiwanese society as disorderly and the Democratic Progressive Party government as authoritarian, oppressive toward critics, and politically biased in its pandemic policies. Furthermore, they aimed to provoke animosity toward Taiwan.

Elevating the Taiwanese Government's Governance Challenges during the Pandemic

In order to address the problem of fake news, the Taiwanese government established the "Special Examination Information" division under the Bureau of Investigation of the Ministry of Justice on August 8, 2019. Investigations before the pandemic found that some fake news originated directly from Chinese social media platforms and other fake news was disseminated by local Taiwanese as part of propaganda coordinated by the CCP. In February 2020, it came to the attention of the Taiwanese government that China had extended its cognitive warfare by disseminating fake news about the pandemic (Ministry of Justice Investigation Bureau 2020).

In order to counter the accusation that China orchestrates disinformation campaigns against Taiwan, the Chinese government claims that Taiwan is the actual aggressor in cognitive warfare. For example, the *Global Times* published an article accusing the Taiwanese government of conducting a large-scale cyberespionage attack on the mainland (Hou 2020).

A prominent example of China's cognitive warfare occurred during Taiwan's COVID-19 surge in 2021. The Chinese media repeatedly emphasized that Taiwan's Democratic Progressive Party refused to purchase the German-made BNT vaccine from the Chinese-owned Fosun distributor in Shanghai because of its anti-China stance. These outlets reported that the Chinese government offered to provide Taiwan with Chinese-made vaccines out of goodwill but the Taiwanese government disregarded the demands of the Taiwanese people and insisted on developing its own vaccine. The Tsai Ing-wen government's purpose in developing Taiwan's vaccine was supposedly not only to further her pro-independence political agenda but to personally profit from sales of the vaccine. Due to the increase in the number of cases of COVID-19 in Taiwan during that time and the lack adequate vaccine doses, such fake news was particularly influential and was readily amplified by Taiwanese opposition party figures.

In fact, since October 2020, the Taiwanese government had been in negotiations to procure the Pfizer-BNT vaccine, a process that experienced Chinese political interference, which caused the original order of 5 million doses to be blocked. In spite of clarifications by the Ministry of Health and Welfare in Taiwan in daily press conferences, the increasing number of infections and the shortage of vaccines generated considerable public dissatisfaction, placing significant pressure on the Taiwanese government. At this critical juncture, Terry Gou, the chairman of Taiwan's Hon Hai corporation and a potential candidate for the 2024 presidential election, who also maintains friendly relations with China, proposed the idea of using his company to purchase vaccines and donate them to the Taiwanese government.

Under the pressure of public opinion, the Taiwanese government agreed to this emergency measure and allowed Hon Hai, the TSMC corporation, and the Tzu Chi Buddhist group to purchase 15 million doses of vaccines and donate them to the Taiwanese government. While this resolved the problem of vaccine shortages, it also highlighted the governance crisis in Taiwan caused by the CCP's international interference, the use of fake news to create dissatisfaction in Taiwan, and the actions of a pro-CCP Taiwanese entrepreneur who intended to enter politics. This case clearly illustrates the difficulty the Taiwanese government faced in managing the pandemic situation under the influence and intervention of the CCP.

In May 2022, during the lockdown in Shanghai, there was another incident in Taiwan involving rumors spread by an entertainer. An actor and television presenter named Guo Yanjun posted a screenshot of a chat with his friend, a medical worker, to Facebook. The friend said, "So many children have passed away", sparking controversy among Taiwanese. While Guo deleted the post and apologized the next day, the story was picked up by the Chinese media and promoted as evidence that the Taiwanese government's coexistence-with-the-virus policy was inhumane and led to the deaths of children, thereby justifying Xi Jinping's zero-COVID policy.

The Taiwanese government believed that such rumors could be the result of cognitive warfare operations and called for an investigation. When the Taiwanese government warned citizens to be careful of fake news and cognitive warfare, the *Global Times* cited Taiwanese netizens' opinions and accused the Democratic Progressive Party of bullying critics and suppressing dissidents under the guise of fighting cognitive warfare (*Global Times* 2022b).

Many Taiwanese entertainers have business dealings with China and become part of the chain of rumor dissemination. There may be several reasons why these entertainers play this role. Perhaps some are recruited by elements of the Chinese propaganda machine or are attempting to gain favor with the CCP, while other may simply be sympathetic to CCP propaganda or other unverified rumors. Whatever the reasons, these rumors increase the difficulty of governance for the Taiwanese government during the pandemic. When the Taiwanese government investigates and clarifies these rumors, it faces criticism from opposition parties, media outlets, and Chinese media, who accuse it of suppressing critical voices and behaving in an authoritarian manner.

Conclusion

This study demonstrates the deep influence of China's intervention on Taiwan's pandemic governance. First, China's combination of external propaganda and internal propaganda has formed a mechanism for producing fake news that can cross borders and influence Taiwan, China, and the globe. Second, these reports are intended to attack Taiwan and strengthen the CCP's regime.

As part of the CCP's long-standing external propaganda efforts in Taiwan, it has cultivated pro-CCP media in Taiwan, such as Taiwan businessman Tsai Yan-ming, who acquired Taiwan's largest media conglomerate, the China Times Group, in 2012. Due to multiple violations, serious factual errors in reporting, and Tsai Yan-ming's significant intervention in news production, the National Communications Commission decided not to re-issue a license for the China Times Group's CTi News TV Channel on November 18, 2020. However, CTi News TV moved to YouTube and opened many political commentary programs on its channel. Therefore, when China's media reports on Taiwan's pandemic news, they can cite pro-CCP Taiwanese media, use content from YouTube channels, and interview pro-CCP political figures, commentators, and others as news sources. They even quote unverified sources such as WeChat messages and Taiwanese social media users to verify Chinese reports on Taiwan's pandemic response. In fact, the research results demonstrate that these reports deliberately portray Taiwan's pandemic situation negatively by exaggerating or fabricating stories about poor governance, officials developing Taiwan's vaccine for personal gain, social chaos, and high child mortality rates. These reports are then circulated back to Taiwan through China's social media platforms or through Taiwanese organizations or individuals, causing unrest in Taiwan among citizens who question the government's pandemic policies. China's combination of internal and external propaganda has built a production mechanism of fake news that can continuously circulate on both sides of the Taiwan Strait.

In addition to propaganda, the Chinese Communist Party also works to suppress Taiwan in the international community, such as preventing Taiwan from joining the World Health Organization and obstructing the Taiwanese government's purchase of vaccines. These efforts have caused difficulties for the Taiwanese government in controlling the pandemic, resulting in issues such as vaccine shortages. When these crises arise, coupled with the CCP's cognitive warfare and fake news attacks, it creates unrest among the Taiwanese people. When the Taiwanese government investigates fake news, it faces criticism from opposition parties, pro-China media in Taiwan, and Chinese media, who accuse the Taiwanese government of suppressing dissidents under the guise of combating the CCP's cognitive warfare.

For the domestic Chinese audience, these reports on the Taiwanese pandemic have three main effects, which help to consolidate Xi Jinping's regime and support his pandemic governance. First, they refute suggestions that Chinese pandemic control is ineffective by portraying such criticisms as rumors spread by hostile foreign forces. Second, by depicting Taiwan's pandemic control as chaotic, they justify Xi Jinping's zero-tolerance policy. For example, in May 2021, a rumor about many Taiwanese children dying was spread to portray the Taiwanese government's policy of coexisting with the virus as cruel and ineffective, thus justifying Xi Jinping's continued zero-tolerance policy. Third, these reports draw on nationalist sentiments to portray Taiwan as a traitor colluding with hostile foreign forces. Since the whole world wants to prevent China's rise, the Chinese people must support the CCP regime and defend China against foreign enemies. Through nationalism, such propaganda shifts people's dissatisfaction with the CCP's pandemic control toward external enemies.

These reports have also stirred up hostility toward Taiwan in Chinese society, and the Taiwan Affairs Office has worked with nationalist outlets such as *Guancha.cn* and *Global Times* to promote this hostility. This means that China is likely to continue to take a hostile attitude toward Taiwan in the future, and geopolitical tensions might continue to run high.

During the pandemic, the Taiwanese government recognized the threat of Chinese cognitive warfare and took specific measures to address it. In August 2019, they established a special investigation team. Throughout the pandemic, the government also conducted press conferences to clarify rumors, increased information transparency, and raised awareness about misinformation. These governance policies that were developed during the pandemic will be valuable in facing new challenges in the post-pandemic era, including the upcoming 2024 Taiwan presidential election. However, in the post-pandemic era, the Taiwanese government and the international community will face a new governance challenge: how to address the hostility injected into Chinese society during the COVID-19 pandemic and prevent its further escalation.

Acknowledgments

This study was supported by the Visiting Scholar Program of the Institute of Sociology at the Academia Sinica.

Conflicts of Interest

The author declares no conflicts of interest regarding the publication of this chapter.

References

Althusser, Louis. 1971. "Ideology and Ideological State Apparatuses." In *Lenin and Philosophy and Other Essays*, edited by Louis Althusser, 127–188. New York: New Left Books.

Bo, Zhiyue. 2004. "Hu Jintao and the CCP's Ideology: A Historical Perspective." *Journal of Chinese Political Science* 9 (2): 27–45. https://doi.org/10.1007/BF02877001

Bondes, Maria, and Sandra Heep. 2013. "Conceptualizing the Relationship between Persuasion and Legitimacy: Official Framing in the Case of the Chinese Communist Party." *Journal of Chinese Political Science* 18 (4): 317–334. https://doi.org/10.1007/s11366-013-9258-y

Brady, Anne-Marie, and Wang Juntao. 2009. "China's Strengthened New Order and the Role of Propaganda." *Journal of Contemporary China* 18 (62): 767–788. https://doi.org/10.1080/10670560903172832

Brown, Kerry. 2012. "The Communist Party of China and Ideology." *China: An International Journal* 10 (2): 52–68. https://doi.org/10.1353/chn.2012.0013

Bu Yi Dao. 2020. "Do the Taiwan Authorities Still Embody Humanity by Treating the Wuhan Pandemic Like This?" *Global Times*, January 28. Accessed August 18, 2022. https://taiwan.huanqiu.com/article/9CaKrnKp6d1

Chen, Titus C. 2022. *The Making of a Neo-Propaganda State: China's Social Media Under XI Jinping*. Leiden: Brill.

Dickson, Bruce J. 2003. *Red Capitalists in China: The Party, Private Entrepreneurs, and the Prospects for Political Change*. New York: Cambridge University Press.

Dickson, Bruce J. 2008. *Wealth into Power: The Communist Party's Embrace of China's Private Sector*. New York: Cambridge University Press.

Dickson, Bruce J. 2010. "Dilemmas of Party Adaptation: The CCP's Strategies for Survival." In *Chinese Politics: State, Society and the Market*, edited by P. H. Gries and S. Rosen, 22–40. London: Routledge.

Ding, Yijiang. 2002. *Chinese Democracy after Tiananmen*. New York: Columbia University Press.

Fewsmith, Joseph. 2003. "Studying the Three Represents." *China Leadership Monitor* 8: 1–11.

Gilley, Bruce. 2004. *China's Democratic Future: How it Will Happen and Where it Will Lead.* New York: Columbia University Press.

Gilley, Bruce, and Heike Holbig. 2010. "Reclaiming Legitimacy in China." *Politics & Policy* 38 (3): 395–422. https://doi.org/10.1111/j.1747-1346.2010.00241.x

Global Times. 2022a. "Pelosi's Plan to Visit Taiwan is 'Postponed' Due to Infection with COVID-19. Expert: Her Visit to Taiwan is Likely to Disturb Biden." April 8, Accessed August 20, 2022. https://world.huanqiu.com/article/47WfG0o8j1s

Global Times. 2022b. "The Pandemic on the Island Caused Severe Encephalitis in Children. The Kuomintang Medical Committee: It is Cruel to Let Children 'Coexist with the Virus.'" May 24, Accessed August 25, 2022. https://taiwan.huanqiu.com/article/488Gu6f2OKt

Goldman, Merle. 2005. *From Comrade to Citizen: The Struggle for Political Rights in China*. Cambridge, MA: Harvard University Press.

Gong, Jiankun, and Amira Firdaus. 2022. "Is the Pandemic a Boon or a Bane? News Media Coverage of COVID-19 in China Daily." *Journalism Practice*. https://doi.org/10.1080/17512786.2022.2043766

Gramsci, Antonio. 1971. *Selections from the Prison Notebooks of Antonio Gramsci*. New York: International Publishers.

Gui, Lili. 2021. "Media Framing of Fighting COVID-19 in China." *Sociology of Health & Illness* 43 (4): 966–970. https://doi.org/10.1111/1467-9566.13271

Han, R., J. Xu, and M. Huang. 2022. "Evaluation of COVID-19 Governance in China: The Effects of Media Use, Pandemic Severity, and Provincial Heterogeneity." *Journal of Asian Public Policy*. https://doi.org/10.1080/17516234.2022.2076551

Han, Rongbin. 2018. *Contesting Cyberspace in China: Online Expression and Authoritarian Resilience*. New York: Columbia University Press.

Heilmann, S., and E. J. Perry. 2011. *Mao's Invisible Hand: The Political Foundations of Adaptive Governance in China.* Cambridge, MA: Harvard University Press.

HKEJ. 2017. "How a Western-educated Fund Manager Became a Democracy Basher." February 14, Accessed January 30, 2022. https://www.ejinsight.com/eji/article/id/1491241/20170214-how-a-western-educated-fund-manager-became-a-democracy-basher

Holbig, Heike. 2009. "Ideological Reform and Political Legitimacy in China." In *Regime Legitimacy in Contemporary China: Institutional Change and Stability*, edited by T. Heberer and G. Schubert, 13–34. London: Routledge.

Holbig, Heike. 2011. "International Dimensions of Legitimacy: Reflections on Western Theories and the Chinese Experience." *Journal of Chinese Political Science* 16 (2): 161–181. https://doi.org/10.1007/s11366-011-9142-6

Holbig, Heike. 2013. "Ideology after the End of Ideology: China and the Quest for Autocratic Legitimation." *Democratization* 20 (1): 61–81. https://doi.org/10.1080/13510347.2013.738862

Hou, Qianjun. 2020. "Authorities: Taiwan Took Advantage of the Pandemic to Launch Large-Scale Cyber-Attacks on the Mainland." *Global Times*. Accessed July 12, 2022. https://taiwan.huanqiu.com/article/3xNkJIFIflh

Huang, Z. A., and R. Wang. 2019. "Building a Network to 'Tell China Stories Well': Chinese Diplomatic Communication Strategies on Twitter." *International Journal of Communication* 13: 2984–3007.

Kuo, H.C., and L. H. Hung. 2007. "An Analysis of the Research, Development, and Preparedness of China's Psychological Warfare." *Fu Hsing Kang Academic Journal* 89: 1–29.

Lieber, Andre. 2013. "The Chinese Ideology: Reconciling the Politics with the Economics of Contemporary Reform." *Journal of Chinese Politics Science* 18 (4): 335–353. https://doi.org/10.1007/s11366-013-9259-x

Liu, Xiaoyan. 2021. "A Few Western Countries Instigated the Holding of Xinjiang-Related Conferences in the United Nations. Hua Chunying: This Is a Blasphemy Against the United Nations!" *Guancha.cn*. Accessed July 18, 2022. https://www.guancha.cn/internation/2021_05_10_590235.shtml

Marx, Karl, and Friederich Engels. 1974. *The German Ideology*. Edited by C. J. Arthur. London: Lawrence and Wishart.

Meadows, C., L. Tang, and W. Zou. 2022. "Managing Government Legitimacy during the COVID-19 Pandemic in China: A Semantic Network Analysis of State-Run Media Sina Weibo Posts." *Chinese Journal of Communication* 15 (2): 156–181. https://doi.org/10.1080/17544750.2021.2016876

Ministry of Justice Investigation Bureau. 2020. "The Mainland Cyber Army's Fake News War Is Escalating, and Taiwanese Should Carefully Discriminate Internet Information." February 29. Accessed August 22, 2022. https://www.mjib.gov.tw/news/Details/1/572

Nathan, Andrew J. J. 2003. "Authoritarian Resilience." *Journal of Democracy* 14 (1): 6–17. https://doi.org/10.1163/9789004302488_005

O'Brien, K., and L. Li. 2006. *Rightful Resistance in Rural China*. New York: Cambridge University Press.

Ogden, Suzanne. 2002. *Inklings of Democracy in China*. Cambridge, MA: Harvard University Press.

Perry, Elizabeth. J. 2015. "The Populist Dream of Chinese Democracy." *Journal of Asian Studies* 74 (4): 903–915. https://doi.org/10.1017/S002191181500114X

Pieke, Frank. N. 2012. "The Communist Party and Social Management in China." *China Information* 26: 149–165. https://doi.org/10.1177/0920203X12442864

Rachman, G. 2020. "Eric Li: 'How Do You Block a Country of 1.4bn People?'" *Financial Times*, February 7. Accessed June 15, 2022. https://www.ft.com/content/60052b56-41eb-11ea-a047-eae9bd51ceba

Reilly, James. 2012. *Strong Society, Smart State: The Rise of Public Opinion in China's Japan Policy*. New York: Columbia University Press.

Sandby-Thomas, Peter. 2011. *Legitimating the Chinese Communist Party since Tiananmen: A Critical Analysis of the Stability Discourse*. Oxford: Routledge.

Sausmikat, Nora. 2006. "More Legitimacy for One-party Rule? The CCP's Ideological Adjustments and Infra-Party Reforms?" *Asien* 99: 70–91.

Shambaugh, David. 2008. *China's Communist Party: Atrophy and Adaptation*. Berkeley, CA: University of California Press.

Shen, Puma. 2021. "The Chinese Cognitive Warfare Model: The 2020 Taiwan Election." *Prospect Quarterly* 22: 1–65.

Shih, Victor C. H. 2008. "'Nauseating' Displays of Loyalty: Monitoring the Factional Bargain through Ideological Campaigns in China." *The Journal of Politics* 70 (4): 1177–1192. https://doi.org/10.1017/S0022381608081139

Sing Bik Ngai, C., Yao, L., & Gill Singh, R. (2022). "A Comparative Analysis of the U.S. and China's Mainstream News Media Framing of Coping Strategies and Emotions in the Reporting of COVID-19 Outbreak on Social Media. " *Discourse & Communication* 16 (5): 572–597. https://doi.org/10.1177/17504813221099191

Su, Xiaobo. 2011. "Revolution and Reform: The Role of Ideology and Hegemony in Chinese Politics." *Journal of Contemporary China* 20 (69): 307–326. https://doi.org/10.1080/10670564.2011.541637

Tai, Yuhui. 2018. "China's Go Global Policy and Capital Flow: Mergers and Acquisitions and the Controversy of New Television Licenses in Hong Kong's Terrestrial TV Industry." *Mass Communication Research* 135: 1–47. https://doi.org/10.30386/MCR.201804_(135).0001

Tai, Yuhui. 2019. "Ideotainment: The Duet of Politics and Popular Culture under Xi Jinping Regime." *Chinese Journal of Communication Research* 36: 193–233. https://doi.org/10.3966/172635812019120036006

Tong, Li. 2020. "There is No Bottom Line! 'Sick Man of China' Appears in the Subtitle of a Taiwan Media Program." *Guancha.cn*, February 25. Accessed July 5, 2022. https://www.guancha.cn/politics/2020_02_25_538356.shtml

Tsai, Kellee S. 2007. *Capitalism without Democracy: The Private Sector in Contemporary China.* Ithaca, NY: Cornell University Press.

Tsai, Lily L. 2007. *Accountability without Democracy: Solidary Groups and Public Goods Provision in Rural China.* New York: Cambridge University Press.

Whyte, Martin. 2010. *Myth of the Social Volcano: Perceptions of Inequality and Distributive Justice in Contemporary China.* Stanford: Stanford University Press

Xinhua News Agency. 2023. "The Standing Committee of the Political Bureau of the CCP Central Committee Held a Meeting, with Xi Jinping Presiding over the Meeting." February 16. Accessed February 18, 2023. http://www.gov.cn/xinwen/2023-02/16/content_5741835.htm

Yang, Guobin. 2009. *The Power of the Internet in China: Citizen Activism Online.* New York: Columbia University Press.

Yang, Suzanne Xiao. 2018. "Soft Power and the Strategic Context for China's 'Media Going Global' Policy." In *China's Media Go Global*, edited by D. K. Thussu, H. de Burgh, and A. Shi, 79–100. London: Routledge.

You Li Er You Mian. 2020a. "The Dream of 'Taiwan Independence' Behind the 'Crazy' Cold-Bloodedness in the Pandemic." *Global Times*, February 4. Accessed July 8, 2022. https://taiwan.huanqiu.com/article/9CaKrnKpbG4

Yu, Yating. 2022. "Resisting Foreign Hostility in China's English-Language News Media during the COVID-19 Crisis." *Asian Studies Review* 46 (2): 254–271. https://doi.org/10.1080/10357823.2021.1947969

Zheng, Y., and L. Lye. 2003. "Elite Politics and the Fourth Generation of Chinese Leadership." *Journal of Chinese Political Science* 8 (1&2): 65–86. https://doi.org/10.1007/BF02876950

12 Health for All? COVID-19, WHO, and Taiwan's Exceptional Governance

Yu-Yueh Tsai

Introduction

Since the World Health Organization's (WHO) constitution was adopted in 1946, the human rights and health movement has grown, but its potential problems remain underdeveloped (Ruger 2018). For example, following the initial outbreak of Coronavirus Disease 2019 (COVID-19) in Wuhan, China, COVID-19 caused a global pandemic that posed a severe challenge to the international authorities responsible for global health governance (GHG), including the WHO. Based on "One China Principle", Taiwan has been excluded from the WHO's ultimate goal of Health for All since 1972. After the outbreak of the COVID-19 pandemic, Taiwan's exclusion from the WHO was reemphasized. Due to its contested statehood, Taiwan's case presents an anomaly during the global COVID-19 crisis, as it has lacked full access to the WHO's information and cooperation.

This chapter examines three related questions. First, why is Taiwan's statehood a problem for WHO's global governance of the COVID-19 pandemic? Second, to what extent does WHO conceal decision-making about Taiwan inside its administrative "black box" and exclude Taiwan experts' participation in fighting infectious diseases? Third, what institutional and organizational problems of WHO as GHG are exposed through Taiwan's case? Drawing on the perspective of GHG and nationalism, this chapter presents Taiwan as an instance of exceptional governance that reveal how the contradictory relationship between nation-states, health rights, and WHO fatally undermines WHO's vision of Health for All.

Literature Review: COVID-19, Nation-States, and GHG

The Reinforcement of Nation-States under New Forms of Global Risk

Observing the transition from the first period of modernity (i.e., industrialization between the 17th and 20th centuries) to the second period of modernity (i.e., reflexive modernization of the global risk society), sociologist Ulrich Beck argues that the global risks of the second period of modernity, such as ozone layer depletion,

DOI: 10.4324/9781003438380-17

global warming, avian influenza, or COVID-19, can no longer be confined to a single nation-state. Transnational sub-political organizations, such as WHO, the European Union (EU), and Médecins Sans Frontières (MSF), must undoubtedly play a more central role in resolving global risks, which necessitates moving beyond governance based only on nation-states (Beck 2000: 91–108). Yet, COVID-19 is like a "demon-revealing mirror" exposing underlying problems of transnational sub-political organizations.

As Sriram Shamasunder et al. (2020) suggest, the pandemic has not only revealed the hollowness of the global health rhetoric of equity and the weaknesses of a health security-driven global agenda, but also highlighted the immediate need to repair the broken systems of global health. In COVID-19, Nationalism, and the Politics of Crisis, Liah Greenfeld et al. point out that globalization is no longer the status quo of human development and that nationalism has not yet been surpassed during the current pandemic (Woods et al. 2020: 4–7). Many scholars note that the global risk of COVID-19 has reinforced the power of the nation-state/nationalism rather than globalization (Yi and Lee 2020; Fidler 2020; Bieber 2020; Woods et al. 2020). The pandemic has also brought nationalist conflicts between the United States and China, as well as within the European Union (EU) to the surface, ruining some scholars' dream that globalization would lead to a global village (Woods et al. 2020). Greenfeld also argues that transnational institutions are most likely to fall victim to the pandemic (Woods et al. 2020). Facing the challenges of COVID-19, many countries implemented border controls to block immigrants and refugees, to reinforce civil surveillance, and to emphasize the importance of state governance (Rachman 2020; Krastev 2020). Both political leaders and citizens agree it is necessary to reinforce state sovereignty to maintain the security of their own nation. Wherever the governments in different countries tend to implement policies that intensify the role of the nation-state itself, it leads to the temporary, unprecedented global phenomenon of "deglobalizaion" (Bieber 2020). The emergence of COVID-19 has reverted us to a nationalist world.

The present literature on nationalism emphasizes nation-building based on language, history, culture, and political ideology (Anderson 1983; Gellner 1983; Hroch 1996; Chatterjee 1986). After the outbreak of COVID-19, some research has focused on the connections between pandemic diseases, biomedicine, and nation-building. For example, Jeremy Youde (2020) argues that during the COVID-19 crisis state medicine is prioritized while medical science is used as a weapon, which in turn leads to the rise of "medical nationalism". Ana Santos Rutschman (2020) further identifies the rise of "vaccine nationalism". Jeroen de Kloet et al. (2020) adopt the term "biopolitical nationalism" to indicate that the pandemic stimulates intense nationalism and localist sentiment when the medical system built by the nation with biopower becomes a benchmark for its national identity, and the citizens take pride in living in a country with the most "effective" governance. As COVID-19 swept over the globe, "us" against the virus ignited a kind of wartime national defense based on "bio-nationalism", ranging from the distribution of medical resources to competition in biotechnology among nation-states. Therefore, COVID-19 has not only expanded the nation-states' administrative capacity to control and reinforced the nationalist idea that they represent "nations", but also weakened the power of transnational governmental organizations such as WHO.

COVID-19, State, and GHG

Globalization has been accompanied by the emergence of GHG since the 1990s. GHG refers to "the use of formal and informal institutions, rules, and processes by states, inter-governmental organizations, and nonstate actors to deal with challenges to health that require cross-border collective action to address effectively" (Fidler 2010: 3). It brings together diverse actors, such as states, international organizations, and non-state actors, to coordinate collective action at the global level. Political scientist Ted Schrecker (2020) suggests that the pressure of global economic integration and domestic policy convergence are making national politics all but irrelevant. This "post-Westphalian" age is characterized by a proliferation of non-state actors. Moreover, through the emergence of a transnational capitalist class, a nascent transnational state which is comprised of a variety of economic and political organizations causes a governance framework such as WHO to emerge. Although these changes lead to many actors appearing to fall under current global governance, this governance is often dependent on states for implementation. Facing new global threats, some studies have reframed the positioning of the state under GHG (Schrecker 2020; Ruger 2018). The role of states is not fading.

The COVID-19 pandemic has revealed deep problems in GHG, with WHO facing obstacles from nationalist governments in controlling the global crisis.

First, as a global governance mechanism, WHO is an ineffective bureaucracy. WHO was already perceived as a troubled agency incapable of responding rapidly to new epidemiological challenges. For example, WHO was initially slow to respond to AIDS, so the Joint United Nations (UN) Program on HIV/AIDS took over the global governance of the disease (Cueto 2020: 32–33). Michael Zürn points out that even though WHO has officially remained an advocate of a universal approach to global health, conflicts among state members lead to a fragmented operating model (Zürn 2018: 191–192). Moreover, since the global governance system consists of the interplay of different spheres of authority, it creates severe legitimation problems, including "technocratic bias" and "absence of a separation of powers" (Zürn 2018: 9–11). Jim Whitman concludes that global governance mechanisms lack consistency and effectiveness with significant vulnerabilitie in WHO (Quah 2006: 19–20).

Second, WHO lacks accountability mechanisms for its authorized powers within its organizational design. Guillermo J. Avilés Mendoza emphasizes that when WHO was established in 1948, the World Health Assembly (WHA) was designated as its decision-making body, with the authority to make recommendations, treaties, and legally binding regulations for Member States (Avilés Mendoza 2005–2006). The ability of WHO to affect national health decisions is limited by nation-states. Nationalist governments prioritize political ideology over epidemiologic reality, violating International Health Regulations (IHR) obligations, failing to share timely and accurate information with WHO. States have further failed to comply with WHO recommendations, weakening global governance (Gostin 2020). Consequently, WHO lacks the legal authority to ensure equitable distribution of medical supplies during a pandemic (Hu 2021: 2).

Third, WHO is negatively affected by geopolitics. The difficulty of global governance is that there are no globally authoritative actors (Whitman 2006: 28). The pandemic has also raised nationalist sentiment. US former President Donald Trump, for example, accused the WHO of promoting the interests of China (Woods et al. 2020). Moreover, the COVID-19 crisis highlights WHO's outdated state-centric design and the conflicts of interest caused by its entanglements in geopolitics. Some also argue that the unfair treatment of Taiwan by WHO is harmful for GHG (Lin et al. 2020a; Chen 2020). After its controversial response to COVID-19, WHO is regarded as a more political and less technical organization (Kuznetsova 2020: 470–471).

COVID-19 has revealed the conflicts of sovereign states in WHO, making it unable to effectively promote global health governance. Jennifer Prah Ruger (2018) points out that after the establishment of WHO, the advancement of Health for All was not a priority for the controlling powerful states. Reflecting on SARS, Ebola, and H1N1, we can see that global health governance has never bypassed state implementations, and states are still the predominant actors.

COVID-19 shatters the myth of Health for All and makes us rethink the vulnerability of WHO as the leading GHG. While the above studies show COVID-19 reinforces state sovereignty and the governance of nation-states, they ignore cases of ambiguous sovereignty, such as Taiwan. Amid the conflict between nationalist and cosmopolitan worldviews, WHO as GHG must accommodate both nationalism and globalism vis-à-vis the contested state of Taiwan. Responding to Taiwan's exceptional governance offers an opportunity to reform the limitations inherent in WHO's GHG.

Research Methods

This chapter is based on multi-qualitative research methods including examination of WHO documents, discourse analysis, and content analysis of COVID-19-related news. First, WHO documents were collected regarding Taiwan and COVID-19, including press releases, situation reports, the meeting minutes of the 73rd and 74th WHA gatherings, press conference transcripts, and pandemic reports. In addition, conference documents and historical archives published on the WHO website were collected. Second, Taiwanese government discourses were collected and analyzed, focusing on speeches by ministerial heads, as well as personal posts on social media platforms. Additionally, ministers' international and domestic media interviews and related news reports were collected and analyzed. Finally, Taiwanese news reports pertinent to the management of COVID-19, as well as foreign coverage of Taiwan's COVID-19 response were also collected.

WHO, GHG, and Taiwan as a Contested State

WHO's "One-China Principle" and the Conflict over Taiwan's Sovereignty

The institutional design of WHO is state-centric governance. Pursuant to Article 3 of the WHO Constitution, "Membership in the Organization shall be open to all States", statehood is the only precondition to join WHO (Burci and Vignes 2004: 21). According to Article 9 of the Constitution, the organs of WHO include WHA, the Executive Board, and the Secretariat. The Secretariat is headed by the Director-General (DG), WHO's chief technical and administrative officer. Currently, there are 194 Member States, one associate member (Faroe Island), and several observers in the WHO.[1]

The Republic of China (ROC) was one of the founding members of WHO in 1948. Nonetheless, on October 25, 1971, the UN General Assembly adopted Resolution 2758 (XXVI), recognizing the PRC government as the only legitimate representative of China to UN.[2] On May 10, 1972, WHA subsequently adopted WHA Resolution 25.1 citing Resolution 2758, stating that it

> ...Decides to restore all its rights to the People's Republic of China (PRC) and to recognize the representatives of its government as the only legitimate representatives of China to the UN, and to expel forthwith the representatives of Chiang Kai-shek from the place which they unlawfully occupy at UN and in all the organizations related to it.[3]

From then on, PRC replaced ROC as the sole Chinese representative at the UN/WHO. Under PRC's "One-China Principle", mainland China and the island of Taiwan are considered a single nation-state, which has significantly impacted Taiwan's participation in WHO's expert/technical activities, *especially during the COVID-19* outbreak.

In reality, there are three ways to become a WHO member: (1) members of the UN can become members of WHO by accepting the Constitution;[4] (2) the founding members of WHO can become members by accepting the Constitution prior to the first WHA session;[5] or (3) if a State does not meet above requirements, its application to join WHO must go through a single majority vote of WHA members,[6] under the premise that this act does not violate the agreements signed between the UN and WHO. Since Taiwan lost its UN membership in 1971, and the first session of WHA had already been held in 1948, it cannot apply to WHO based on Article 4 or Article 5. If Taiwan wishes to become a member based on Article 6, its application also requires a simple majority vote from WHO Member States (Gau 2013: 145–147).

Due to the PRC's "One-China Principle", which has been accepted by most Member States, the names and national identities under which Taiwan should participate in WHO/WHA often trigger controversies. Beginning in 1997, Taiwan former President Lee Teng-hui (李登輝) proactively advocated that Taiwan rejoin WHO, but this has been consistently obstructed by China. On May 5, 1997, two WHO Member States with diplomatic relations with Taiwan, Nicaragua (尼加拉瓜) and Honduras (宏都拉斯),[7] submitted to the General Committee of WHA a supplementary agenda requesting Taiwan's participation in the Assembly under the name "Republic of China" as an observer.[8] The General Committee rejected the proposal. The decision was later submitted to WHA for review, and the agenda item was rejected through a 128:19 vote.[9] This process was repeated from 1998 to 2002.

Using the name ROC to participate in WHO raises the issue of the legitimate representation of China (Crawford 2007). To avoid this dispute, the Democratic Progressive Party (DPP), after winning the presidency, used the name "Taiwan" as a "health entity" to apply for WHA observership in 2002 but did not succeed.[10] In 2003, Taiwan reapplied under the name "health authorities of Taiwan", but China's delegate accused Taiwan of politicizing SARS to serve its separatist activities and rejected the concept of "health entity". The application was eventually denied by WHA.[11] In 2004, Taiwan's diplomatic allies resubmitted the proposal under the name "Taiwan" and the US and Japan supported Taiwan for the first time. Finally, the proposal was rejected by WHA through a 133:15 vote.[12]

Although UN Resolution 2758 and WHA Resolution WHA25.1 recognize the PRC as the only legitimate representative of China, neither addresses the issue of Taiwan's sovereignty. Therefore, some legal scholars argue that Taiwan is theoretically eligible to apply to become a Member State representing a country distinct from China based on Article 6 of the WHO Constitution (Lin et al.2020b: 103). On April 11, 2007, former President Chen Shui-Bian (陳水扁) sent a letter to WHO DG Margaret Chan (陳馮富珍) to apply to become a full WHO member, using "Taiwan" as the name of a country independent from PRC. He also sent a letter to UN Secretary-General Ban Ki Moon later on July 19, 2007, to apply for UN Membership. These applications marked a shift in the Taiwanese government's attitude on Taiwan's sovereignty. The General Committee reached consensus in not accepting Taiwan's application, and this decision was rejected at WHA by a vote of 148:17.[13]

After President Lee Tung-hui's claim of "special state-to-state relations" and President Chen Shui-bian's "one country on each side" concept, the tension in cross-strait relations eased under President Ma Ying-jeou's advocacy of the "One China, different interpretations" concept when the KMT returned to power in 2008. On April 30, 2009, DG Margaret Chan sent a letter to Taiwan Department of Health Minister Yeh Chin-chuan (葉金川) to invite Taiwan to participate in WHA as an observer under the name "Chinese Taipei" (Yeh 2009).

From 2009 to 2016, Taiwan used the name "Chinese Taipei" to avoid the sovereignty disputes and participate as an observer in WHA through the DG's invitation. In 2017, President Tsai Ing-Wen (蔡英文) of the Democratic Progressive Party (DPP) took office and refused to affirm the "One-China Principle". Since them, the DG has ceased sending invitations to "Chinese Taipei", and WHA continues to oppose proposals by Taiwan's diplomatic allies.

The Taiwan Issue Resurfaced after the COVID-19 Outbreak

While COVID-19 raged worldwide, *Taiwan* emerged as a successful case in the early years of the pandemic. Meanwhile, Taiwan's political elites and experts utilized the success of the Taiwan model of governance to challenge the denial of ROC's statehood under WHO/WHA's state-centric framework, fighting for WHO membership to gain international recognition.

On May 11, 2020, at a WHO press conference, a journalist from the British *Telegraph*, raised questions about how WHO would respond to Taiwan's accusation that WHO blocked Taiwan under Beijing's pressure. Steve Solomon, the legal officer of the WHO, replied: (1) The WHO Secretariat works according to regulations determined by its 194 Member States, including the WHA resolution passed 49 years ago to identify the PRC as the only legitimate representative of China and to expel Chiang Kai-shek from WHO. (2) The Director-General makes decisions according to the Constitution; only Member States have the right to make the final decision. From 2009 to 2016, the DG invited Taiwan to attend WHA under the title of "Chinese Taipei", following the consensus of Member States at that time. Currently, the Member States show divergent stances; the DG thus lacks a legitimate basis to invite "Chinese Taipei". (3) While 13 states propose Taiwan's inclusion, the proposal should be decided by all 194 WHA Member States, as stipulated by the constitution.[14] Meanwhile, the US and Japan have shown support for Taiwan's meaningful participation in WHA. On May 19, 2020, Alex Azar, the US Health and Human Services (HHS) Secretary, emphasized that "... It is important for Taiwan to be invited to participate as an observer to WHA, for they can share their exemplary experience in disease prevention with the globe".[15]

On March 28, 2020, a Radio Television Hong Kong reporter asked Bruce Aylward, senior advisor to the DG of WHO, several times whether WHO would reconsider Taiwan's membership on a video call. Aylward pretended he didn't hear the question and later requested to skip it. When the journalist asked for Aylward's comment on Taiwan's disease prevention, he remarked that each region of China overall performed very well.[16] In response, Foreign Minister Wu posted on Twitter, "Wow, can't even utter 'Taiwan' in WHO?" and suggested that WHO "should set politics aside when dealing with a pandemic".[17] On March 29, 2020, WHO issued a press release on "Information sharing on COVID-19", re-emphasizing that Taiwan's membership issue should be decided by Member States, not WHO staff.[18]

On November 9, 2020, the first day of WHA's 73rd session, Taiwan's application was discussed, and the General Committee adopted a "two-against-two" closed-door meeting, where delegates of Taiwan's diplomatic allies debated with delegates of China and Cuba. Nauru's (諾魯) delegate argued:

> ...The WHO Constitution acknowledges the highest attainable standard of health as one of the fundamental rights of every human being and it should live up to that vision by recognizing Taiwan and its people, and their right to participate in the global health security system.

The representative of China in turn claimed that as an agency of the UN, WHO should follow the "One-China Principle". The authorities of Taiwan refused to recognize the 1992 consensus, and thus the political foundation for Taiwan to participate in WHA had ceased to exist.[19] The General Committee eventually rejected the proposal. At the end of WHA plenary meeting, WHO published a news statement stressing that "this is the 15th time since 1997 where such proposal has been submitted", and WHA made a decision in accordance with Resolution 2758 and WHA Resolution 25.1, rejecting Taiwan's application.[20]

The 74th WHA was held in Geneva on May 2021 via video conference, and Taiwan's 14 diplomatic allies submitted a proposal similar to the previous year's to the General Committee. During the WHA plenary meetings, Nauru's (諾魯)

Year	Formal title used to apply for WHA participation	Name-Status
1946	The WHA passed the WHO Constitution; the R.O.C. was one of the founding member states.	
1971	The R.O.C. expelled from the UN and WHO.	
1997 - 2001	Inviting Republic of China (Taiwan) as an observer in the WHA	Republic of China - Observer Failed
2002	Inviting Taiwan as an observer in the WHA	Taiwan -Observer Failed
2003	Inviting Health Authorities of Taiwan as an observer in the WHA	Health Authorities of Taiwan -Observer Failed
2004 - 2006	Inviting Taiwan as an observer in the WHA	Taiwan -Observer Failed
2007	Inviting Republic of China (Taiwan) as a member in the WHO	Taiwan -Member Failed
2008	Inviting Taiwan as an observer in the WHA	Taiwan -Observer Failed
2009 - 2016	Taiwan was invited to attend the WHA as an observer under the title of Chinese Taipei.	Chinese Taipei- Observer
2017 - 2022	Inviting Taiwan as an observer in the WHA	Taiwan -Observer Failed

Figure 12.1 A Summary of Titles of Taiwan's Application for Participation in WHO (1946–2022)

Source: Compiled by the author based on relevant WHO documents.

delegate stated that "… The political pressure from one country should not legitimize the continued exclusion of Taiwan, which ultimately destabilizes global health efforts". Belize's (貝里斯) delegate also said: "The inclusion of all nations is imperative in the preparation and response of global health emergencies…, the Government of Belize supports the inclusion of Taiwan as an observer of WHA".[21] WHA again decided to reject the proposal. In response, Minister of Foreign Affairs Joseph Wu (吳釗燮) argued that (Figure 12.1)

> The PRC has never ruled over Taiwan, but it constantly misinterprets the UN Resolutions 2758 and WHA25.1 and misleads the international society. Only the democratically elected government of Taiwan is eligible to represent the 23.5 million Taiwanese people in WHO and other international organizations.[22]

The essence of nationalism is about "Who am I?" The problem of "Who am I?" is related to name and identity. The names "Chinese Taipei" or "Taiwan, Province of China" have replaced the names "Taiwan" or "ROC" under the "One-China principle" in WHO's state-centric design. After the outbreak of COVID-19, the disagreements between "Taiwan/ ROC" and "China/ PRC" in WHO have become even more contentious. The focus on state sovereignty runs counter to the need for cooperation in fighting a global pandemic and GHG in totality. To some extent, WHO as a centralized nation-state-based model of GHG may crowd out important actors operating in a contested state or territory. Constantly excluded from WHO, the Taiwan government urges the adoption of the name of Taiwan as an equivalent sovereign state – a sovereignty made more clearly visible in the international community through Taiwan's success in controlling COVID-19.

The Silencing of Taiwan by WHO

In the face of emerging communicable diseases, the establishment of a network for emergency notification, information sharing, and mutual communication has become the focus of GHG. Although infectious diseases can break out anywhere, Taiwan has become a gray area in WHO's GHG and has not been able to enjoy the right to health guaranteed to other countries.

Taiwan Listed as a Province of China in WHO's Reports and Taiwan's One-Way Communication Under the International Health Regulations (IHR)

In March 2003, Taiwan confirmed its first case of SARS, and Taiwan Centers for Disease Control (CDC) immediately reported it to WHO's Western Pacific Regional Office (WPRO).[23] Former Vice President Chen Chien-jen (陳建仁), a PhD epidemiologist from John Hopkins University, referred to as "Taiwan's Weapon Against Coronavirus" by the *New York Times,*[24] commented in an interview with a Japanese journalist, "Before the case broke out at Hoping Hospital, we had requested assistance from WHO to give us samples of the SARS virus strain to develop instant diagnostic tools … but WHO ignored us".[25] Taiwan, despite its proximity to China, could not obtain any information from WHO because Taiwan was not a Member State (Taiwan CDC 2004).

Under China's oppression, "Taiwan" has also become a sensitive keyword at WHO. From SARS to COVID-19, both Taiwan's name and experts have been excluded from WHO's global information network. During the initial outbreak of COVID-19, WHO listed Taiwan as a province of China. This caused problems for Taiwan when Italy and Vietnam banned Taiwanese flights from entering their borders in 2020.[26]

The map on WHO's official website still marks Taiwan as a part of China.[27] On May 14, 2005, WHO's DG Margaret Chan signed the "Implementation of the Memorandum of Understanding between the WHO Secretariat and China" (MOU), requiring that documents or information which is published, incorporated or referred to in WHO publications or documents, whether electronic or in hard copy, must use the terminology "the Taiwan Province of China".[28] In the nine journals officially published by the WHO, Taiwan is often referred to as "Taiwan, China". From January 2020 to March 2022, WHO's reports on COVID-19 used "Taiwan, China", "Taiwan, Special administrative region of China", and "Taipei Municipality" instead of Taiwan. The Independent Panel for Pandemic Preparedness and Response (IPPR) established by the WHO DG published the report "COVID-19: Make it the last pandemic", which again refers to Taiwan as "Taiwan, China".[29] The request to correct the inappropriate designation from Taiwan's Ministry of Foreign Affairs was, unsurprisingly, ignored by the IPPR.[30]

After the SARS epidemic, WHA revised IHR to prevent the spread of new infectious diseases, and adopted it in May 2005. The revised IHR, which entered into force in June 2007, covers new and emerging diseases, expands the power of the DG to announce COVID-19 Public Health Emergency of International Concern (PHEIC), and obliges States to establish IHR National Focal Points (NFPs). The goal of the new IHR is to reinforce global emergency responses and to provide guidance on effective measures to tackle infectious diseases. Although IHR only covers its State Parties,[31] Article 3 paragraph 3 in the IHR stipulates that "The implementation of these Regulations shall be guided by the goal of their universal application for the protection of all people of the world from the international spread of disease".[32] This article left open the possibility of including Taiwan in the application of IHR, since the IHR should apply to every corner of the world (Chen 2018). In May 2006, Taiwan preliminarily implemented the IHR before it entered into force. Simultaneously, Taiwan unilaterally established its own NFP and set up the NFP email account **ihrfocalpoint@cdc.gov.tw**,[33] hoping to use it to share information with other countries' NFPs, the WPRO, and the Program for Monitoring Emerging Diseases (ProMed).[34] Although not acknowledged by WHO or WPRO, this email has been used to exchange disease information with some countries.[35]

On May 15, 2007, China established the WHO China Country Office in accordance with Article 4 of the IHR and claimed that it should be used as the contact point for Taiwan.[36] However, as cross-strait relations eased during President Ma Ying-jeou's presidency, Taiwan CDC received a letter on January 13, 2009, from Dr. Bernard P. Kean, Executive Director of the WHO Office of the DG, which detailed the proposed arrangements by WHO for Taiwan's participation in the implementation of IHR.[37] The concrete measures proposed by WHO are as follows: (1) WHO should accept Taiwan's NFP and allow it to directly contact the WHO Secretariat. WHO also provided Taiwan access to the Event Information Site (EIS), a website that contains information on global endemic and epidemic diseases, and information about other States' NFPs; (2) when a PHEIC occurs in Taiwan, WHO can send experts to assist Taiwan or invite representatives of Taiwan to attend the WHO emergency committee in accordance with Article 48 of the IHR; (3) Taiwan can appoint its own health expert to join the IHR Expert Roster under Article 47 of the IHR.[38] In contrast to the SARS outbreak during which Taiwan could not directly obtain WHO information, Taiwan can now access EIS for epidemic information and other States' contact information. However, other States cannot directly communicate with Taiwan.

The dangers of Taiwan's partial participation in IHR became apparent during the COVID-19 pandemic. As early as December 31, 2019, a Taiwanese CDC physician happened upon information concerning a viral outbreak in Wuhan on PTT, the largest online bulletin board system in Taiwan. Taiwan CDC subsequently emailed WHO via the IHR contact point to request further information. Liu Li-ling (劉麗玲), the Technical Superintendent, Ministry of Health and Welfare (MOHW), explained that "we proactively reported to WHO on December 31, 2019, and treated COVID-19 as a human-to-human transmitted disease in early January 2020. Nevertheless, this was not taken seriously by WHO" (MOHW 2020). Further, the first COVID-related official report published by WHO on January 5, 2020, the organization evidently ignored Taiwan's warning.[39] It was not until January 30 that the Emergency Committee advised the DG to announce COVID-19 as PHEIC.[40] Former Vice President Chen Chien-jen commented in an interview with France 24 on May 9, 2020: "…So I think that in light of our information provided to WHO, WHO should have discovered it was quite likely that there was human-to-human transmission".[41] He also stated that "While the IHR's internal website provides a platform for all countries to share information on the epidemic and their response, none of the information from Taiwan CDC is being put up there".[42]

While the IHR 2005 represents a shift toward a collective governance strategy that integrates different actors and places in governing infectious disease outbreaks, the COVID-19 pandemic reveals that IHR 2005 can neither compel State Parties to fulfill their obligations, nor provide a mechanism for accountability. As evidenced by IHR requirements early on, the lack of national capacity to report and manage outbreaks, China's political unwillingness to fulfill its obligations to notify the WHO, and WHO ignoring Taiwan's timely warnings, all pose threats to the capacity of the WHO to implement IHR 2005 effectively.

Taiwan's Participation in WHO Meetings through China's Approval

Information sharing and transparency are at the heart of GHG of infectious diseases. Currently, there are three types of WHO technical meetings: (1) expert technical meetings, including 41 "Expert Advisory Panels and Committees" (five of which hold annual meetings), WHO disease prevention network systems, and expert meetings and task forces held by WHO;[43] (2) expert technical meetings held by the WPRO; and (3) emergency committees and review committees comprised of health experts pursuant to Articles 48 and 50 of the IHR.[44]

Taiwan is not able to join any WHO Expert Advisory Panels and Committees, nor is it eligible for participation in WPRO meetings. Moreover, based on an MOU[45] with China in 2005, WPRO acknowledged the PRC government's power over the participation of the ROC's experts in WHO/WHA. Among several important WHO disease prevention networks, Taiwan can only participate in the Global Influenza Surveillance and Response System (Taiwan CDC 2017).

Established by WHO in 2000, the Global Outbreak Alert and Response Network (GOARN, 全球疫情警報與反應網路) comprises technical and research institutions, universities, international health organizations and technical networks. Its goal is to help countries around the world initiate disease control measures. During the revision of IHR in 2005, Taiwan actively pursued its goal of "meaningful participation" in GOARN, hoping to establish its own NFP based on the IHR principle of universality. Nevertheless, the Director of the Office of the WHO DG, Denis Aitken, publicly said Taiwan's application to join GOARN was rejected because of political reasons.[46]

In theory, the DG could accept Taiwanese experts into IHR expert groups and let them join emergency committees and review committees in accordance with Article 47 of the IHR.[47] However, Taiwan has not been able to enjoy the rights and obligations shared among IHR State Parties. Addressing the attention toward Taiwan's successful COVID-19 response from foreign media, WHO issued a statement on March 29, 2020, stating that it had been cooperating with Taiwan, which is a member of the Training Programs in Epidemiology and Public Health Interventions Network (TEPHINET). WHO also stated it shares GOARN alerts and requests for assistance with TEPHINET and that Taiwanese public health experts also participated in the Global Research and Innovation Forum convened by WHO on February 11–12, 2020, alongside other scientists.[48]

The next day, Taiwan's Ministry of Foreign Affairs (MOFA) criticized WHO for stating a partial fact. First, although Taiwan can access the EIS for relevant information, it is limited to one-way communication since Taiwan cannot share any information with other countries. During the COVID-19 pandemic, Taiwan was the very first to notify WHO through the NFP, but WHO Secretariat never published such information on EIS, nor did it provide this information in its first "COVID-19 Situation Report". Second, though it is a member of TEPHINET, Taiwan has never participated in GOARN. Lastly, the Global Research and Innovation Forum only allows Taiwan to participate online, and never grants it a chance to exchange ideas with other delegates. From 2009 to 2019, Taiwan submitted 187 applications to participate in WHO technical meetings, and it was only invited to 57 meetings, a rejection rate of approximately 70%. Geographically, WHO WPRO is responsible for Taiwan's health issues, but Taiwan has been constantly excluded from WPRO meetings. In addition, although Taiwanese experts are allowed to join the clinical management and infection control networks, they are still not eligible for participation in the laboratory network.[49]

When giving a keynote speech at the conference *Taiwan and the COVID-19 Pandemic: Lessons for the World* at Stanford University in 2020, former Vice President Chen Chien-jen explained Taiwan's incomplete participation in WHA. He said,

> This lack of timely information exchange has become a hidden risk in the global public health system … we call on WHO to stand up for its self-declared ideals of professionalism and neutrality by inviting Taiwan to attend WHA as an observer, and grant Taiwan full participation in WHO, without political preconditions.[50]

Chen further expressed his concern when interviewed by *The New York Times* in 2020, stating, "although WHO says that Taiwan has participated, our participation is fragmented and limited, not complete … Our participation is very conditional, and only with China's agreement".[51]

Although the spread of COVID-19 and its variants in one place can have repercussions everywhere, Taiwan, with its contested statehood, has been erased in WHO's reports and meetings even as the WHO calls for global cooperation to fight COVID-19. Several important heads of government in Taiwan, especially technocrats with medical backgrounds such as Chen Chien-jen, Chen Chi-mai, and Chen Shih-chung, have become Taiwan's internationally visible spokespersons. By actively using foreign media and international platforms to speak out, they take advantage of Taiwan's early achievements in pandemic governance and its special geographical position to accuse WHO of its likely prioritization politics over health. They also use Taiwan's model in controlling the pandemic to condemn WHO for recklessly blocking Taiwan's participation in expert meetings and improperly categorizing Taiwan's pandemic data under China. These efforts expose "the black box" in which WHO, WHA, and IHR make politically charged decisions about Taiwan while emphasizing the information gap between Taiwan and WHO/WHA. Utilizing the discourse of Health for All, Taiwanese leaders have attempted to regain international attention during the COVID-19 pandemic by highlighting that Taiwan cannot obtain the latest information from WHO/WHA, and WHO/WHA cannot obtain the latest information from Taiwan (Figure 12.2).

Lessons from Taiwan's Exceptional Governance: How to Fix the Vulnerabilities in WHO'S GHG

Article 25 of the 1948 Universal Declaration on Human Rights adopted by the UN stipulates that "Everyone has the right to a standard of living adequate for the health and well-being of himself and of his family".[52] In the same year, the WHO Constitution reaffirmed that health is a universal human right.[53] In 1978, the International Conference of Primary Health Care adopted the Alma-Ata Declaration, which for the first time promoted the concept of Health for All as WHO's goal to

Year / Expert/ technical meetings and networks	1971 – 2008	2009 - 2016	2017 - 2021
1 Expert meeting networks built by WHO			
1.1WHO Expert Advisory Panels and Committees	Not able to participate	Not able to participate	Not able to participate
1.2 Epidemic prevention network systems affiliated with WHO	Not able to participate	Limited participation	Limited participation
1.3. Expert meetings and task forces organized and established by WHO	Limited participation	Limited participation	Limited participation
2 WPRO technical expert meetings	Limited participation	Limited participation	Not able to participate
3 IHR point of contact and expert group meetings	Not able to participate or communicate	Limited participation and communication	Limited participation and communication

Figure 12.2 Taiwan's Participation in WHO Communications and Expert/Technical Meetings from 1971 to 2021

Source: Compiled by the author based on relevant WHO documents.

resolve health inequalities.[54] In 2000, the Committee on Economic, Social and Cultural Rights of the UN made General Comment No. 14, stressing that States need to take joint and separate actions in order to fully realize the right to health. The Committee also points out that States should respect the right to health of other countries and refrain from interfering with their rights.[55] Despite its contested statehood, legal scholar James Crawford suggests that Taiwan is still an entity under international law and is thus entitled to relevant rights (Crawford 2007: 219–221).

From SARS in 2003 to the current COVID-19 pandemic, Taiwan has been an exceptional case in GHG because of the geopolitics between Taiwan and China. The risks of new communicable diseases highlight the significance of Taiwan's case, through which we can reflect on the discrepancy between the universal value of Health for All and the state-centric design of WHO.

Contested Statehood Is a Security Flaw in WHO's GHG

WHO's Constitution stipulates that only "States" can become WHO members. Nonetheless, there have been some examples of areas with contested "statehood" that eventually became WHO members. For instance, the Federal Republic of Germany applied and became a WHO member in 1951. After the division of East and West Germany, the German Democratic Republic was also invited by the DG in 1971 and became a WHA observer. Its membership application was later approved in 1973. Timor-Leste, once colonized by Portugal and then invaded by Indonesia, officially became an independent State through a referendum in 2002 and joined WHO as a Member State in the same year.[56] These cases demonstrate that statehood is subject to change. Moreover, some areas with contested "statehood" have also become WHO observers. For instance, the UN General Assembly made Resolution 3118 XXVIII),), requiring all UN-specialized agencies to contact and cooperate with the national liberation movements of colonial territories in Africa.[57] Subsequently, WHA adopted Resolution 27.37 in 1974, requesting the DG to invite the representatives of African national liberation movements. This resolution later became the basis for the DG to invite contested states like Palestine to become WHA observers (Burci and Vignes 2004: 36–39).

The history of WHO demonstrates that "statehood" is not necessarily an obstacle to participating in WHO. The major barrier to Taiwan in participating WHO is China's interference. Gian Luca Burci and Claude-Henri Vignes (2004) stressed there are two types of WHO observers. The first is observers invited for a limited period, which includes States and territories that have applied to become members and associate members of WHO. The second is quasi-permanent observers, which include three circumstances: (1) Non-Member State observers such as the Holy See; (2) An observer (Palestine) invited by the DG in accordance with WHA Resolution 27.37; (3) Normal observers like the Order of Malta, the International Committee of the Red Cross (ICRC), etc. Of all three circumstances, only non-Member State observers meet the requirement of "statehood", indicating that areas of contested statehood such as Taiwan can become WHA observers if the DG invites them.

Currently, there are areas like Taiwan and Kosovo that are not included in WHO's GHG.[58] As shown, WHO as GHG is flawed because its governance is based on nation-states that perpetuate power inequalities at the expense of Heath for All. The power of a few sovereign States within WHO can overshadow the universal right to health. Taiwan is not able to participate effectively in WHO's pandemic safeguarding community due to the political intervention of China. Placed in the middle of a political power struggle between national governments, WHO faces a predicament that can emerge when powerful Member States define the limits of acceptable action.

WHO Should Reinforce Its Transparency and Legitimacy

WHO's DG signed a secret MOU[59] with China in 2015. It emphasizes that the implementation of MOU must be in conformity with WHA Resolution 25.1 and regulates Taiwan's participation in three major ways. First, based on MOU Articles 5–7, Taiwanese experts' participation in WHO technical expert meetings must be considered on a case-by-case basis, and must be approved by China's delegate. The Taiwanese experts participating in the meetings must not exceed the level of the "DG", and their designation must be "Taiwan, China". Second, according to Articles 8–12, the dispatch of WHO staff members and experts to Taiwan for crises must be approved by China's delegate, and the staff dispatched must also be under the level of Director and cannot be current or former government officials. Third, pursuant to Articles 13–16, in case of an acute public health emergency in Taiwan, WHO can dispatch staff members or experts after gaining approval from the China Ministry of Health. If the duration of the dispatch exceeds eight weeks, WHO shall regularly consult the Chinese Mission and report their activities in Taiwan. Health issues not covered by the MOU are handled on a case-by-case basis through consultations between WHO and China. The MOU also requires WHO to prevent Taiwanese authorities from sending NGOs to participate in WHO meetings.

This secret MOU between WHO and China does not only limit Taiwan's participation in WHO expert and technical meetings, but also clandestinely gives China the power to control Taiwan's activities in WHO. It violates the principle of good governance and exposes potential vulnerabilities in WHO's GHG, including the legitimacy of the MOU, the transparency of the information shared about communicable diseases, and the appropriateness of the DG's excessive decision-making power.

First, under international law, an MOU usually is not legally binding (Aust 2007: 52–53). The WHO Constitution does not contain any provision empowering the DG to sign an MOU with any State government. Furthermore, this MOU is not approved by WHA or Executive Board. Despite creating an illegal and illegitimate black box, this document is the guiding principle of how WHO handles Taiwan. China and WHO should have abided by their obligations to promote the right to health as interpreted by the UN Committee on Economic, Social, and Cultural Rights.[60] Under the MOU, however, WHO can only provide Taiwan emergency assistance with China's approval. This clandestinely created governance instrument again demonstrates that the unjustified intervention of political force has undermined the right to health of 23.5 million Taiwanese people, violating the universal value of health equity. In the aftermath of this MOU, other States might exploit similar approaches to serve their own interests, reducing the credibility of WHO as a transnational health organization.

Second, WHO aims to keep track of infectious diseases threatening the international community in a timely manner through a mechanism established in the IHR 2005. It also seeks to share information about pathogens, vaccine development, and disease prevention measures through global cooperation between technical personnel and health experts. Taiwanese experts' participation in these meetings, as well as WHO's provision of emergency assistance to Taiwan, are subject to the agreement of China. Taiwan is thus unable to access relevant networks such as GOARN and excluded from equal access to the global system of pandemic information sharing.

Finally, the way the DG secretly signed an MOU with China reveals the excessively centralized power of the DG and calls the appropriateness of WHO's decision-making process into question. As the chief officer of WHO, the DG's main responsibility is to make administrative decisions. The term of office of the DG is five years, and he/she can be reappointed once, making the total term up to ten years.[61] Legal scholars Gian Luca Burci and Claude-Henri Vignes point out that the DG can participate in any WHA meetings and committees, and the WHA rules of procedure also grant the DG the power to make statements during the meetings. These statements often alter the attitudes of States toward specific matters. Therefore, the political responsibilities and capacity of the DG usually go beyond the scope authorized by the laws, and the leadership and personality of the DG can exert significant influence in WHO (Burci and Vignes 2004: 50).

Moreover, the WHO DG has the additional power to decide whether he/she wants to invite Taiwan to become a WHA observer. Clearly, the discretionary power is overly centralized in the office of the DG. Past examples of WHA observers such as Palestine did not fall under the scope of Rule 3 of the WHA Rules of Procedure or Article 18(h) of the Constitution. But Palestine and others successfully participate in WHA as observers with the DG's invitation. In other words, the DG has discretionary power in complex issues such as contested statehood (Burci and Vignes 2004: 37–38).[62] From 2009 to 2016, under the approval of China, Taiwan was proactively invited by the DG as a WHA observer. Since 2017, the invitation ceased after President Tsai Ing-wen was elected. Further, the current WHO DG, Dr. Tedros Adhanom Ghebreyesus, was elected with Chinese support (Rowen 2020) and has been criticized for his biased policies toward China during the pandemic. With excessive power and authority, he has further impeded Taiwan's participation in WHO.

Conclusion

COVID-19 has posed new challenges to globalization while reinforcing the growing power of nationalism and nation-states. Facing the global COVID-19 crisis, WHO has a mandate to be the directing authority on international health affairs;[63] however, nation-states have actively limited WHO's autonomy to further their own national interests. WHO's treatment of Taiwan contradicts its mission to promote Health for All.

Moreover, the vulnerability of WHO to political interference became even more apparent after the outbreak of the COVID-19 pandemic. Due to its state-centric design, WHO prioritizes the interests of nation-states and thus exacerbates geopolitical competition among Members States. The thorny problem of Taiwan's status poses a challenge for WHO to free itself from the political intervention of Member States and build good governance for the health affairs of an interdependent world.

Through the structural obstacles inherent in an infective system of the coronavirus, Taiwan's exceptional governance reveals broader problems with the institutional primacy of nation-states in WHO/WHA, the excessive centralization of power in the hands of the Director-General, and contested states in obtaining timely information during the pandemics crisis that might heighten the risk of future pandemics, which will further jeopardize GHG.

Acknowledgments

An earlier version of this paper was presented at the Harvard STS Program, Academia Sinica, and 4S annual meetings. I would like to thank Professor Shelia Jasanoff, Professor Richard Madsen, Professor Jia-shin Chen, and Professor Wen-yuan Lin for their valuable suggestions. This research is part of the project funded by the Thematic Research Program at Academia Sinica (AS-TP-111-H02) and Taiwan's National Science Council (NSC112-2410-H-001-034-MY2).

Notes

1 WHO.2021. "Seventy-Fourth WHA List of Delegates and Other Participants." See https://apps.who.int/gb/ebwha/pdf_files/WHA74/A74_Div1Rev1-en.pdf. Accessed December 17, 2021.

2 UN. 1971. "Restoration of the lawful rights of the People's Republic of China in the UN." See UN Digital Library, https://digitallibrary.un.org/record/192054/files/A_RES_-2758%28XX-VI%29-EN.pdf. Accessed April 12, 2022. In 1945, the ROC government began exercising jurisdiction over Taiwan following Japan's surrender at the end of World War II. When the Chinese Communist Party won the Chinese Civil War in 1949, the Chinese Nationalist Party (KMT) led by Chiang Kai-Shek retreated to Taiwan.

3 WHO. 1972. "WHA25.1 Representation of China in the WHO" See https://apps.who.int/iris/handle-/10665/85850. Accessed November 26, 2020.

4 Article 4 of the WHO Constitution.

5 Article 5 of the WHO Constitution.

6 Article 6 of the WHO Constitution.

7 They have diplomatic relation with Taiwan at that time.

8 MOFA. 1997. "The Foreign Relations Yearbook 1997 Republic of China (Taiwan)." See https://multilingual.mofa.gov.tw/web/web_UTF-8/almanac/almanac1997/32.html. Accessed November 16, 2021.

9 WHO. 1997. "Fiftieth WHA: Provisional Verbatim Record of the Third Plenary Meeting" See https://apps.who.int/iris/bitstream/handle/10665/179800/WHA50_VR3_eng.pdf?seq-uence=1&isAllowed=y. Accessed December 17, 2021.According to WHA Rules of Procedure, the supplementary agenda item can be proposed to the General Committee, and the Committee can decide whether it will adopt it into the WHA official agenda. If the Committee decides to reject the proposal, the WHA will later review the decision at the plenary meeting. During the reviewing process, Member States can call for a vote on whether the WHA would accept or reject the Committee's decision.

10 WHO. 2002. "Executive Board 109th session, Geneva, 14–21 January 2002: summary records." See https://apps.who.int/iris/handle/10665/259565. Accessed May 13, 2020.

11 WHO. 2003 "Fifty-Seventh WHA, Geneva, 17–22 May 2004: Summary Records of Committees and Round Tables Reports of Committees." See https://apps.who.int/irisbitstream/handle/10665/260147/-WHA57-2004-REC-3eng.pdf?sequence-=1&isAllowed=y. Accessed December 17, 2021.

12 WHO. 2004 "Fifty-Seventh WHA, Geneva, 17–22 May 2004: Verbatim Records of Plenary Meetings and List of Participants." See https://apps.who.int/iris/bittreamhandle/10665/-260146/WHA57-2004-REC-2-eng-fre.pdf?sequence=1&isAllowed=y. Accessed December 17, 2021.

13 WHO. 2007. "Sixtieth WHA, Geneva, 14–23 May 2007: Summary Records of Committees and Ministerial Round Tables Reports of Committees." See https://apps.who.int/iris/bitstream/handle-/10665/-22640/A60_REC3en.pdf?sequence=1&-isAllowed=y. Accessed December 17, 2021.

14 WHO. 2020. "Virtual Press Conference 11 May 2020." See www.who.int/docs/default-source/coron-aviruse/transcripts/who-audio-emergencies-coronavirus-press-conference11may2020.pdf?sfvrsn=4f7-8bd0_0. Accessed November 24, 2020.

15 MOHW. 2020. "U.S. Statement on Taiwan's Participation at the World." See https://www.mohw.gov.tw/cp-16-53984-1.html. Accessed May 9, 2022.

16 Hong Kong Free Press. 2020. "Video: Top WHO Doctor Bruce Aylward Ends Video Call after Journalist Asks about Taiwan's Status." See https://hongkongfp.com/2020/03/29/video-top-doctor-bruce-aylward-pretends-not-hear-journalists-taiwan-questions-ends-video-call/. Accessed April 22, 2022.

17 MOFA. Twitter. (March 29, 2020). See https://twitter.com/mofa_taiwan/status/124407665635-3935361. Accessed December 6, 2021.

18 WHO. 2020. "Information Sharing on COVID-19." See https://www.who.int/-news/item/29-03-2020-information-sharing-on-covid-19. Accessed December 6, 2021.

19 WHO. 2020. "Seventy-Third WHA: Summary Records of Committees, Reports of Committees." See https://apps.who.int/iris/bitstream/handle/10665/46063/73_REC3eng.pdf?sequ-ence=1&isAllowed=y. Accessed December 6, 2021.

20 WHO. 2020. "Health Policy Watch. 2020. WHA Puts Aside Rivalry Over Taiwan to Move Ahead on WHO Reform and COVID-19 Pandemic Agendas." See https://health-policy-watch.news/78728-2/. Accessed December 6, 2021.

21 The 74th WHA plenary meeting does not produce a verbatim record, instead, it was recorded live and is accessible through the website. Taiwan MOFA made a transcript of those States that supported Taiwan during the meeting. See, https://subsite.mofa.gov.tw/igo/News.aspx?n=6052&sms=1678. Accessed July 14, 2022.

22 MOFA. 2021. "Foreign Minister Jaushieh Joseph Wu and Health and Welfare Minister Chen Shih-chung Express Deep Displeasure at Taiwan's Exclusion from the Virtual 74th WHA." See https://en.mofa.gov.tw/News_Content.aspx?n-=1329&s=95895. Accessed: April 25, 2022.

23 WPRO was established by the WHA in 1950. It mainly translates WHO global health initiatives into regional plans, facilitating contact between governments in the region and WHO.

24 New York Times. 2020, "Coronavirus Crisis Offers Taiwan a Chance to Push Back Against China" on April 22, 2020. See https://www.nytimes.com/2020/04/22/world/asia/coronavirus-china-taiwan.html Accessed May 21, 2022.

25 Chen, Chien-Jen 2020 Facebook. (2020, February 27). See https://www.facebook.com/story.php?-story_fbid=2770125159734955&id=937931539621002&refid=52&tn=-R. Accessed April 22, 2020.

26 The official press release provides that Italy and Vietnam banned Taiwanese flights at the beginning of the outbreak. See the website of Taipei representative office in Italy at https://www.roc-taiwan.org/it/post/7591.html. Accessed May 21, 2020.
27 WHO. 2020. "Number of COVID-19 cases reported to WHO." See https://covid19.who.int/region/wpro-/country/cn. Accessed December 6, 2021.
28 Liberty Times. 2011. "WHO Document Was Revealed, Taiwan Listed as a Province of China." On May 9, 2011. See https://news.ltn.com.tw/news/focus-/paper/490829. Accessed May 21, 2022.
29 WHO. 2021. "The Independent Panel for Pandemic Preparedness & Response. 2021. COVID-19: Makes it the Last Pandemic." See https://theindependentpanel.org/wp-content/uploads/2021/05/CO-VID-19-Make-it-the-Last-Pandemic_final.pdf. Accessed December 6, 2021.
30 MOFA. 2021. "List of China Prevents Taiwan from Participating in International Community Events." See https://www.mofa.gov.tw/cp.aspx?n=2585. Accessed: March 12, 2022.
31 Article 64 paragraph 1 of the IHR.
32 WHO. 2005 "IHR Third Edition." See https://www.who.int/publications/i/item/9789241580496. Accessed April 22, 2022.
33 Article 4 of the IHR.
34 MOFA.2007. See https://www.mofa.gov.tw/News_-Content.aspx?n=96&sms=74&s=70076. Accessed December 6, 2021.
35 Taipei Economic and Cultural Center in India. 2018. See https://www.roctaiwan.org/in/post-/5060.html. Accessed December 6, 2021.
36 National Health Commission of the People's Republic of China. 2007. See http://en.nhc.gov.cn/about.html. Accessed April 21, 2022.
37 Taiwan CDC. 2009. "WHO Agrees to Include Taiwan in the Implementation of IHR." See https://www.cdc.gov.tw/Category/ListContent/AHwuigegBBBmuDcbWkzoGQ?uaid=HgWO7_umIHYNi44tL7DI0g. Accessed: February 16, 2022.
38 Taiwan CDC. 2009. See https://www.cdc.gov.tw/En/Bulletin/Detail/ijDOgFLf8UnPhk-PCa7y-Yeg?typeid=158. Accessed December 6, 2021.
39 WHO, 2020. Pneumonia of unknown cause – China. See https://www.who.int/emergencies/disease-outbreak-news/item/2020-DON229. Accessed December 6, 2021.
40 WHO. 2020. "Statement on the Second Meeting of the IHR (2005) Emergency Committee regarding the outbreak of novel coronavirus (2019-nCoV)." See www.who.int/news/item/30-01-2020-statement-on-the-second-meeting-of-the-international-health-regulations-(2005)-emergency-committee-regarding-the-outbreak-of-novel-coronavirus-(2019-ncov). Accessed December 6, 2021.
41 Office of the President. 2020. "Vice President Chen interviewed by France 24." See https://www.president.gov.tw/News-/25306. Accessed April 25, 2020.
42 Office of the President. 2020. "Vice President Chen interviewed by Nihon Keizai Shinbun." See https://www.president.gov.tw/News/25241. Accessed April 25, 2020.
43 WHO. 2022. "Expert Advisory Panels and Committees." See https://www.who.int/about/collabor-ation/expert-advisory-panels-and-committees. Accessed May 3, 2022.
44 Article 48 paragraph 2 of the IHR.
45 MOU. 2005 "Implementation of the Memorandum of Understanding between the WHO Secretariat and China." See https://link.springer.com/content/pdf/bbm%3A978-3-658-05527-1%2F1.pdf. Accessed April 26, 2022.
46 Taiwan News. 2006. "WHO Official Says Taiwan Receives Adequate Benefits." See https://www.tai-wannews.com.tw/en/news/104021. Accessed April 21, 2022.
47 According to Article 47 of the IHR, "The Director-General Shall Establish a Roster Composed of Experts in All Relevant Fields of Expertise…"

48 WHO 2020. "Information Sharing on COVID-19." See https://www.who.int/news/item/29-03-2020-information-sharing-on-covid-19. Accessed March 3, 2022.
49 MOFA. 2020. "MOFA Calls on WHO to Take Neutral, Professional Stance Facilitating Taiwan's Full Participation and Contributions." See https://en.mofa.gov.tw/News_Content.aspx?n=1329&s=91670. Accessed April 25, 2022.
50 Office of the President Republic of China (Taiwan). 2020. "Vice President Chen Delivers Speech at Videoconference Hosted by Stanford University's Hoover Institution." See https://english.president.gov.tw/NEWS/5998. Accessed: April 25, 2020.
51 Office of the President Republic of China (Taiwan). 2020. "Vice President Chen interviewed by The New York Times." See https://www.president.gov.tw/News/25288. Accessed April 25, 2020.
52 UN. 1948. "Universal Declaration of Human Rights." See https://www.ohchr.org/sites-/default/files/UDHR/Documents/UDHR-_Translations/eng.pdf. Accessed April 21, 2022.
53 WHO. 1946. "Constitution of the WHO." See https://www.who.int/governance/eb/who_constit-ution_en.pdf. Accessed December 17, 2021).
54 WHO. 1978. "WHO called to return to the Declaration of Alma-Ata." See https://www.who.int/teams/social-determinants-of-health/declaration-of-alma-ata. Accessed April 15, 2022).
55 Office of the High Commissioner for Human Rights. 2000. "CESCR General Comment No. 14: The Right to the Highest Attainable Standard of Health (Art. 12)." See https://www.refworld.org/pdfid-/4538838d0.pdf. Accessed April 15, 2022.
56 Timor-Leste. Department of State. See https://hist-ory.state.gov/countries/timor-leste. Accessed April 21, 2022.
57 UN. 1973. "Implementation of the Declaration of the Granting of the Independence to Colonial Countries and Peoples by the Specialized Agencies and the International Institutions Associated with the UN." See https://digitallibrary.un.org/record/191599/files/A_RES_3118%28XX-VIII%29-EN.pdf. Accessed May 18, 2022.
58 Kosovo declared independence in 2008 and is currently recognized by 112 States. However, if Kosovo applies for WHO membership, the United States is afraid that Palestine will follow course, leading to the US pressuring Kosovo not to apply. Prishtina Institute for Political Studies. 2020. "Kosovo's Membership in the WHO." In Prishtina Institute for Political Studies, See https://pips-ks.org/en/Detail/ArtMID/1446/ArticleID/4172/Kosovos-membership-in-the-World-Health-Organization-WHO. Accessed 11 April 2022.
59 MOU. 2005 "Implementation of the Memorandum of Understanding between the WHO Secretariat and China." See https://link.springer.com/content/pdf/bbm%3A978-3-658-05527-1%2F1.pdf. Accessed April 26, 2022.
60 Economic and Social Council. 2000. "General Comment No. 14: The right to the highest attainable standard of health (Article 12 of the International Covenant on Economic, Social and Cultural Rights)." See https://digitallibrary.un.org/record/425041/files/E_C.12_2000_4-EN.pdf. Accessed: April 15, 2022.
61 WHO. 2020. "Basic Documents. 2020. Rules of Procedure of the WHA." See https://apps.who.int/gb/bd/pdf_files/BD_49th-en.pdf#page=179. Accessed April 21, 2022.
62 Aside from the case of the Holy See, all other observers are invited by the WHO Director-General without consulting with the WHA first.
63 WHO. 1946. "Constitution of the WHO." See https://www.who.int/governance/eb/who_constitu-tion_en.pdf. Accessed December 17, 2021).

References

Anderson, Benedict. 1983. *Imagined Communities: Reflections on the Origin and Spread of Nationalism*. London: Verso.

Avilés Mendoza, Guillermo J. 2005–2006. "New International Health Regulations: Platform for Global Health Governance." *Ethos Gubernamental* (4): 79–99, 2006–2007.

Aust, Anthony. 2007. *Modern Treaty Law and Practice.* 2nd ed. Cambridge: Cambridge University Press.

Beck, Ulrich. 2000. "Risk Society Revisited: Theory, Politics and Research Programmes." Pp. 211–229 in *The Risk Society and Beyond: Critical Issues for Social Theory*, edited by Barbara Adam, Ulrich Beck and Joost Van Loon. London: Sage.

Bieber, Florian. 2020. "Global Nationalism in Times of the COVID-19 Pandemic." *Nationalities Paper* 50(1): 13–25.

Burci, Gian Luca, and Claude-Henri Vignes. 2004. *World Health Organization.* London: Kluwer Law International.

Chatterjee, Partha. 1986. *Nationalist Thought and the Colonial World: A Derivative Discourse?* London: Zed Books.

Chen, Ping-Kuei. 2018. "Universal Participation Without Taiwan? A Study of Taiwan's Participation in the Global Health Governance Sponsored by the World Health Organization." Pp. 263–281 in *Asia-Pacific Security Challenges*, edited by Anthony J. Masys and Leo S.F. Lin. Switzerland: Springer International Publishing AG.

Chen, Yen-Fu 2020. "Taiwan and the World Health Assembly/World Health Organization: Perspectives from Health Services and Research." *International Journal of Taiwan Studies* 3:10–27.

Crawford, James. 2007. *The Creation of States in International Law.* New York: Oxford University Press.

Cueto, Marcus. 2020. "The History of International Health: Medicine, Politics, and Two Socio-Medical Perspectives, 1851 to 2000." Pp. 19–36 in *The Oxford Handbook of Global Health Politics, edited by* C. McInnes, K. Lee and J. Youde. New York: Oxford University Press.

De Kloet, Jeroen, Jian Lin, and Yiu Fai Chow. 2020. "We Are Doing Better': Biopolitical Nationalism and the COVID-19 Virus in East Asia." *European Journal of Cultural Studies* 23(4): 635–640.

Fidler, David. 2010. "The Challenges of Global Health Governance." Council on Foreign Relations Working Paper. See https://www.researchgate.net/publication-/26523284_The_Challenges_of_Global_Health_Governance. Accessed July 15, 2022.

Fidler, David. 2020. "Vaccine Nationalism's Politics." *Science* 369(6505): 749.

Gellner, Ernest. 1983. *Nations and Nationalism.* Ithaca, NY: Cornell University Press.

Gau, Sheng-ti. 2013. "Taiwan and WHO: A Study on the Legal Feasibility of the Government of the Republic of China to Participate in Various Mechanisms Meetings of WHO." *Chengchi Law Review* 133:133–224.

Gostin, Lawrence, O. 2020. "Reimagining Global Health Governance in the Age of COVID-19." *American Journal of Public Health* 110:1615–1619

Hroch, Miroslav. 1996. "From National Movement to the Fully-Formed Nation: The Nation-Building Process in Europe." Pp. 60–78 in *Becoming National: a Reader*, edited by Geoff Eley and Ronald Grigor Suny. New York and London: Oxford University Press.

Hu, Zhang. 2021. "Challenges and Approaches of the Global Governance of Public Health under COVID-19." *Frontiers in public health* 9:727214.

Krastev, Ivan. 2020. "Seven Early Lessons From the Coronavirus, Views From the Council." in *European Council on Foreign Relations.* See www.ecfr.eu/article-/commentary_seven_earlylessons_from_the_coronavirus. Accessed November 6, 2020.

Kuznetsova, L. 2020. "COVID-19: The World Community Expects the World Health Organization to Play a Stronger Leadership and Coordination Role in Pandemics Control" *Frontiers in Public Health* 8:470.

Lin, Ching-Fu., Chien-Huei Wu, and Chuan-Feng Wu. 2020a. "Reimagining the Administrative State in Times of Global Health Crisis: An Anatomy of Taiwan's Regulatory

Actions in Response to COVID-19 Pandemic." *European Journal of Risk Regulation* 11 (Special Issue 2: Taming COVID-19 by Regulation): 256–272.

Lin, Ching-Fu, Han-Wei Liu, and Chien-Huei Wu. 2020b. "Breaking State-Centric Shackles in the WHO: Taiwan as a Catalyst for a New Global Health Order." *Virginia Journal of International Law* 61:99–114.

Ministry of Health and Welfare. 2020. *In the Progress of Combatting COVID-19: Recording Key Moments of Combatting the Pandemic.* Taipei: Ministry of Health and Welfare.

Quah, Stella R. 2006. "Governance of Epidemics: Is there a Reason for Concern?" Pp. 11–23 in *Crisis Preparedness: Asia and the Global Governance of Epidemics*, edited by Stella R. Quah. Stanford,CA: Walter H. Shorenstein Asia-Pacific Research Center; Baltimore,MD: Brookings Institution.

Rachman, Gideon. 2020. "Nationalism Is a Side Effect of the Coronavirus." *Financial Times*, See www.ft.com/content/644fd920-6cea-11ea-9bcabf503-995cd6f. Accessed November 6, 2020.

Rowen, Ian. 2020. "Crafting the Taiwan Model for COVID-19: An Exceptional State in Pandemic Territory." *The Asia-Pacific Journal, Japan Focus* 18(9): 1–12.

Ruger, Jennifer Prah. 2018. *Global Health Justice and Governance*. New York: Oxford University Press.

Santos Rutschman, Ana. 2020. "The Reemergence of Vaccine Nationalism." *Georgetown Journal of International Affairs* (online), Saint Louis U. Legal Studies Research Paper No. 2020-16. DOI:10.2139/ssrn.3642858.

Schrecker, Ted. 2020. "The State and Global Health." Pp. 281–299 in *The Oxford Handbook of Global Health Politics*, edited by Colin McInnes, Kelley Lee, and Jeremy Youde. New York: Oxford University Press.

Shamasunder, Sriram et al. 2020. "COVID-19 Reveals Weak Health Systems by Design: Why We Must Remake Global Health in This Historic Moment. "*Global* Public Health 15(7): 1083–1089.

Taiwan Centers for Disease Control. 2004. *Recording Key Moments in Combatting SARS: Building Strong Foundations in Public Health and Epidemic Prevention*. Taipei: Ministry of Health and Welfare.

Taiwan Centers for Disease Control. 2017. "Building a Virus Database for Taiwan in Contributing to Manufacture Influenza Vaccines: An Annual Report." Project Leader Peter Lin. Centers for inspecting and developing vaccines. Project Number: MOHW106 CDC C 315 000110.

Whitman, Jim. 2006. "The Global Governance of Epidemics: Possibilities and Limitations." Pp. 25–46 in *Crisis Preparedness: Asia and the Global Governance of Epidemics*, edited by Stella R. Quah. Stanford: Walter H. Shorenstein Asia-Pacific Research Center; Baltimore, MD: Brookings Institution.

Woods, Eric Taylor et al. 2020. "COVID-19, Nationalism, and the Politics of Crisis: A Scholarly Exchange." *Nations and Nationalism* 26(4): 807–825.

Yeh, Chin-Chuan. 2009. "Planning and Progress of Taiwan's Participation in the World Health Organization." *Journal of Healthcare Quality* 3(4): 50–53.

Yi, Joseph, and Wondong Lee. 2020. "Pandemic Nationalism in South Korea." *Society* 57(4): 446–451.

Youde, Jeremy. 2020. "How 'Medical Nationalism' Is Undermining the Fight Against the Coronavirus Pandemic." *World Politics Review*, See https://www.worldpoliticsreview.com/how-medical-nationalism-is-undermining-the-fight-against-the-coronavirus-pandemic/. Accessed November 6, 2020.

Zürn, Michael. 2018. *A Theory of Global Governance: Authority, Legitimacy, and Contestation*. Oxford: Oxford University Press.

Index

Note: **Bold** page numbers refer to tables; *italic* page numbers refer to figures and page numbers followed by "n" denote endnotes.

Kolibri 360 GmbH
Ferdinand-Jühlke-Straße 7
99095 Erfurt, Deutschland
produktsicherheit@kolibri360.de